Fitness For Dummies, 3rd Edition

W9-BTA-584

Keys to Fitness Success

The following tips can help you meet your fitness goals (see Chapter 3 for ideas on setting goals for yourself).

- **Set specific, realistic goals.** Instead of vowing to "get in shape," commit to walking three times a week.
- **Get your fitness tested.** Testing pinpoints the area(s) you need to work on, such as your aerobic conditioning, strength, flexibility, or body fat.
- **Dress the part.** You don't have to become a fitness clothing or equipment junkie, but having the right stuff keeps you safe, makes you comfortable, and gets you fired up to work out.
- **Keep a daily exercise diary.** Record the details of your workouts, such as how far you walked, how hard you pushed, how many sets or weights you did, and how you felt during your workout.
- **Pace yourself.** Don't do three hours of exercise or lift 250 pounds your first time out. You'll burn out fast and may even get injured.
- **Work out with a buddy or join a club.** You'll gain more motivation — and fitness — than if you exercise alone.
- **Join an Internet fitness community.** On fitness Web-site forums or discussion groups, visitors chat with like-minded exercisers and develop strong bonds with one another. See Chapter 28 for a section on Internet fitness sites.
- **Educate yourself.** Keep up with exercise trends and techniques by reading magazines, the Internet, and books like this one!

Money Matters to Consider When Choosing a Gym

Getting a good deal on a gym membership can be tricky (see Chapter 18). Before committing, consider the following:

- **Beware of hidden costs.** The monthly membership may be reasonable, but will you pay up the wazoo for parking, towel fees, and specialty classes? Is there a start-up fee or a large down payment upfront?
- **Don't be afraid to bargain.** Many clubs make special deals if you ask, especially during slow periods or if you join with a friend.
- **Steer clear of long-term memberships.** Don't even think about it. You don't know where you're going to be in three years — or whether the club will even be in business.
- **Ask about the club's cancellation policies.** If you change your mind within three days, most state laws require the club to refund your money in full.

Words of Wisdom for Buying Fitness Products

Remember these caveats when shopping for fitness products (and check out Chapter 26 for more fitness rip-offs):

- **Don't be suckered by the infomercial audience or "real people" offering testimonials.** These people are paid! And the fine print always says, "results are not typical."
- **Don't be swayed by seemingly scientific terminology like *zero-carb dieting* and *thermogenic fat burners.*** Many impressive-sounding terms have no accepted scientific meaning.
- **Beware of celebrity or "expert" endorsements.** Don't think that some three-time Mr. Universe built his biceps with a plastic contraption that looks like a model of the Starship *Enterprise.*
- **Don't be awed by the fact that a product was "awarded a U.S. patent."** To get a patent, you need to have an *original* idea, not necessarily a *good* one.
- **Beware of the term *proven.*** In fact, don't assume that any scientific studies were conducted at all.

For Dummies: Bestselling Book Series for Beginners

Fitness For Dummies,
3rd Edition

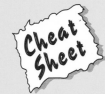

Judging Fitness News Reports

Don't believe everything you hear or read. Keep in mind these tips when evaluating fitness news (and check out Appendix A for more tips):

- **Look for context.** Does the news report mention how the latest research compares to the studies that came before it? One new study may be an aberration.
- **Consider the source.** A health study is more likely to be legit if it comes out of a major university or government agency rather than some mysterious private institute.
- **Don't assume cause and effect.** If a study says oat bran is "associated with" low cholesterol, this doesn't mean eating oat bran *causes* low cholesterol.
- **Look at the number of subjects.** If the sample size of a research study is no larger than the friends you eat breakfast with, beware.
- **Don't make too much of animal studies.** The way an obese mouse responds to a diet drug may not be the same way humans do.

Fitness Myths Debunked

Don't believe these common fitness myths:

- *Myth:* You must exercise for 30 consecutive minutes.
  Reality: Three 10-minute sessions of exercise burn as many calories and provide nearly the same health benefits as one 30-minute session.
- *Myth:* Lifting weights will turn you into a World Wrestling Federation contender.
  Reality: Virtually all women and most men can't develop huge muscles without spending hours a day in the gym lifting very heavy weights.
- *Myth:* If you stop exercising, your muscles will turn to fat.
  Reality: They'll just shrink. Fat and muscle are two different entities; you can't turn one into the other.
- *Myth:* By focusing on abdominal exercises, you can lose that beer gut.
  Reality: You can't selectively zap fat off a particular part of your body. To lose a beer gut, you need to lose weight and exercise (and you need to cut down on the brewskis).
- *Myth:* Exercising during pregnancy increases the rate of miscarriage or birth defects.
  Reality: With a doctor's approval, prenatal exercise is very healthy for you and your baby. In fact, studies show that labor and delivery are easier for women who exercise during pregnancy, as is getting back to your pre-pregnancy weight.

For Dummies: Bestselling Book Series for Beginners

Praise for the first editions of Fitness For Dummies

"Hey who are you guys calling a dummy? When it comes to fitness, like most male American slugs, I'm actually more of a complete blathering moronic idiot. This book will come in handy for those of us who don't know a fat gram from Phil Gramm or a donut from a bagel. Now all I need to know is how to look cool and studly in the gym while sweating profusely."

> —Steve Elling, *Raleigh News & Observer*

"This book is a joy to read — written with wit and style, it comes as a welcome reassurance that both razor-sharp accuracy and first-rate writing can co-exist in the same package."

> —Jonathan Bowden, M.A.C.S.C.S., Senior Faculty, Equinox Fitness Training Institute and Contributing Editor, *Fitness* magazine

"*Fitness For Dummies* is a smart buy for the exercise enthusiast. It's the fitness equivalent of carbo-loading."

> —*Orange County Register*

"This is one of the most comprehensive, authoritative — and entertaining — fitness books I've ever seen."

> —*Men's Fitness* magazine

"No one is more of a dummy when it comes to exercise than I am. Until I read *Fitness For Dummies,* I thought taking a book like this off the shelf counted as a workout. Now I know better. It's only a warm-up!"

> —Phil Rosenthal, Columnist, *Los Angeles Daily News*

"The exercise content and evaluations in this book are outstanding. Liz and Suzanne are the ultimate professionals, and *Fitness For Dummies* will help all exercisers maximize their potential."

> —*Fitness* magazine

"*Fitness For Dummies* is the definitive book for people who would like to achieve a stronger, healthier body."

—Mark Allen, Six-Time Ironman Champion

"Suzanne and Liz have created an insider's guide through the maze of mis-information about fitness. Before you buy an exercise gadget, a gym membership, or a fitness video, read this book!"

—*Women's Sports & Fitness* magazine

"*Fitness For Dummies* is a real rarity: a fitness book written by fitness writers — two of the best. It's full of smart, jargon-free, common-sense advice for anyone who's interested in fitness. These two are not afraid to tell the truth. It's like getting the word from a trusted friend."

—*Shape* magazine

"I am duly impressed with the newest entry into the *For Dummies* series. From dispelling myths such as how we really burn fat to a comprehensive look at every choice of equipment on the market today, this book becomes a trustworthy, truly helpful guide to getting in shape."

—Diana Nyad, World Record Holder, Longest Swim in History, and TV Broadcaster

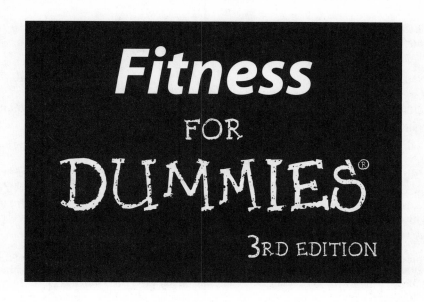

Fitness
FOR
DUMMIES®

3RD EDITION

**by Suzanne Schlosberg and Liz Neporent, M.A.,
with Tere Stouffer Drenth**

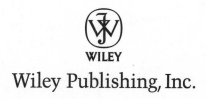

WILEY

Wiley Publishing, Inc.

Fitness For Dummies,® 3rd Edition

Published by
Wiley Publishing, Inc.
111 River St.
Hoboken, NJ 07030-5774
www.wiley.com

Copyright © 2005 by Wiley Publishing, Inc., Indianapolis, Indiana

Published simultaneously in Canada

For general information on our other products and services, please contact our Customer Care Department within the U.S. at 800-762-2974, outside the U.S. at 317-572-3993, or fax 317-572-4002.

For technical support, please visit www.wiley.com/techsupport.

Wiley also publishes its books in a variety of electronic formats. Some content that appears in print may not be available in electronic books.

Library of Congress Control Number: 2005920303

ISBN: 0-7645-7851-0

Manufactured in the United States of America

10 9 8 7 6 5 4 3 2 1

3B/RV/QT/QV/IN

WILEY

About the Authors

Suzanne Schlosberg is a magazine writer known for her humorous approach to health and fitness. She is a contributing editor to *Shape* and *Health* magazines and coauthor of *Weight Training For Dummies* and *Kathy Smith's Fitness Makeover.* She is also the author of *The Ultimate Workout Log,* Second Edition, and an instructor in UCLA Extension's Certificate in Journalism Program.

Suzanne writes frequently about her fitness adventures — from her failed tryout for The American Gladiators to her record-setting victory in Nevada's Great American Sack Race, a quadrennial event in which competitors run 5 miles while carrying a 50-pound sack of chicken feed on their shoulders. Suzanne also has chronicled her two bicycle treks across the United States. She never travels without her weight-lifting gloves and has put them to good use at gyms in Zimbabwe, Morocco, Guam, and the Micronesian island of Yap.

A Los Angeles native, Suzanne refuses to walk anywhere, including the Starbucks 0.4 miles from her house — to which she commutes daily in her SUV.

Liz Neporent is a certified trainer and president of Plus One Health Management, a fitness consulting company in New York City. Her job is to make sure the members of more than a dozen fitness centers in hotels and corporations throughout New York are happy, motivated, and exercising on a regular basis.

Liz holds a master's degree in exercise physiology and is certified by the American Council on Exercise, the American College of Sports Medicine, the National Strength and Conditioning Association, and the National Academy of Sports Medicine. She is coauthor of *Abs of Steel, Buns of Steel: Total Body Workout,* and *Weight Training For Dummies.* She also wrote *Fitness Walking For Dummies.* Additionally, she is the Gear Editor for *Shape* magazine and a regular contributor to *The New York Times.* She appears regularly on TV and radio as an authority on fitness and exercise.

Liz is an avid runner and has competed in more than two dozen marathons and ultra-marathons. She's also a devoted sports climber, walker, hiker, and weight trainer. She lives in New York City with her husband, Jay Shafran, and her greyhound, Zoomer.

Tere Stouffer Drenth is a fitness writer and retired professional runner who now spends her days hiking, walking, and snowshoeing with her workout partner, a chocolate Lab named Maxine. She is the author of *Marathon Training For Dummies* and coauthor of *Fit Pregnancy For Dummies.*

Authors' Acknowledgments

The authors are indebted to Mitchel Gray, our photographer, and all the models depicted throughout this book: Nancy Ngai, Shel Bibbey, Terry Certain, Aja Certain, Annemarie Scarammucia, Melody Fadness, Yvonne Mitchell, Chris Stothard, Stacy Collins, Val Towne, James Jankiewicz, Jay Shafran, Doris Shafran, Melissa Saxon, Patty Buttenheim, Sunshine Hopkins, and Jane Scott.

Thanks, also, to our agent, Felicia Eth, for staying on the ball. At Wiley, we'd also like to thank Acquisitions Editor Tracy Boggier, whose vision guided this project, and Project Editor Elizabeth Kuball, who managed our book project with grace, humor, and exceptional skill. Technical Editor Randall Broderdorf added tremendous value to the book with his spot-on recommendations and additions.

From Suzanne:

I'm grateful for input from Sarah Bowen Shea, Mary Duffy, Daryn Eller, Daniel Hernandez, Jim Kraft, John Lehr, Wendy Niemi Kremer, Jennifer Schlosberg, and Dana Sullivan. Nancy Gottesman performed her usual function of allowing me to kvetch whenever I felt like it.

Special thanks to my family — particularly my parents, my grandparents, and my sister — for understanding my absence from various events while I worked to meet my deadline. And thanks Mom, Dad, Espy, Jen, and John for helping me move in the middle of all of this!

Finally, I couldn't have a better coauthor than Liz Neporent, a good friend, a great wit, and the supreme maven of all things fitness.

From Liz:

Many thanks to my Plus One partners, Jay Shafran, Mike Motta, and Bill Horne.

Thanks also to the entire Plus One staff, with special gratitude to Grace De Simone, Holly Byrne, Baze Amiri, Lemont Platt, Bob Welter, Jamie Macdonald, and Tom Maraday. And, as always, I'm grateful to the individual site managers for making my job so easy and giving me the time to do all my extracurricular projects: John Buzzerio, Shel Bibbey, Kathleen Troy, Jason Ferrara, Terry Certain, Nancy Ngai, Nancy Belli, Mary Franz, Laura Girodano, Tom McCann, and Carrie Wujick.

To my parents, sister, brothers, nieces, nephews, and all of my in-laws: Thanks for your encouragement. Ditto to my good friends Patty Buttenheim, Gina Allchin, Norman Zinker, and Mary Duffy. I also appreciate Frank Tirelli, Lucy McGovern, Pam DiPietro, and David Wildstein for helping out with organization and proofreading.

A very special thanks to my husband, Jay Shafran, who is without a doubt the most supportive person on the face of the earth. And a very special thank-you to my coauthor Suzanne Schlosberg. It is always fun, entertaining, and enlightening to work with you.

Publisher's Acknowledgments

We're proud of this book; please send us your comments through our Dummies online registration form located at www.dummies.com/register/.

Some of the people who helped bring this book to market include the following:

Acquisitions, Editorial, and Media Development

Project Editor: Elizabeth Kuball

(Previous Edition: Wendy Hatch)

Acquisitions Editor: Tracy Boggier

Copy Editor: Elizabeth Kuball

(Previous Edition: Donna Love)

Technical Editor: Randall Broderdorf

Editorial Supervisor: Carmen Krikorian

Editorial Manager: Michelle Hacker

Editorial Assistants: Courtney Allen, Nadine Bell

Cover Photos: ©Royalty-Free CORBIS

Cartoons: Rich Tennant, www.the5thwave.com

Composition

Project Coordinator: Emily Wichlinski

Layout and Graphics: Carl Byers, Lauren Goddard, Joyce Haughey, Stephanie D. Jumper, Barry Offringa

Proofreaders: Leeann Harney, Jessica Kramer, Joe Niesen, Carl William Pierce,

Indexer: TECHBOOKS Production Services

Publishing and Editorial for Consumer Dummies

Diane Graves Steele, Vice President and Publisher, Consumer Dummies

Joyce Pepple, Acquisitions Director, Consumer Dummies

Kristin A. Cocks, Product Development Director, Consumer Dummies

Michael Spring, Vice President and Publisher, Travel

Kelly Regan, Editorial Director, Travel

Publishing for Technology Dummies

Andy Cummings, Vice President and Publisher, Dummies Technology/General User

Composition Services

Gerry Fahey, Vice President of Production Services

Debbie Stailey, Director of Composition Services

Contents at a Glance

Table of Contents

Introduction

Some things in life never change, like the traffic in Los Angeles or the weather in Tahiti. But fitness doesn't fall into that category. In the exercise world, there's something new in equipment, research, classes, gadgets, videos, and Web sites just about every day. In fact, so much has changed since the first two editions of *Fitness For Dummies* were published that we felt compelled to overhaul the book, adding several chapters and substantially revamping the others.

So what exactly is new in fitness? Health clubs are offering innovative new classes, like circuit training, cardio kickboxing, and firefighter boot camp, and nifty new machines, like the elliptical trainer. Yoga, Pilates, and other "mind-body" workouts have become so popular that we've devoted additional space to them. Technology has transformed fitness in many ways, too. And many clubs have invested in fancy entertainment systems so you can watch your own personal TV — or even surf the Internet — while running on the treadmill.

Of course, this being the fitness industry, the last few years have also seen the invention and marketing of new schlock — like pills that claim to eliminate cellulite or burn extra carbohydrates and machines that purport to tone your thighs "without any effort on your part." And there's no shortage of hokey books, Web sites full of misleading fitness information, and magazine ads posing as articles. We help you sort through all of that.

About This Book

Fitness For Dummies, 3rd Edition, updates you on all the latest — the good, the bad, and the totally weird. But our main mission remains the same as it was the first two times around: to tackle your fears, whether you worry that operating a stair-climber requires a degree in mechanical engineering or fret that no matter what exercise routine you start, sooner or later you'll end up back in the recliner.

We don't want you to become a fitness statistic. The fact is, among people who start an exercise program, half quit within eight weeks. This book gives you the knowledge and motivation to stick with fitness for the rest of your life.

Fitness For Dummies, 3rd Edition, tells you the stuff you really want to know, such as:

- ✔ Will you burn more fat if you exercise at a slower pace?
- ✔ Which brands of home exercise equipment are most reliable?
- ✔ How do you know if a health club is trying to rip you off?
- ✔ Can you actually become "Rock Solid in 6 Weeks," like the magazines say?
- ✔ Which weight-training exercises are best for beginners?
- ✔ What the heck is Pilates, and how do you pronounce it?
- ✔ How many days a week do you really need to work out?
- ✔ Is low-carb eating right for you?

The book is basic enough for the fitness rookie to understand, but it's also useful for workout veterans who want to brush up on the latest fitness concepts, gadgets, or training techniques.

Conventions Used in This Book

We use few conventions in this book, because we want you to be able to pick it up and start anywhere. Two conventions to keep in mind are the following:

- ✔ New fitness jargon appears in italics, *like this,* along with a brief definition. Use these terms to impress your friends.
- ✔ Web sites appear in a special font, `like this`, to distinguish them from other text. Jump on over to your computer and check them out.

We also use the terms *fitness routine, workout, exercise,* and *activity* to mean the same thing: whatever you're doing to raise your heart rate, build strength, or both.

Foolish Assumptions

We make few assumptions about you, dear reader, but the first and most important is that you want to improve your fitness. You may be brand-new to working out and have questions ranging from how to get started to what shoes to buy. Or you may have been working out for years and are looking for advice on how to reinvigorate your routine. Or you may be returning to a healthier lifestyle after a few years in the recliner.

Whatever your situation, this guide helps you make the best choices for your goals, lifestyle, and current fitness level. We give you step-by-step instructions and explain fitness terminology so you don't feel overwhelmed when talking to the salesperson trying to sell you a treadmill or a gym membership. (***Added bonus:*** These terms come in handy if you find yourself at a dinner party with a bunch of personal trainers.) And we let you know when your situation may benefit from the advice of a personal trainer, physician, or specialized publication.

How This Book Is Organized

Fitness For Dummies, 3rd Edition, is divided into eight parts, and the chapters within each part cover specific topic areas in detail. You can read each chapter or part without having to read what came before, although we may refer you to other sections for more information about certain topics. Here's a brief look at the eight parts.

Part 1: Getting Your Butt off the Couch

In this part, we give you the tools to start a fitness program. First, we give you an overview of the entire book, so you have a fast and easy way to understand the basics. Then, we discuss the important first steps in any fitness program, such as getting your fitness tested and setting realistic goals. We present strategies for making exercise a habit and explain the basics of healthy eating so you steer clear of fad diets and useless supplements. We also show you how to choose a personal trainer, should you decide to take that popular option.

Part 11: Enjoying Total-Body Health: Eating Well and Staying Injury-Free

This part covers everything everyone hopes to ignore about fitness: injuries, stretching, and nutrition. Sure, getting off the couch is critical to getting fit, but if you end up with an injury, you'll be benched again before you know it. Stretching may not be pretty or exciting, but it's one of the surest ways to ensure the long-term health of your muscles and joints. Finally, with so many differing opinions today about how to eat — low-carb, low-fat, carbo-loading, raw-foods-only — this part gives you the lowdown.

Part III: Getting to the Heart of the Matter

This part is devoted to cardiovascular exercise — the kind that strengthens your heart and lungs, burns lots of calories, lowers your stress level, and gives you the energy to chase down your cat for a bath. We tell you how long, how often, and how hard you need to work out in order to slim down, live longer, or train for a 10K run. We cover the most popular cardiovascular options, both indoor and outdoor, and offer tips on how to combat boredom when you're walking, climbing, or pedaling in place.

Part IV: Lift and Curl: Building a Stronger Bod with Weights

In this part we explain why everyone — whether you're 18 years old or 80, male or female — ought to strength-train. We give you the know-how to get started and answer questions such as:

✔ What's the difference between weight machines, dumbbells, and barbells?

✔ How much weight should I lift?

✔ How many exercises should I do?

✔ What's a deltoid, and why should I care?

We also updated the book by including a complete weight-training routine you can perform either at home or at the gym.

Part V: Cardio-Strength Workouts: Getting the Best of Both Worlds

If you can combine cardio workouts with strength building, you've managed to get two workouts in one. One of the most popular cardio-strength workouts is circuit training, in which you set up strength-building and cardio exercise stations, and walk or briskly run between each, giving you a total-body workout; in this part, you find a chapter devoted to circuit training. Yoga, one of the oldest forms of exercise in the world, is also discussed here, in its many forms and varieties. You also find out about hot, hot Pilates, a strength-and-cardio workout phenomenon.

Part VI: Conquering the Gym (Even at Home)

Walking into a health club can be a terrifying proposition, sort of like landing cold in some foreign country where you don't know a soul, don't speak the language, don't know the customs, and feel like everyone's staring at you. This part gives you the information you need to enter a gym with confidence. We explain how to choose a good club, fill you in on locker-room etiquette, and tell you how to get through an exercise class when you feel like you have two left feet that are tied together. We also update you on the latest in exercise classes, from spinning to treading to kickboxing.

Health clubs aren't for everyone, so in this part, we also help you choose the best fitness equipment for your budget, your goals, and the size of your living room. We cover a wide range of equipment, from space-age treadmills to $3 rubber exercise tubes. We offer tips for designing your home gym so you'll actually use the stuff you buy. And we tell you everything you ever wanted to know about exercise DVDs and videos.

Part VII: Exercising for All Ages and Stages

Worried about continuing your workouts during your pregnancy? Don't be. This part helps calm your fears and gives you the basics on what to do — and what not to do — to keep you and your baby healthy. And to help get your kids off on the right fitness foot, this part shares some ways you can involve the whole family in fun activities, whether you're the parent of a toddler or a teenager. If you're moving into your senior years, this part is for you, too. Here, we show you how to get and stay fit into your 90s, so you can enjoy this golden time in your life.

Part VIII: The Part of Tens

Every *For Dummies* book has a Part of Tens. These chapters give you a different spin on some of the information already presented in the other parts. For example, scattered throughout this book are many reasons to get and stay fit; in Chapter 24, you find a whole chapter of reasons. In Chapter 25, we tell you which low-priced fitness products we consider to be the best bargains. Conversely, in Chapter 26, we give you our picks for the worst fitness products and pills. Finally, in Chapter 27, we present ten tips for staying motivated.

Icons Used in This Book

Icons are small pictures in the margins of this book that flag certain material for you. The following icons highlight information you want to pay special attention to.

This icon flags great strategies for getting in shape, such as recording your workouts in a daily log. We also use the target for money-saving tips, such as asking your health club to waive its initiation fee. It also highlights first-rate exercises and fitness products, from treadmills to stretching devices to nutrition newsletters.

When information is just too good to forget, this icon helps you remember. This is the stuff you want to jot down and attach with a magnet to your fridge.

We use the Myth Buster superhero to dispel popular fitness myths. For example, in Chapter 8, we explain that exercise doesn't have to hurt in order to be good for you. In Chapter 26, we explain that you can't sweat off excess fat by wearing vinyl workout suits.

This icon warns you about hucksters who offer false promises, sell bogus products, or try to snare you with slimy sales tactics. We also use this icon to caution you about common exercise mistakes, such as neglecting to adjust the seat on an exercise machine.

We use this icon when we tell a story about our own adventures in fitness or recount the experiences of people we know. The anecdotes range from the wacky to the inspirational to the just plain helpful.

Where to Go from Here

You can dive into this book in two ways:

- ✔ **If you want a crash course in fitness, read the book cover-to-cover.** You'll get a thorough understanding of what it takes to get in shape. And you'll come across topics you may not have thought to look up, such as proper etiquette in the gym, how to judge the accuracy of fitness Web sites, and how often you need to buy new running shoes.

- ✔ **If you want to find out about a specific topic, you can flip to that section and get your answers right away.** Use the book as a reference every time you boldly enter uncharted territory, like a yoga class or the exercise aisle at your video store.

Part I
Getting Your Butt off the Couch

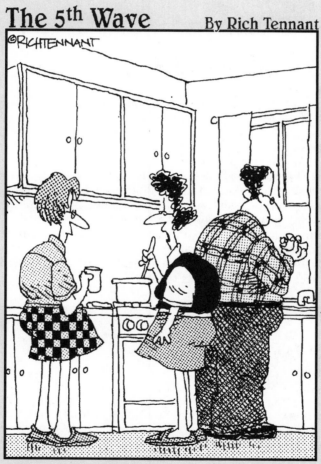

The 5th Wave   By Rich Tennant

"Nutritionally, we follow the Food Guide Pyramid. When I first met Philip, he ate from the Food Guide Stonehedge. It was a mysterious diet and no one's sure what its purpose was."

In this part . . .

We help you get going on a fitness program, no matter what shape you're in.

Chapter 1 gives you a brief overview of the entire book, so that, if you're short on time, you can get the quick-and-dirty lowdown on fitness. Chapter 2 explains the important first step toward getting fit: having your fitness tested. (Don't worry — you can't flunk!) Chapter 3 helps you devise a game plan: You find out how to set goals, track your progress, and use strategies to make exercise a habit. And because personal trainers are all the rage these days, Chapter 4 tells you how to choose one for yourself — and how much you can expect to pay.

Chapter 1

Fitness 101: Getting the Scoop

In This Chapter

▶ Getting ready for your first fitness test

▶ Deciding among your many choices of exercise routines

▶ Stretching well and eating right

▶ Working out while pregnant, in childhood, and into your senior years

*I*f you're reading this chapter, you've decided to get fit. (Or, like wannabe home remodelers who do nothing more than sit on the couch watching *Home Time* or *This Old House,* you're pretending to get fit by reading this book!) While transforming yourself from couch potato to buff hottie doesn't take a Ph.D. in physiology or kinesiology, you do need to follow a few rules of the road.

This chapter outlines the very basics of getting fit. If you want to find out more, each section tells you which chapters to read for all the juicy details.

Yes, This Class Has Tests

In order to best determine how to reach your fitness goals, you first need to figure out where you are, physically. And the best way to do this is to sign up for a fitness evaluation (see Chapter 2), including a full health/fitness history and other important measures, such as the following:

✔ **Resting heart rate:** Also known as pulse, this test measures the number of times per minute your heart beats while you're sitting down or in some other way relaxing. As you exercise more and more, your resting heart rate will likely drop.

✔ **Heart rate after physical activity:** Generally, you exercise for about 15 minutes on a treadmill or stationary bicycle and test your pulse. Cardio exercises (discussed in Chapter 8) can gradually lower this number.

✔ **Blood pressure:** This test measures how hard your heart has to work to pump blood through your blood vessels. Cardio activities (see Chapter 8) can help alleviate high blood pressure (hypertension), which can lead to health problems.

✔ **Percentage of body fat:** Instead of measuring how much you weigh, which doesn't necessarily indicate how fit you are, measuring your body fat tells you how much of you is fat and how much is muscle, bones, blood, organs, and other tissues. Up to a point, the lower the number, the better; reducing your body fat is often a matter of eating better (discussed in Chapter 7) and burning calories through cardio workouts (see Chapter 8) and lifting weights (see Chapter 11).

✔ **Strength:** This tests measures the strength of your upper body, abdominal muscles, and lower body by doing sit-ups, push-ups, leg extensions (on a weight machine), and so on. Weight lifting, described in Chapter 11, helps improve your strength.

✔ **Flexibility:** Because flexibility is the downfall of even the super-fit, make sure your evaluation measures the range of motion of your joints and muscles. Chapter 6 gives you the lowdown on stretching, which is one of the best ways to improve your flexibility.

Each of these tests can be done by a physician, a personal trainer, or a fitness professional working at a gym. But don't spend any time studying for them: You can't fail these tests. Think of them more as baseline measurements that help you decide where to put your emphasis: improving the health of your heart, losing weight and reducing body fat, building strength, improving your flexibility, and so on.

Choosing Your Weapon

With so many workout options available these days, you have plenty of fitness weapons from which to choose. Your workout options tend to fall into three categories, however: cardio, strength, and combination workouts. The three following sections give you a brief overview of each.

Seeing into the heart of the matter

Workouts that get your heart pumping are known as *cardio* (short for cardiovascular) exercises, and these improve the health of your heart and blood vessels. Cardio workouts also burn calories, which helps you lose weight. Check out Chapter 8 for a cardio primer.

The simplest — and, perhaps, the cheapest — cardio exercise is walking. Other popular cardio exercises include running, cycling, in-line skating, swimming, rowing, and (if you live in a snowy winter climate) snowshoeing and cross-country skiing. Chapter 10 discusses many of these outdoor cardio activities and gives you pointers for developing good techniques for each.

You don't have to brave the outdoors to get a cardio workout, however. Chapter 9 discusses indoor cardio machines, including treadmills, elliptical trainers, stationary bikes, stair-climbers, and rowing machines.

Getting buff with weights

Many men focus heavily on weight training, while some women shy away from it. The truth is that both men and women need to do some strength training (along with some cardio workouts, discussed in the preceding section, to get the heart and blood vessels into tip-top shape) for one important reason: to help burn more calories. Strange as it seems, weightlifting improves your resting metabolism, which means you turn into a fat- and calorie-burning machine. Chapter 11 shares this and many other reasons to start pumping iron.

Cardio and strength together: Two for the price of one

A few activities combine cardio and strength training into one workout. One of the most popular, circuit training (see Chapter 15), combines a cardio warm-up and cooldown with a series of weight-lifting and other strength stations. Not only can circuit training save you time, but it's also a lot of fun, because you move from station to station every 30 or 40 seconds.

Two other popular strength-cardio exercises are yoga and Pilates, which tend to focus on *core strength,* the strength and flexibility of your midsection. Discussed in Chapters 16 and 17, respectively, yoga and Pilates can be high-energy, revved-up workouts or soothing, mind-body workouts that leave you feeling refreshed.

Stretching Your Mind (and Body)

Don't let recent headlines claiming there's no correlation between stretching and injuries fool you: If you stretch properly and do it after (not before) you work out, studies show that you reduce your risk of injury. (But do take care that you perform some flexibility movement prep before your workout — see Chapter 6.) And the bottom line is that you want to avoid injuries, because they keep you from working out as often and as intensely as you'd like. We offer you an entire chapter on stretching (see Chapter 6), plus a short chapter on avoiding common injuries (see Chapter 5).

Yoga, discussed in Chapter 16, is an excellent way to improve your flexibility.

What Are You Eating?

The link between exercise and nutrition has been clear for decades, and you're likely to have trouble improving your fitness if you make poor nutritional choices. But how do you know which choices to make? Low fat? High carb? Low carb? High protein? Low calorie? Food pyramids? Hydration? Vitamins? It's enough to make your head spin.

Knowing what to eat for optimal fitness has never been a murkier proposition. Fortunately, in Chapter 7, we guide you through the haze, giving you a clear picture of the benefits of a low-fat, low-bad-carb, high-good-carb, moderate-protein, Mediterranean-food-pyramid, lots-o-water, balanced diet. Flip to that chapter when you're ready to get the final scoop on nutrition — final for based on current scientific research, that is.

At Home or at the Gym — Choosing What's Best for You

To join or not to join, that is the fitness question everyone asks himself at some point. Joining a gym can be a big financial investment, and many people choose not to join for that reason, opting for the free activities (walking, running, cycling) available just by walking out your front door.

But gyms have plenty to offer, including the latest and greatest workout equipment, fun and invigorating classes, the opportunity to schedule time with a personal trainer, and the infectious energy of other gym members. Chapter 18 gives you step-by-step instructions for how to scout out and decide whether to join a local gym and offers a basic lesson in gym etiquette. Chapter 19 offers practical advice on deciding whether to join an exercise class or purchase a DVD to use at home.

A gym isn't the only place to use exercise equipment. If you have the money to invest in your own equipment, you can set up your own home gym in your basement, spare room, garage, or any other convenient area. Chapter 20 helps you plan your space and make the most of your fitness equipment shopping excursions; Chapter 25 offers ten low-cost fitness investments for your home.

Special Exercises for Special People

Fitness isn't only for those buff, 20-something gyms gods. In fact, you can start exercising in your 80s and still reap the benefits of a healthier, longer life. And the earlier in life you start working out, the more likely it will become a lifelong habit. Chapter 23 offers some tips and advice for beginning an exercise program in your senior years.

How early is early enough? How about the womb? One study shows that women who exercise during pregnancy have leaner babies who turn into leaner kids. The benefits aren't only for the kids, however. From reducing back pain and encouraging better sleep patterns to encountering an easier delivery to slipping back into your old jeans more quickly, exercising during pregnancy offers incredible health benefits. See Chapter 21 for a short tutorial on getting and staying fit during pregnancy. For an in-depth look at pregnancy workouts, check out *Fit Pregnancy For Dummies* by Catherine Cram and Tere Stouffer Drenth (published by Wiley).

Kids, perhaps more than any other age group, understand that being active is fun. If you can tap into their natural love of activities, especially games, sports, and dancing, you can help your kids avoid the alarming rates of obesity that plague children today. Without emphasizing "exercise" or "workouts," you can introduce your child to all sorts of healthy activities that encourage a lifelong fitness. Keep the emphasis on fun, without pushing your child into competitions or activities she doesn't enjoy, and you'll help your child become an adult with a strong body and a healthy heart.

Chapter 2

Testing Your Fitness

*W*e've never been fond of tests that you can't study for. Nevertheless, we think the first step toward getting in shape is having your fitness evaluated. Don't panic. This test isn't like your driver's license renewal exam: You can't flunk, and you don't have to stand in line for three hours listening to people rant and rave about government bureaucracy. A fitness test simply gives you key information about your physical condition.

We constantly hear people say, "I'm so out of shape. I need to lose weight." But that's like telling a travel agent, "I'm in Europe. I need to go to Africa." Your travel agent needs to know the specifics: Are you in Rome? Berlin? Moscow? Do you want to go to Cairo? Cape Town? The Kalahari Desert? Before you embark on a fitness program, you need to know your starting point with the same sort of precision. A fitness evaluation gives you important departure information, such as your heart rate, body fat, strength, and flexibility. Armed with these facts, you or your trainer can design an intelligent plan to get you to your fitness destination. And when you get there, you'll have the numbers to prove just how far you've come.

In this chapter, we describe what to expect when a professional tests your fitness. We also explain how to test your fitness on your own. However, even if you do most of the testing yourself, consider getting certain aspects of your fitness evaluated at a sports medicine clinic or fitness center. As you complete the various tests, record your results on the chart found at the end of this chapter.

What's Your Health History?

When you join a gym, one of the first things you should be asked to do —
after signing your check, of course — is to fill out a health-history questionnaire. Your answers to these questions give a snapshot of your overall well-
being, including your eating and exercise habits, your risk for developing
cardiovascular disease, and any orthopedic limitations or medical conditions
that you may have. Typical questions include: Do you have any chronic joint
problems such as arthritis? Do you have a high stress level? Are you currently
taking any over-the-counter or prescription medications?

If you don't belong to a gym, ask yourself the following questions, which are
designed to indicate your risk of developing heart disease:

- ✔ Are you inactive?

- ✔ Do you have a history of heart disease?

- ✔ Do you have diabetes or high blood sugar?

- ✔ Do you have a history of high blood pressure?

- ✔ Did your mother, father, sister, or brother develop any form of
  heart disease before age 50?

- ✔ Do you smoke cigarettes, or have you quit within the last two years?

- ✔ Do you have high cholesterol — either total cholesterol higher than 200
  mg/dl or HDL less than 40 mg/dl?

If you answer "yes" to at least one question and you're over age 35, see a
physician for a complete medical evaluation before you even pursue a fitness
testing session. A physician is the only one who can accurately determine
whether exercising puts you in any danger. If you answer "yes" to two or more
questions, get a checkup no matter how old you are.

Some gyms request that you be tested by a physician if a staff member feels
you may have a medical problem. Don't groan; a request like this indicates
that your gym is on the ball. Some health clubs just want your money. They
may not require any testing — other than the test that determines whether
you can sign your name on a credit-card slip. If that's the case, you need to
take responsibility for getting tested.

After you fill out your questionnaire, your tester should discuss the answers
with you and ask for more information if necessary. If you're a smoker, for
example, he may ask you how much you smoke. Respond honestly and thoroughly. Don't say that you run 5 miles a day if you haven't broken a sweat
since high school — or if you intend to run every day but just haven't gotten
around to it.

Let your tester judge what's important. Liz tested two men who failed to tell her that they'd each had a lung removed. Another client neglected to mention that he had serious congenital heart problems. Two weeks later, he passed out while running on the treadmill and hit his head on the way down, causing a life-threatening head injury. Lucky for him, an ambulance arrived within five minutes, and the paramedics were able to save him.

What's Your Heart Rate?

Your *heart rate,* also known as your *pulse,* is the number of times your heart beats per minute. Your fitness evaluation should include a measure of your resting heart rate — your heart rate when you're sitting still. Ideally, your resting heart rate should be between 60 and 90 beats per minute. It may be slower if you're fit or genetically predisposed to a low heart rate; it may be faster if you're nervous or have recently downed three double cappuccinos. In addition to caffeine, stress and certain medications can speed up your heart rate. To be sure, take your heart rate first thing in the morning for three consecutive days and find the average to determine your heart rate.

After a month or two of regular exercise, your resting heart rate usually drops. This means that your heart has become more efficient. It may need to beat only 80 times per minute to pump the same amount of blood (or more) than it used to pump in 90 beats. In the long run, this saves wear and tear on your heart.

The simplest place to take your own pulse is at your wrist. Rest your middle and index fingertips (not your thumb) lightly on your opposite wrist, directly below the base of your thumb. Most people can see the faint bluish line of their radial artery; place your fingertips here. Count the beats for 1 minute. Or, if you have a short attention span, count for 30 seconds and multiply by 2. For a really, really short attention span, count for 6 seconds and multiply by 10. An even easier and faster way to measure your pulse is to strap on a heart-rate monitor, an extremely useful gadget we describe in Chapter 8.

What's Your Blood Pressure?

Have a professional test your blood pressure. Home blood-pressure machines tend to be inaccurate, as do those contraptions in the mall that charge a quarter for a reading.

Blood pressure is a measurement of how open your blood vessels are. Low numbers mean that your heart doesn't have to work very hard to pump the blood through your blood vessels. Ideally, your blood pressure should read 115/75 or below, a lower standard than the old standby of 120/80. If it's slightly higher, don't get stressed (that only increases it even more). However, if your blood pressure is higher than 140/90, you are considered *hypertensive,* a fancy term for having high blood pressure. In case you're wondering, the top number, called your *systolic blood pressure,* measures pressure as your heart ejects blood. The bottom number, your *diastolic blood pressure,* measures pressure when your heart relaxes and prepares for its next pump.

If you get a high blood-pressure reading, ask your tester to try again. The numbers can be affected by many factors, such as illness, caffeine, nervousness, or racing into your test because you were late. But if you repeatedly get high readings, see a doctor.

How Fit Is Your Heart?

Most reputable clubs perform something called a *submax test.* That's short for *submaximal test,* fitness jargon for a test that evaluates your heart rate when you're working at less than your maximum effort. Typically, this test takes you to about 75 to 85 percent of your maximum heart rate. A *maximal test* — in which you go all-out — should only be performed by a physician or in the presence of a physician.

Submaximal tests are usually performed on a stationary bicycle, treadmill, or step bench. (If you're a runner, request a treadmill; if you're a cyclist, ask to be tested on a bike. You're best at what you practice most.) The test usually lasts about 15 minutes. During this time, you increase your intensity every three or four minutes while the tester monitors your heart rate and blood pressure. The test shouldn't be very hard. On a bike, the worst it should feel like is pedaling up a moderately steep hill for a few minutes.

If you don't belong to a health club, you can test your aerobic fitness using a watch with a second hand and a course that's exactly 1 mile long. Warm up with a slow walk for five to ten minutes, and then time yourself as you walk or run the mile as briskly as you can. Take your pulse right before you stop, and make a mental note of the number. Also note your time as you complete your mile.

One minute after you finish the mile, take your pulse again. See how far it has dropped from the pulse check you did right at the end of your walk. Try this test again in two months and see how much faster you can complete the mile and how much more quickly you recover. If a mile sounds like too much for you right now, do a half-mile or even walk around the block. Just choose a distance that you can measure again at a later date.

Schedule a second fitness evaluation in six weeks. Those first weeks of training can bring about some dramatic changes, and it's really motivating to see how well you've done. After that, changes tend to be steady but somewhat slower. Get tested again every three to six months. Don't go longer than a year without reevaluating your progress. You don't want to waste time with a workout program that's not getting results.

How Much of You Is Fat?

During your evaluation, your tester will probably weigh you. Just know that your weight is of limited value. When you hop on a scale, you learn the grand total weight of your bones, organs, blood, fat, muscle, and other tissues. This number can be misleading because muscle weighs more per square inch than fat.

Consider two men who stand 5'8" and weigh 190 pounds. One guy may be a lean bodybuilder who has a lot of muscle packed onto his frame. Another guy may be a couch potato whose gut hangs 4 inches over his belt buckle. Even a low weight doesn't necessarily indicate good health or fitness. It may simply mean that you have small bones and little muscle.

More helpful than your body weight is your *body composition* — how much of your body is composed of fat and how much is composed of everything else. Your body composition is also called your body-fat percentage. If you score a 25 percent on a fat test, this means that 25 percent of your weight is composed of fat.

Like your weight, your body-fat percentage is not necessarily a measure of your health. True, cardiovascular disease, diabetes, and certain cancers are more prevalent among overweight people — men who have more than about 20 percent body fat and women who have more than about 30 percent body fat. However, some researchers believe that these health problems are not caused by the extra fat itself but rather by a lack of exercise and a poor diet. In other words, if you exercise regularly and eat well, extra body fat may not compromise your health. So consider your body-fat score in a context with other health measures, such as your cholesterol levels, blood pressure, and other gauges of fitness, such as a submaximal test and your resting heart rate.

An additional number to consider is the circumference of your waist. Excess abdominal fat — the type that lies deep in your belly, clumped around your organs — is linked to increased risk for heart disease. Heavy thighs, on the other hand, do not appear to be related to health problems. (In other words — to use terms we can all relate to — a beer belly is more harmful to your health than saddlebags.) Men with waist measurements greater than 40 and women with waist measurements greater than 35 should consult a physician.

Although body fat testing has its limits, your results can give you great insight into how your fat-loss and exercise program is coming along. Sure, your scale can tell you that you lost 7 pounds. But a body-fat test can tell you that your 7-pound loss means that you lost 10 pounds of fat and gained 3 pounds of muscle, results that are probably more motivating.

Body-fat testing also can tell you if you have too *little* fat. Maybe you can never be too rich, but you definitely can be too thin. For women, super-low body fat — below about 16 percent — may lead to problems such as irregular menstrual periods, permanent bone loss, and a high rate of bone fractures.

Keep in mind that every body-fat testing method has room for error. At a recent fitness convention, Suzanne had her body fat measured by two different methods — and appeared to have gained 11 percent body fat in a matter of 15 minutes. You may even get wildly different readings using the same test, depending on the skill of the tester or the condition of the equipment.

The only way to measure body fat with complete accuracy is to burn yourself up and take a carbon count of the ashes. Because that technique doesn't draw too many volunteers, scientists have developed a number of other methods. Here's a look at the ones you're most likely to come across.

Pinching an inch

The most common body-fat test uses the *skinfold caliper,* a gizmo that resembles a stun gun with salad tongs attached (see Figure 2-1). When your tester fires, the tongs pinch your skin, pulling your fat away from your muscles and bones. (You feel moderate discomfort, like when your great aunt pinches your cheek on the holidays.) Typically, the tester pinches three to seven different sites on your body, such as your abdomen, the back of your arm, and the back of your shoulder. The thickness of each pinch is plugged into a formula to determine your body-fat percentage. Your tester should pinch each site two or three times to verify the measurement.

Many things can go wrong with a caliper test. The tester may not pinch exactly the right spot, or he may not pull all the fat away from the bone. Or he may pinch too hard and accidentally yank some of your muscle. Also, research suggests that certain formulas are more accurate for certain ethnic groups, age ranges, and fitness levels.

Experts give this test a margin of error of four points, meaning your actual body-fat percentage could be four points higher or lower than it actually is. Be sure to get tested before your workout. When you exercise, blood travels to your skin to cool you down. This can cause your skin to swell, and you may test fatter than you really are. Plus, calipers can slip if your skin is wet from sweat.

If you want to try this method on your own, you can purchase calipers such as Accu-Measure (available for about $20 through Collage Video, a company you can visit at www.collagevideo.com and that's described in Chapter 19). These calipers come with a decent booklet that explains how to test yourself and interpret the results. For better accuracy, you may want to have a friend perform the test on you.

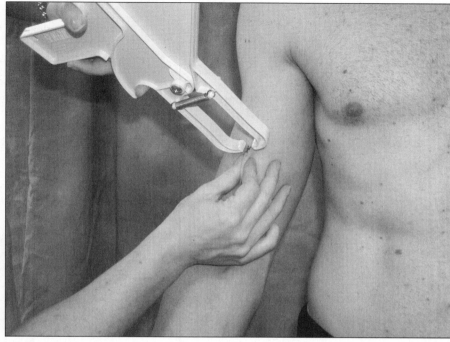

Figure 2-1:
Getting
pinched
with
calipers.

Photograph by Jennifer Lawler

Taking your measurements

A less precise but also helpful way to keep track of your body fat is to take your measurements. You don't get a percentage, but you can use the numbers to keep track of inches lost (or gained, if you're trying to pack on muscle), which can be motivating in and of itself. If you're losing inches, chances are, you're dropping body fat. Some common places to measure include across the middle of your chest, the center of your upper arm, the smallest part of your waist, the widest part of your hips, the widest part of your thigh, and the widest part of your ankle. You can write these numbers on the chart at the end of this chapter.

Calculating your body mass index

Yet another method of estimating how "fat" you are is *body mass index* (BMI), a number derived from your height and weight. To determine your BMI, turn to Table 2-1, locate your height in inches, and then move across that row until you find your weight. The number at the top of that column is your BMI.

Table 2-1   **Body Mass Index**

BMI	19	20	21	22	23	24	25	26	27	28	29	30	31	32	33	34	35
Height (inches)	Body Weight (pounds)																
58	91	96	100	105	110	115	119	124	129	134	138	143	148	153	158	162	167
59	94	99	104	109	114	119	124	128	133	138	143	148	153	158	163	168	173
60	97	102	107	112	118	123	128	133	138	143	148	153	158	163	168	174	179
61	100	106	111	116	122	127	132	137	143	148	153	158	164	169	174	180	185
62	104	109	115	120	126	131	136	142	147	153	158	164	169	175	180	186	191
63	107	113	118	124	130	135	141	146	152	158	163	169	175	180	186	191	197
64	110	116	122	128	134	140	145	151	157	163	169	174	180	186	192	197	204
65	114	120	126	132	138	144	150	156	162	168	174	180	186	192	198	204	210
66	118	124	130	136	142	148	155	161	167	173	179	186	192	198	204	210	216
67	121	127	134	140	146	153	159	166	172	178	185	191	198	204	211	217	223
68	125	131	138	144	151	158	164	171	177	184	190	197	203	210	216	223	230
69	128	135	142	149	155	162	169	176	182	189	196	203	209	216	223	230	236
70	132	139	146	153	160	167	174	181	188	195	202	209	216	222	229	236	243
71	136	143	150	157	165	172	179	186	193	200	208	215	222	229	236	243	250
72	140	147	154	162	169	177	184	191	199	206	213	221	228	235	242	250	258
73	144	151	159	166	174	182	189	197	204	212	219	227	235	242	250	257	265
74	148	155	163	171	179	186	194	202	210	218	225	233	241	249	256	264	272
75	152	160	168	176	184	192	200	208	216	224	232	240	248	256	264	272	279
76	156	164	172	180	189	197	205	213	221	230	238	246	254	263	271	279	287

Source: National Heart, Lung, and Blood Institute (NHLBI)

If you're in the mood to pull out your calculator, you can determine your BMI by following these steps:

1. **Multiply your height in inches times your height in inches.**
2. **Divide your weight by the number you arrived at in Step 1.**
3. **Multiply the number you came up with in Step 2 by 705.**

   The result is your BMI.

So what does your BMI mean? The National Institutes of Health has issued the BMI guidelines shown in Table 2-2.

Table 2-2	Understanding Your Body Mass Index
BMI	*Weight Status*
Less than 19	Underweight
19 to 24.9	Healthy
25 to 29.9	Overweight
30 or greater	Obese

People with a BMI of 25 or above are considered at higher risk for heart disease, stroke, hypertension, diabetes, gallbladder disease, cancer, and death. But these guidelines are controversial. Even members of the government panel that issued the guidelines believe that setting the low point for overweight at a BMI of 25 is somewhat arbitrary. Keep in mind that BMI, like body-fat percentage, is only one factor in assessing your health. Also know that BMI measurements for extremely muscular athletes and pregnant women are not very accurate.

You may wonder: If BMI has so many limitations, why are we including it in this book? Because it's the simplest way — no fees, no equipment, and no schlepping to the health club — of estimating whether you may be in the overweight ballpark.

Getting zapped (also body-fat scales and handheld testers)

Another common method of body fat testing is called *bioelectrical impedance analysis* (BIA). You lie on your back while a signal travels from an electrode on your foot to an electrode on your hand. The slower the signal, the more fat you have. This is because fat impedes, or blocks, the signal. The signal travels quickly through muscle because muscle is 70 percent water and water conducts electricity. Fat, on the other hand, is just 5 to 13 percent water.

Similar technology is used in body-fat scales and handheld gadgets that resemble a car steering wheel and are even less accurate than BIA.

Bioelectrical impedance can have a huge margin of error, especially if you're extremely fat or extremely lean. In one study, world-class female distance runners were found to average 20 percent body fat, when more reliable methods actually show that they were closer to 10 percent. Dehydration also can skew the results wildly; the signal slows down, and you appear to have more fat than you really do. Don't drink alcohol or caffeine for at least 24 hours before the test because they can lead to dehydration.

Getting dunked (underwater weighing)

Underwater weighing is the most cumbersome method of body-fat testing, but it's also the most accurate method that's anywhere near affordable. You sit on a scale in a tank of warm water about the size of a Jacuzzi. (When Suzanne did this, she felt like a giant piece of tortellini floating in a big pot.) Then comes the unnerving part: You blow all the air out of your lungs and bend forward until you're completely submerged. If there's air trapped in your lungs, you score fatter than you really are. Knowing this fact makes you try really, really hard to blow out your air, which makes you feel like you're about to explode. You stay submerged for about five seconds while your underwater weight registers on a digital scale. The result is then plugged into a mathematical equation.

This method of testing is based on the premise that muscle sinks and fat floats. The more fat you have, the more your body wants to float when dunked under water. The denser you are, the more you sink, and the more water your body displaces.

The margin of error for this test is 2 to 2.5 percent for young to middle-aged adults. The results are less accurate for children, older adults, and extremely lean people. This is because lean body tissue is made up of other things besides muscle. Bone, for example, isn't fully formed in children, and it may be somewhat porous in older adults and somewhat denser in super-fit people. You can get this test done at sophisticated sports-medicine clinics or labs for $50 to $100.

BOD POD: The cutting edge of body-fat testing

Underwater weighing has long been the standard for body-fat testing, but a sophisticated contraption called the *BOD POD* may one day replace it. The BOD POD is a 5-foot-tall fiberglass chamber that looks like a giant egg with a tinted window. You sit in the chamber for two or three 50-second tests while computerized pressure sensors determine how much air your body displaces — in other words, how much space you take up. (Underwater weighing determines the same information, just in a way that's less convenient.)

Research suggests that the BOD POD may be as accurate as underwater weighing, but the technology is so new that only a few studies have been conducted. Although the machine costs about as much as a luxury car, at universities, fitness expos, and some health clubs around the country, you can get a BOD POD test for about $25.

DEXA: X-ray vision

Another method is Dual-Energy X-ray Absorptiometry (DEXA). Not only does it measure how much fat you have, but it also determines where the fat is located on your body, a more relevant health indicator. Originally developed to scan bone density, DEXA is available at hospitals and in doctors' offices; it usually requires a physician's referral. (The test costs from $150 to $200.) You lie on a bed while low doses of two different X-ray energies scan your body from head to toe.

How Strong Are You?

Fear not: You won't be required to do one-arm push-ups or lift a barbell that weighs more than your dad. Strength tests, like the other tests that we describe in this chapter, are simply designed to give you a starting point. If you get started on a good weight-lifting program and stick to it, you're likely to see dramatic changes when you take another fitness test in two or three months.

Most health clubs don't take true strength measurements; in other words, they don't measure the absolute maximum amount of weight you're capable of lifting. Going for your "max" can be dangerous and can cause more than a little muscle soreness. Instead, gyms test your muscular endurance: how many times you can move a much lighter weight. You can do many of these tests at home. Having a friend count for you and make sure you're doing the exercise correctly is a help. Here are some common muscular endurance measures.

Measuring your upper-body strength

Count how many push-ups you can do without stopping or losing good form. For this test, men do military push-ups, with their legs out straight and toes on the floor. Women do modified push-ups, with their knees bent and feet off the floor. Lower your entire body at once until your upper arms are parallel to the floor. Pull your abdominals in to prevent your back from sagging. Do this test correctly! One guy we watched didn't have the strength to lower his body all the way, so he just bobbed his head up and down.

Use Table 2-3 or Table 2-4 to find out how you stack up against other people of your age and gender.

Table 2-3		Push-Ups — Men			
Age:	*20–29*	*30–39*	*40–49*	*50–59*	*60+*
Excellent	55+	45+	40+	35+	30+
Good	45–54	35–44	30–39	25–34	20–29
Average	35–44	25–34	20–29	15–24	10–19
Fair	20–34	15–24	12–19	8–14	5–9
Low	0–19	0–14	0–11	0–7	0–4

Table 2-4		Push-Ups — Women			
Age:	*20–29*	*30–39*	*40–49*	*50–59*	*60+*
Excellent	49+	40+	35+	30+	20+
Good	34–48	25–39	20–34	15–29	5–19
Average	17–33	12–24	8–19	6–14	3–4
Fair	6–16	4–11	3–7	2–5	1–2
Low	0–5	0–3	0–2	0–1	0

Some health clubs also measure upper-body strength on a free-weight bench press or a chest-press machine. (In Chapter 12, we explain the difference between free weights and machines.) The amount of weight doesn't matter, as long as you use the same weight every time you get tested. You simply do as many repetitions as you can.

Measuring your abdominal strength

The strength of your abdominal muscles is usually measured by a crunch test. (However, this test isn't recommended if you have a history of lower-back problems.)

Place two pieces of masking tape about halfway down the length of a mat, one directly behind the other, about 2½ inches apart. Lie on your back on the mat with your arms at your sides and your fingertips touching the rear edge of the back piece of tape. Bend your knees and place your feet flat on the floor. Curl your head, neck, and shoulder blades upward, sliding your palms along the floor until your fingertips touch the front edge of the front piece of tape. Return to the starting position and keep going until you're too tired to continue or you can't reach the tape. Don't cheat by sliding your arms without moving your body or by moving only one side of your body. See Figure 2-2 for an example of the crunch test.

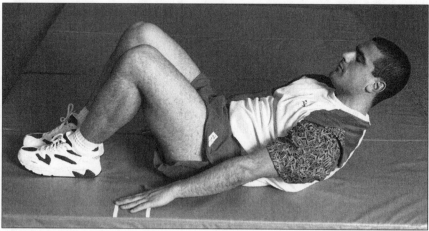

Figure 2-2:
The crunch test.

Photograph by Sunstreak Productions, Inc.

Use Tables 2-5 and 2-6 to gauge the results of your crunch test.

Table 2-5	Crunches — Men		
Age:	*Under 35*	*36–45*	*Over 45*
Excellent	60	50	40
Good	45	40	25
Marginal	30	25	15
Needs work	15	10	5

Table 2-6	Crunches — Women		
Age:	*Under 35*	*36–45*	*Over 45*
Excellent	50	40	30
Good	40	25	15
Marginal	25	15	10
Needs work	10	6	4

Measuring your lower-body strength

The strength of your lower-body muscles is often measured on a leg-extension machine, which targets your front-thigh muscles. (This machine is sort of like a big chair with a high back.) Some clubs test lower-body strength on other machines; others don't test your lower-body strength at all.

You can test the strength of your thigh and butt muscles at home by doing an exercise called a squat, described in Chapter 14. We suggest that, if you're a woman, you hold a 5-pound dumbbell in each hand with your arms hanging down at your sides, and if you're a man, use 15-pound dumbbells. If you're a novice, skip the weight and place your hands on your hips.

There are few standard norms for this test, so just use your results as a basis of comparison for future evaluations.

How Flexible Are You?

How come gymnasts can wrap their legs around their shoulders while you have trouble touching your toes? Because gymnasts are more flexible than you are. *Flexibility* refers to how far you can move around a joint's axis (your range of motion) and how easily you can move it. Because your muscles attach to your bone and bones move around a joint's axis (therefore, muscles move the bones around a joint), flexibility also refers to the mobility of your muscles.

Flexibility tests sometimes feel like a cross between circus tryouts and an IQ test. The tester asks you to twist yourself into some strange positions, and you have to figure out what he's talking about. Then you have to see whether your body agrees to follow along.

One common test is the sit-and-reach, which measures the flexibility of your lower-back and rear-thigh muscles. You sit with your legs out straight and place your feet flat on the side of a special metal box. Keeping your legs straight, you lean forward and reach toward the box as far as you can. Along the top of the box, a scale in inches measures how far you reach forward. We find it amusing that the special box costs $200. You can do this same test with the carton that the box comes in.

Some clubs don't get that sophisticated with flexibility measurements; don't hold it against them. As a measure of lower-back and hamstring flexibility, they may simply ask you to bend over and try to touch your toes. Estimating your flexibility instead of measuring it to the exact degree is okay. At least you find out which joints are tight, so you emphasize them when you stretch. For details about how to stretch properly, see Chapter 6.

Table 2-7 describes flexibility tests you can do at home. You may also encounter these tests during a health-club evaluation.

Table 2-7	Testing Your Flexibility			
The Test	*What to Do*	*You Have Good Flexibility If . . .*	*Your Flexibility Needs Work If . . .*	*Your Flexibility Needs A Lot of Work If . . .*
Rear thigh and lower back (toe touch)	Take off your shoes and stand with your feet together and your knees straight but not locked. Bend forward and reach for the floor.	You can touch the floor with little effort and no discomfort in your rear thighs or lower back.	You can just touch your toes with little or no discomfort.	You can't touch your toes, or you feel considerable pain when you try. You may be susceptible to lower-back problems.

(continued)

Table 2-7 *(continued)*

The Test	What to Do	You Have Good Flexibility If . . .	Your Flexibility Needs Work If . . .	Your Flexibility Needs A Lot of Work If . . .
Shoulder	Reach your right hand behind your back and your left hand across your back toward your right shoulder blade. Try to clasp your hands together behind your back.	You can clasp your hands together.	Your fingertips almost touch.	You aren't within an inch of touching your fingertips together. This means you're susceptible to shoulder and neck pain.
Calf and ankle	Sit on the floor with your legs straight out in front of you. Flex your foot so your toes move toward you.	Your toes move enough toward you so that they are beyond perpendicular to the floor.	Your toes bend so they are just in line with your ankles (exactly perpendicular to the floor).	You can barely bend your toes toward you. You may be susceptible to ankle injuries.
Shin	Sitting in the same position as the calf-and-ankle test, point your toes and stretch them toward the floor.	Your toes touch or nearly touch the floor.	Your toes come to within an inch or so of the floor.	Your toes barely move toward the floor. You may be susceptible to shin splints (see definition, Chapter 24).
Top, front of hip; buttocks	Lie on your back and hug one knee to your chest; clasp your hands around your shin just below your knee. Keep the other leg straight.	Your straight leg rests on the floor directly in line with your hip, and you can easily hug your bent knee to your chest.	Your leg, when straight, rests along the floor but to the outside of your hip, and you can almost hug your knee to chest.	Your straight leg doesn't touch the floor, and you can't bring your knee to within a few inches of your chest. You may be susceptible to upper-back and shoulder pain.

The Test	What to Do	You Have Good Flexibility If . . .	Your Flexibility Needs Work If . . .	Your Flexibility Needs A Lot of Work If . . .
Upper back	Lie on your back with your legs out straight, and lift your arms straight overhead. Now drop your arms back behind you toward the floor.	Your arms easily fall to the floor without your lower back arching up.	Your hands almost touch and your lower back remains in contact with the floor.	Your arms don't come within an inch of touching the floor, and your back arches up. You may be susceptible to upper-back and shoulder pain.
Front thigh	Lie on your stomach with one leg straight, and bend the other knee so that your heel moves toward your buttocks.	Your heel easily touches your buttocks.	Your heel comes close to but doesn't quite touch your buttocks.	Your heel doesn't come within a few inches of your buttocks. You may be susceptible to knee pain.

Your Fitness Test Results

Need a place to store your score? Table 2-8 gives you spaces to jot down the results of all the tests described in this chapter.

Table 2-8	Your Fitness Test Results			
Test	Your Score (Test #1)	Your Score (Test #2)	Your Score (Test #3)	Goal
Resting heart rate				
Resting blood pressure				
Aerobic endurance				

(continued)

Table 2-8 *(continued)*

Test Goal	Your Score (Test #1)	Your Score (Test #2)	Your Score (Test #3)
BMI			
Body-fat percentage			
Measurements			
Upper-body strength			
Middle-body strength			
Lower-body strength			
Flexibility			

TIP

What to do with your results

At the end of your fitness evaluation, your tester should not simply say, "Well, your resting heart rate is 72, you did 23 sit-ups, and your body fat is 28 percent." He may explain how your results stack up against other people who are your age and your gender, and he should tell you which areas need the most improvement. A conscientious tester will also help you use the results of tests to customize cardiovascular, strength-training, and flexibility workouts.

Your test results should be detailed on a piece of paper (sort of like a report card) that you can take home. Save this piece of paper so you can see how much you've improved later. One day, it may mean more to you than your high school diploma.

Chapter 3

Establishing Your Plan of Attack

*Y*ou wouldn't start or expand a business without a plan — a clear-cut idea of where you want to take your company and how you propose to get there. Instead, you would assess your cash flow and expenses, choose a location for your office, decide on your hours of operation, and develop strategies to overcome obstacles.

Your workout program deserves the same level of attention, whether you're just beginning to map out your fitness plan or looking to expand and improve your current fitness routine. This chapter helps you develop your plan of attack. We show you how to set realistic goals and track your progress, and we offer strategies for sticking to your plan so that your workout program is as successful as any of those upstart Internet companies run by 20-year-old CEOs.

Setting Goals

Before you embark on a new exercise program — or attempt to invigorate your existing one — clarify why you want to get fit. Maybe heart disease runs in your family, and you want to avoid carrying on that tradition. Maybe you can't keep up with your grandkids. Maybe your pants split as you got up to greet your blind date, and you thought, "I really ought to do something about this." Whatever the reason, make sure you're doing this for yourself — not simply to please your doctor or to lure back the spouse who left you for someone much younger.

Then, after you evaluate your current fitness level (see Chapter 2 for details about fitness testing), start setting specific goals. Research shows that goal-setting works. In typical studies, scientists give one group of exercisers a specific goal, such as doing 60 sit-ups. Meanwhile, they tell a second group of exercisers simply, "Do your best." The exercisers with specific goals tend to have significantly more success than the comparison groups. This approach can work for you, too.

When you start an exercise program, you need to set a few different types of goals. Look at the big picture while giving yourself stepping stones to get there. Having mini-goals makes your long-term goals seem more feasible. Here's a look at the different types of goals you should set.

Long-term goals

Give yourself a goal for the next three to six months. Some people get really creative with their long-term goals. One Ohio woman Suzanne interviewed set a long-term goal to walk to a friend's house — in Birmingham, Alabama. No, she didn't literally hoof it 697 miles. She charted the route on an auto-club map, and for every 20 minutes that she spent doing an aerobic exercise video, she gave herself credit for 1 mile. At the end of each week, she added up her "mileage" and used a yellow highlighter to mark the ground she covered on the map.

Make sure your long-term goals are realistic. If you start your swimming program today, jumping into the frigid waters of the English Channel and swimming all the way to France is not exactly what we recommend for a six-month goal. On the other hand, don't be afraid to dream. Choose a goal that really sparks you — something that may be out of reach at the moment but is not out of the realm of possibility. People are often surprised by what they can accomplish. Liz has a client who was 60 years old when he started training for a trek up Alaska's Mount McKinley. Liz eventually had the guy walking uphill for up to 90 minutes on the treadmill with a heavy pack and hiking boots. After six months of training, the man successfully completed his trek. He was the oldest one on the trip, but he wasn't the slowest. His success inspired him to train for many other hiking events.

Judge for yourself what's realistic. Some people rise to the occasion when they set goals that seem virtually impossible. Other people get discouraged by setting extremely high expectations. If you're a beginner, we recommend setting moderately challenging goals. If you reach your goals earlier than you expect, that's the time to choose more ambitious ones. Here are some concrete examples of long-term goals that may spark your imagination:

- Complete a 50-mile bike ride that's four months away.
- Drop 3 percent body fat in 10 weeks.

- ✔ Do one full pull-up.
- ✔ Drop 20 points from cholesterol count.
- ✔ Fit into that pair of jeans.
- ✔ Walk 1 mile in under 15 minutes.

Short-term goals

Six months is a long time to wait for feelings of success. In order to stay motivated, you need to feel a sense of accomplishment along the way. When Suzanne was bicycling from the West Coast of the United States to the East Coast, she didn't dream about the Atlantic Ocean every day; she focused on a goal that seemed more manageable, like getting across North Dakota. Set short-term goals for one week to one month. Here are some examples:

- ✔ Take two step aerobics classes a week for one month.
- ✔ Improve your 1-mile walk time by 20 seconds.
- ✔ Use the stair-climber four times this week for 30 minutes each time.
- ✔ Bicycle 60 miles a week for the next four weeks.

Immediate goals

Immediate goals refer to goals for each week, day, or workout. This way, when you walk into the gym, you don't waste any time figuring out which exercises to do. Here are examples of immediate goals:

- ✔ Spend a full ten minutes stretching at the end of a workout.
- ✔ Do upper-body weight exercises and 20 minutes on the stair-climber.
- ✔ Run 2 miles.
- ✔ Bike a hilly 20-mile course.

Backup goals

You always need a Plan B, in case something happens and you're not able to reach your primary goal as soon as you want to. By setting backup goals, you have a better chance of achieving something, and you don't feel like a failure if your long-term goal doesn't work out. Suppose your long-term goal is to lose 10 pounds by eating healthier and walking 3 miles a day. Your backup goal could be increasing your stamina enough to walk 3 miles in less than an hour. Or say that you're training for a 10K run in the spring, but you sprain an ankle and have to stop running. If one of your backup goals is to strengthen your upper body, you can still keep on track while your ankle heals.

Finding Ways to Reward Yourself

You let your kids watch their favorite video when they bring home good grades, right? You give your golden retriever a doggy treat when he fetches the Frisbee. Be nice to yourself, too. Attach an appropriate reward to each of your goals. If you drop 3 percent body fat over the next two months, buy yourself a nifty sports watch. If you lift weights three days a week for a month, treat yourself to a massage. Sure, it's bribery, but it works. Short-term rewards are particularly important because there's always a chance that you may not make it all the way to your long-term goal. You need to give yourself credit for making it even halfway. (By the way, triple-decker fudge cake isn't what we have in mind for a reward. Try to make sure your reward is as healthy as your goal.)

As with your goals, you can get pretty creative with your rewards. We know a guy who asked a friend to hold $500 for him. If he reached his goal of losing 25 pounds, he'd get the money back and buy new clothes. If he didn't reach his goal, the money would become a charitable contribution to the Young Republicans. Considering that this guy made Edward Kennedy look like Rush Limbaugh, this was a very good incentive, indeed. The guy lost his 25 pounds.

Writing Everything Down

Setting goals and rewards is pretty easy; forgetting what they are is even easier. To keep yourself honest — and motivated — consider tracking your goals and accomplishments on paper. One friend of ours tapes his goals to the inside of his gym locker. Some people program their computers to flash their goals on-screen twice a day. A member of Liz's Thursday night Internet chat group posts her fitness and weight-loss accomplishments on the message board every week, along with a note thanking other members for their encouraging notes. (And this idea of sharing your goals with others, even someone in the cubicle next door, is a powerful motivator and may keep you from giving up.) Losing 30 pounds was a big milestone for the woman and touched off quite a bit of buzz among the regulars. Other members of the group read these messages avidly and live vicariously through her progress; many have been inspired to start their own fitness programs. Here are some other ways that you can monitor your progress.

Making a goal sheet

Write down your goals on a piece of paper or index card and put it somewhere so that you can see it every day, like taped to your desk or on your
refrigerator. Next to every goal, write down the corresponding reward. This
strategy isn't just for amateurs. Many world-class athletes use it, too. Figure
3-1 shows a sample goal sheet that you can fill out each week. Underneath
each heading, write down your goal and your target date.

Long-Term Goals	Long-Term Rewards
Backup Long-Term Goals	
Short-Term Goals	Short-Term Rewards
Weekly Goals	Weekly Rewards
Workout Goals	Daily Rewards

Figure 3-1:
Make a goal
sheet like
the one
here (or
photocopy
this one).

Keeping a workout log

Whatever your goals are, keeping track of your workouts in a *workout log* (also called a *workout diary* or *training diary*) can help you get better results. You can look back at the end of each week and say, "I did that?" And you may be inspired to accomplish even more. Keeping a log shows you whether your goals are realistic and gives you insight into your exercise patterns. If you're losing weight, building strength, or developing stamina, you won't have to wonder what works, because you'll have a blow-by-blow description of everything you've done to reach your goals.

On the other hand, if you get injured or stuck in a rut, you can turn to your diary for clues as to why. You may discover that if you don't eat before you cycle, you cover your usual route five minutes slower. Maybe you pull a hamstring every time you run over a certain hilly course. Maybe you're more susceptible to catching a cold if you don't rest at least one day each week.

A workout diary keeps you honest. You may think that you're working out four times a week. But when you flip through your log, you may realize that you've been overestimating your efforts.

Bookstores and sporting-goods stores carry a variety of logs, some aimed at walkers, others at weight lifters; others have space to chart any activity you can think of. You also can buy nifty computer software to monitor your progress or use a Web-based tracking program. In Chapter 25, we mention some of our favorite products for recording your workouts. You can also use Figure 3-2 (photocopying the page) to see whether you enjoy tracking your workouts on paper.

Here are some suggestions for filling in the blanks.

Day, date, and conditions

Don't forget to note the day and date. This information helps you assess what you've done in a week; when you look back, you'll know whether you ran those 20 miles in one week or two. Also, you may discover that you always have a bad workout on Fridays because you stay up late Thursday nights to watch *ER*. Maybe Friday is the day for you to take off. Note the day and date of your rest days, as well. This way you know how much recovery time you're giving yourself.

In the Conditions box, you may also want to note the weather conditions, including the wind and the temperature, because you work much harder when it's raining or hot. Describe the course you cover (was it hilly or flat?); who you worked out with ("Marge talks too much"), and how you feel before, during, and after your workout. These notes may help you trace the root of any training problems that crop up.

Day of the Week	Date		Conditions	
Goals				
Cardiovascular Training	Time		Distance	Difficulty Rating
Strength Training		Weight	Sets	Reps	Notes
Notes					

Figure 3-2:
A sample
workout log.

Goals for the workout

Write down what you hope to accomplish during your workout, like completing the 20-minute Roller Coaster program on the stair-climber or swimming a half mile. Rather than scribbling a few lines while you're running from the locker room into an aerobics class, fill in this section the night before or, better yet, immediately following your last workout. This makes you stop and think about just what it is that you're trying to achieve. If you keep your goals in mind, you may have more enthusiasm for your workout.

Cardiovascular training

Write down the type of activity, whether it's stationary cycling, walking, skating, rowing, and so on. In the Time and Distance sections, note how long your aerobic session lasted and (when applicable) how far you went — for example:

> ✔ **Cardiovascular Training:** "Jogged on treadmill"
>
> ✔ **Time:** "20 minutes"
>
> ✔ **Distance:** "1.8 miles"

In the Difficulty Rating box, rate your workout on a scale from one to ten. Don't base this assessment simply on the number of miles you walked or the number of calories you burned. Instead, rate your workouts according to how hard you push yourself. A 1 rating is an extremely easy day; a 10 is an all-out workout. (See Chapter 8 for details on rating your exertion.) The purpose of the difficulty rating is to remind you to aim for a healthy mix of numbers. If you rate a 9 on Monday, Tuesday is a good day for a 2 workout. Log a 0 for the days you don't exercise.

Strength training

Jot down the name of each exercise, the amount of weight you lifted, and the number of sets you did. (If you need any of these terms defined, see Chapter 14.) If you don't know the name of an exercise, make it a point to find out. Writing down "bicep curl" may reinforce the idea that this exercise strengthens your biceps. (If you're not sure where your biceps are, see Chapter 12.) You may also want to note what changes you need to make during your next weight-lifting session. Suppose you use 50 pounds on the leg-press machine and have a pretty easy time of it. In your diary, write that you want to try 60 pounds the next time. Also, note which exercises are particularly easy and which need more attention.

Stretching

Simply note whether you stretched or not. You may also jot down a few words about which muscles felt the tightest and which stretches felt the best.

Notes

Here's your chance to record any details that don't seem to fit into the other categories. For example, you may describe a new leg exercise you tried. Or you may elaborate on which yoga poses you found most difficult. Or you may realize that you always feel great when you work out with a certain friend. Write down whatever you feel is important.

Making Exercise a Habit

As we mention in the introduction to this book, 50 percent of new exercisers quit within eight weeks. Of course, we want to make sure that you're among the other 50 percent. The following tips can help you get over the hump and boost the odds that you'll stick with your new program. We discuss several of these topics in detail throughout the book, but we want you to keep them in mind from the start.

Expect to feel uncomfortable at first

Exercise doesn't need to be painful, but if you've neglected your body, don't expect a free ride. Despite what you hear on infomercials — "just five minutes a day, and you can do this on the couch while watching TV!" — exercise is a serious commitment. You can't get into shape without exerting some real effort and, perhaps, without experiencing some (but not a lot of) discomfort.

Pace yourself

Don't buy every exercise video on the market or try every weight machine in the gym the first day. You'll kill your enthusiasm and flame out fast. Always keep yourself hungry for more.

Work out with friends or join a club

An exercise buddy can push you to new heights — or get your butt outside for a walk on the days when you'd rather stay home and watch reruns of *Bewitched.* If you make a date to meet a friend at the gym, you're a lot more likely to show up than if you make a date with yourself.

Take the initiative to find workout buddies by joining an exercise class at your community center or YMCA, a Sierra Club hike, a local running group, or a charity event or race that has a training program.

Mix it up

One common complaint about exercise is that it's boring. But if you change your workouts every couple of months, or even every time you exercise, that excuse pretty much flies out the window. This book is filled with ideas for varying your workouts — experimenting with different weight-training equipment, trying new stretches, and changing the intensity of your cardiovascular program, doing full-body or body-part workouts, training energy systems, varying reps, sets, times, intensity techniques, and so on.

Not only does this strategy keep you motivated, but it also keeps you healthy. Many injuries are the result of repeating the same movement patterns. So if you alternate, say, swimming with running, you're less likely to develop the knee problems that are common to runners or the shoulder injuries that crop up among swimmers.

Buy the right gear and equipment

Cycling isn't going to be fun if you're riding an old clunker that doesn't shift properly. Walking isn't going to be comfortable or safe if you're doing it in sandals. You don't need to spend megabucks on top-of-the-line equipment, but investing in the right gear and equipment can sometimes be the difference between success and failure.

Liz had a client who went out hiking in a 20-year-old pair of aerobics shoes and had a miserable time. She kept twisting her ankles because the shoes had poor ankle support, and her feet were blistered and bruised because the thin padding didn't protect her from the rocks underfoot. Upon returning from her hike, the client announced to Liz that she hated hiking. Liz suggested that she buy a new pair of hiking boots and give it another try. The next time out, outfitted in a comfy, sturdy pair of boots, the woman sailed to the head of the group and leapt from rock to rock like a mountain goat. She then reported to Liz that she loved hiking.

In Chapter 10, we discuss gadgets and apparel you need for a number of different outdoor activities. But here are some general tips on shoes, one of the most important fitness purchases:

✔ **Buy the right shoe for your sport.** Walking shoes are more flexible and have firmer heel support than running shoes. Shoes for tennis, golf, and basketball have their own special designs; even sprinters and distance runners have different footwear needs. If you dabble in a variety of activities — walking one day, biking the next, and lifting weights the next — *cross-training shoes* may suffice (ask for them at your favorite sporting-goods store), but if you spend a lot of time doing one particular activity, invest in shoes designed for that activity.

✔ **Don't cheap out.** Bargain brands may look the same, but today's fitness shoes are highly technical. Beneath those swooshes, stripes, and flashy colors, a lot of biomechanical engineering is going on to protect your feet, ankles, and other joints. A decent pair of athletic shoes may cost you at least $40, and in some cases more than double that. But you save money down the line: One thing that's always more expensive than a good pair of shoes is a visit to an orthopedist.

- ✔ **Shop at a specialty store where the salespeople are fitness enthusiasts themselves.** In New York, runners are blessed with a fine chain of equipment shops called Super Runners, and many other cities and suburban areas have at least one running and/or walking store. If you're a tennis player, look for a tennis specialty store. Same with cycling, yoga, and so on. When you find a shoe you're comfortable with, you can save money on future pairs by shopping through a catalog or by joining a frequent-buyers club at your local shop.

- ✔ **Make sure the shoes feel good from the moment you put them on.** Forget this "breaking in" business. Try on several pairs of shoes, and take each one for a test run around the mall. Bounce up and down in them; mime a few quick volleys.

Cut yourself some slack

Recognize that people come in all shapes and sizes, and everyone improves at a different pace. Getting inspiration from other people is great, but don't let anyone else's accomplishments diminish your own. Be proud that you've worked up to walking 3 miles every other day, even if your neighbor runs 10 miles a day.

And don't get mad at yourself if you miss a few days — or even a few months — of exercise. Expect to be up and down a bit in your motivation, which means you won't always exercise with the same consistency and frequency. If you fall off the wagon, just try again. You have the rest of your life to get this right.

Chapter 4

Hiring a Trainer

*O*perating exercise equipment isn't nuclear physics, but neither is it something you should attempt to figure out on your own. We recommend signing up with a trainer — for at least one session — to get yourself started on a strength and cardiovascular program suited to your goals. Even workout veterans have plenty to gain from a session or two with a trainer.

A trainer can teach you the subtleties of using exercise equipment: how to grip a barbell, how far to pull down a rope, and how to adjust a machine to fit your body — stuff that's tough to glean from a book or video. We know a woman who hired a trainer just to teach her how to use the new technology in her gym, like the computerized weight machines, the wireless TV/radio headphones, and the fancy treadmill programs.

A good trainer can teach you all this and more. Unfortunately, the industry has its share of quacks. This chapter explains how you can benefit from a trainer and discusses how to find a qualified one.

Five Smart Reasons to Hire a Trainer

Trainers do a lot more than just whip wimpy actors into shape for their next action movie, and they don't all charge $200 an hour. (We tell you more about how much you should expect to pay in the "Trainer fees" section later in this chapter.) Consider hiring a trainer if you're in any of the following situations:

✔ **You're totally out of shape (or *deconditioned,* as the politically correct like to say).** If climbing the ropes in high school gym class was the last time you worked out, a personal trainer is a great way to bring you into the modern age. A lot has changed over the years, from the equipment to the lingo to proper stretching and strength-training techniques. A trainer can get you comfortable in your new environment and start you on a program that's appropriate for your fitness level, so your new foray into fitness doesn't end a week later with a trip to the orthopedist. You don't need to sign up for life; five to ten sessions can get you up and running.

✔ **You want to update your program.** You can hire a trainer for a session or two to reevaluate your workout regimen. If you're feeling stagnant, a new routine can give you a jump-start and ultimately improve your fitness level. (Of course, you actually have to work out for this to happen.)

✔ **You're training for a specific goal.** Say you want to run your first 10K race, but you aren't sure how long, how far, how often, or how hard to train. A qualified trainer can design a workout program that'll get you to the finish line. Look for a trainer who specializes in the area you want to work on, such as losing weight, building strength, or getting fit for ski season. We know a trainer who works only with runners, designing their running schedules and appropriate strength-training and stretching routines. Many of her clients are people who want to run their first marathon without getting injured.

✔ **You're coming back from an injury or illness.** If you have a specific condition such as lower back pain, or if you've just had surgery on your knee, a trainer can help you get back on your feet. Check with your doctor; she may want you to visit a physical therapist first. Still, more and more physicians are giving the okay for trainers to participate in a patient's rehabilitation. Screen the trainer carefully, so you don't make matters worse. A growing number of trainers specialize in conditions such as multiple sclerosis or breast cancer.

✔ **You need motivation.** If you won't exercise unless a trainer is standing there counting your repetitions, consider the money well spent.

Weeding Out the Poseurs

Currently, few states have legal requirements for fitness trainers (and even those laws have loopholes). At the same time, a behind-the-scenes scramble is underway among the various professional organizations vying to be declared the official certifying body. In the meantime, however, anyone who can hoist a dumbbell and print a business card on a home computer can call himself a personal trainer.

Screen a potential trainer with the same care that you use to screen a potential employee. And don't be afraid to try someone new if you don't hit it off with the first trainer. It's your time, your money, and your health we're talking about. Our friend Daniel was thoroughly demoralized by his first trainer. "The guy kept looking at himself in the mirror and then pulling up his shirt and showing me his abs," Daniel recalls. "Then he'd stick me on some machine without showing me any technique and leave me there while he'd go talk to some girl." It took Daniel four years to muster the courage to hire another trainer. "I should never have waited so long," says Daniel, who's now a confident lifter and a regular in the weight room.

The following sections tell you what to consider when investigating trainers.

Certification

As with many other occupations and professions, the fitness industry offers certification tests. A certification is by no means a guarantee of competence, but getting certified by quality organizations is a time-consuming, pain-in-the-butt process. You have to study for at least a few months and then spend a full day taking a test. At the very least, going through this process shows commitment: You know that the trainer isn't just doing this job because it pays better than her old job as a bike messenger. And by getting the certification, trainers surely pick up enough to have a basic level of competence.

Still, some mighty unqualified people show up for these exams. While proctoring a recent certification test, Liz asked one candidate to demonstrate a thigh stretch. He sat down on the floor and twisted one of his legs behind him, then began scooting himself forward on the floor. When Liz asked why he was doing that, the candidate explained that the maneuver shocks the muscle into stretching. He admitted that the stretch was indeed as painful as it looked, but said that was an unfortunate but necessary part of the exercise. Although Liz was technically not allowed to offer candidates her opinion, she felt compelled to tell the guy that he should never, ever, *ever* use that technique with a client.

High-quality certifying organizations weed out bozos like that. However, some organizations certify any breathing body. These schools are sometimes advertised on late-night TV or in the back of fitness magazines (alongside the ads for legitimate schools). You definitely don't want a trainer who graduated from the National Correspondence School of Diesel Mechanics, TV Repair, and Personal Training. If you're skeptical, ask to see a copy of the actual certificate.

The following are among the best organizations that certify trainers. Their Web sites can refer you to certified trainers in your area. And make sure that your trainer's certification is current; most expire after a year or two unless the trainer takes continuing education classes.

- **Aerobics and Fitness Association of America (AFAA):** This organization offers a variety of certifications, including Personal Trainer and Advanced Personal Trainer. The Personal Trainer exam, which includes both a practical and written portion (and many other tests are written-only), covers a wide range of topics but require less knowledge than ACSM or ACE certification tests. If the AFAA Personal Trainer is your trainer's only certification, your trainer may be a former aerobics instructor making the switch to personal trainer without enough education or experience. Or, the trainer may have taken the exam out of convenience, because it's offered in many rural areas where other exams aren't available. See the organization's Web site at www.afaa.com.

- **American College of Sports Medicine (ACSM):** The ACSM offers several certification levels and usually requires that the trainer possess a graduate degree in one of the exercise sciences. The certification we recommend is the Health/Fitness Instructor. The test is very tough, so many trainers avoid it, but it's the gold standard for personal trainers. Visit www.acsm.org.

- **American Council on Exercise (ACE):** This organization certifies both personal trainers and group trainers (such as aerobics instructors); we prefer the certification geared toward personal trainers. The ACE Personal Trainer certification is the most popular in the industry, and although the test is easier than the ACSM Health/Fitness Instructor test, it's still plenty challenging. The certification is more practical than most, emphasizing the trainer's ability to design appropriate programs for a wide variety of fitness levels and medical conditions. Visit www.acefitness.org.

- **International Sport Science Association (ISSA):** ISSA has ten different certification programs, including Youth Fitness, Personal Fitness Trainer, and Senior Fitness. Most of its programs are similar in the information they contain, with sections devoted to the specific area of certification. ISSA has more of a bodybuilding emphasis and focus from its founders, educators, and information. Its certification process is actually more stringent than many, requiring case studies and written papers as part of the process, in addition to the written test. Although not quite at the level of the other certifying organizations, ISSA has become much more widely recognized. Check out www.issaonline.com.

- **National Academy of Sports Medicine (NASM):** This group, now affiliated with Reebok, offers a well-respected and practical Personal Trainer certification. Trainers must attend a workshop and pass an exam; trainers need strong physiology, anatomy, and biomechanics backgrounds going into the workshop, which provides the education, solutions, and tools needed by fitness professionals to systematically progress any client through specific phases of training in order to reach any goal. NASM trainers have a strong emphasis on understanding the in-depth workings of the body as a functional unit. Check out `www.nasm.org`.

✔ **National Strength and Conditioning Association (NSCA):** This organization offers two tough certifications: the Certified Strength and Conditioning Specialist (CSCS), geared toward training high-level athletes in team sports, and the Certified Personal Trainer (CPT), designed for trainers who work in gyms. All trainers must pass a three-part written exam that includes a video analysis of exercises. Trainers certified by the NSCA usually know a lot about strength training and conditioning; the NSCA asks candidates to identify every muscle involved in a particular exercise and requires them to know precisely what role each muscle is playing at which point in the movement. Visit the NSCA Certification Commission at `www.nsca-cc.org`.

✔ **Specialty certifications:** Some specialty fields, such as yoga (see Chapter 16), Pilates (see Chapter 17), and kickboxing (discussed in Chapter 19) do have certifications. Others, such as boxing, don't. Don't expect a boxing instructor or a country-and-western line-dancing teacher to be certified as a trainer. But if he does have a diploma from one of the organizations we list, that's a plus.

These organizations aren't the only ones that offer certifications and certificates. Many colleges and universities offer their own extensive programs. And while some health clubs put their employees through rigorous training courses, trust courses from recognized organizations and universities above all else.

University degrees

Most trainers don't have degrees in physiology or related fields, so don't hold it against them. But a master's degree (M.A. or M.S.) is usually even better than a certification, and a fitness-related B.A. or B.S. can be a big plus. Look for degrees in exercise physiology, exercise science, physical therapy, occupational therapy, fitness management, sports medicine, physical education, or kinesiology. If the trainer has a fitness-related university degree but not an industry certification, ask whether she keeps up with the latest techniques by going to conferences and seminars. Opinions and facts change quickly in the health and fitness field; if your trainer earned his Ph.D. in 1973 and hasn't attended a workshop since, he needs to join the modern world.

Many registered nurses and physical therapists are getting into the training business. They tend to know a lot about how muscles work; what's more, they may be able to accept insurance reimbursement if a doctor recommends training for treatment or rehab purposes.

Experience

Choose a trainer who has at least two years of experience at a club or on her own. Be sure to check references. The best way to get the lowdown on a trainer is from other clients. Also consider your own needs: If you're looking to have a detailed program designed, you have medical conditions or injuries that require experience, or you have specific athletic goals you want to reach, look for someone with many years of experience.

Brochures

An in-home trainer should have a brochure or packet describing her background and experience as well as her focus and philosophy. (Trainers employed by a single health club probably won't have brochures, although clubs may post information about their trainers' qualifications.) The packet also should clearly explain fees, payment schedules, and cancellation policies. Printed materials show a degree of professionalism. Many trainers also have their own Web sites. Clients can go on the Net and peruse the trainer's bio, photo, and sample workouts.

Liability insurance

Make sure your trainer has insurance to cover any mishaps that may occur. Many trainers have you sign a release, but this doesn't absolve them from responsibility and from using safe and appropriate judgment, like asking you to bench-press 250 pounds during your first workout.

Lawsuits against trainers are unusual but not unprecedented. The widower of a health-club member who died of a stroke filed a $40 million suit against his wife's trainer for giving dangerous nutritional advice. (The club was also named in the suit.) According to the suit, the trainer recommended ephedra, an herbal supplement that has been linked to dozens of deaths and should never be taken by people with high blood pressure. At the time, the woman was taking prescription medicine for hypertension.

An interview

To make sure that you're compatible with your trainer, talk with him at length and ask questions before hiring him. A trainer may look good on paper but may not be able to speak in complete sentences. Or you may have a personality conflict — the trainer may have too much or too little enthusiasm for your taste. Liz knows a woman who won't work with a particular trainer because the trainer laughs too loudly; she's afraid he'll draw too much attention to her when she already feels self-conscious about working out.

Don't judge your potential trainer by looks alone. Just because someone's a chiseled workout god doesn't mean he knows which exercises are best for you or even how to teach them to you. A great teacher can live in a less-than-godlike body.

A trial session

Before you commit to several sessions with a trainer, ask for a free or discounted trial workout. Also look for a money-back guarantee if you're not fully satisfied with your trainer or the session. Many trainers will comply in the hopes of getting a long-term client. Most gyms that offer personal training either offer a first session free or a discounted session before making you commit to a package of sessions.

Trainer fees

Fees vary from region to region, and from big cities to small towns. In Des Moines, you may pay $30 an hour; in New York, the going rate is between $85 and $105 per hour, and trainers charging as much as $120 per hour is not uncommon. (Charges depend on experience and popularity; the more experienced and popular a client, the higher the fee.) Ask friends or call gyms to get a sense of rates in your area, so you know if a trainer's fees are way out of the ballpark.

On the off chance that someone is charging too little, watch out. Your so-called trainer may just be a pizza-delivery guy who happens to work out in his spare time and thinks he can make extra cash on the side.

If you belong to a health club, you'll probably save money by hiring a trainer through the club. Good gyms thoroughly screen their trainers and keep an eye on them. However, follow the rules we list in the preceding section for weeding out bad trainers: Don't assume that the club hires trainers who are certified and experienced.

You also can cut costs by signing up for joint sessions with a friend. The trainer may charge slightly more than the regular hourly fee, but split two ways, your session is still a deal. You won't get quite as much attention from the trainer, but teaming up with a friend may make a session affordable. Try to choose a friend who's at the same fitness level as you or who has similar fitness goals. If you're training for a marathon and your friend is a linebacker getting ready for football season, the trainer is going to have a tough time serving both your needs at once.

Another way to save money is to do a half-hour of cardio exercise on your own (see Part III of this book) with a program designed but not supervised by your trainer, and then hook up with the trainer for a half-hour of weight training. This is a service primarily offered by gym trainers, as opposed to trainers who come to your home.

Cybertrainers

If you're not big on human contact, if you want to save money, or if you just can't get enough of technology, you may be interested in hiring an Internet trainer. We can't really call these "personal" trainers, because you never actually come face-to-face with a person, but many of these Web sites offer more individualized advice than you can get from a book or a video (or a lousy human trainer). But watch out: Some of these sites are a rip-off.

Most programs start by asking you questions about your health, your goals, and your current workouts. The better ones also ask you to perform some basic at-home fitness tests, similar to those we describe in Chapter 2, and then enter the results online. The really bad ones ask you for little more than your credit-card number.

After you plug in all this info, your cybertrainer sends you a workout routine with suggested exercises, sets, and repetitions. Usually, you can download videos demonstrating how to perform each recommended exercise. Or, you can go to an exercise database, click on any number of exercises for a particular muscle group, and watch a demonstration. You can print out the routine and take it with you to the gym, or tack it up on the wall at home. If you plug in your workouts, you get feedback — allegedly from an actual human being — on how you're progressing. For example, the trainer may suggest that you increase your weight or try a new shoulder exercise.

The Internet training program Web sites we like best, `http://personaltraining.org` and `www.physicalgenius.com`, offer workouts designed by trainers who seem to know what they're doing. Physical Genius lets you download programs into a handheld device that you can carry to the gym. You have to pay a couple hundred dollars for the device, which you order through the site.

Expect to pay up to $500 for four months of cybertraining. Watch out for programs that charge $100 a session and those with exercise descriptions written in jargonese. Pay attention to the credentials of the trainers who are supposed to have designed the routines.

To find an Internet trainer other than the two we list, enter "online personal trainer," "workout programs," or "weight-training programs" into Google or some other search engine.

Finally, ask whether your trainer charges by the hour or by the session. Typically, sessions last 45 to 90 minutes, including discussion and consultation time (not just workout time). If you're paying by the hour and your session runs over, you may wind up paying a lot more than you expected.

Knowing a Quality Trainer When You See One

Trainers have different philosophies and use a variety of techniques. Some come from the drill-sergeant school of motivation; others prefer the cheer-leading approach. Still, there are some characteristics that all trainers should share. Choose a trainer who:

✔ **Evaluates your fitness and goals:** Before anything else, your trainer should assess your current physical condition. (See Chapter 2 to find out what's included in a fitness evaluation.) Then your trainer should have a long talk with you about your expectations for the training sessions — your hopes, your dreams, and your specific goals. All this information is crucial: To really be of help to you, a trainer must know where you're starting from and where you want to go.

✔ **Gives you a balanced program:** Unless you specifically request otherwise, your sessions should include three components: cardiovascular exercise, strength training, and flexibility exercises. Some trainers prefer that you do the cardiovascular portion on your own, but if you ask, your trainer should help you design a program and keep tabs on your workout and intensity. *Heads up:* Many trainers also skip the stretching and cool-down portions of a workout.

✔ **Watches you closely:** Your trainer should pay attention to your form and give you pointers throughout the session. On the other hand, you don't want a trainer who blabs incessantly. Your trainer also should *spot* you — in other words, stand poised to grab the weight and give you some help if your muscles give out.

✔ **Reassesses your goals and measures your progress:** A good trainer retests you after the first six weeks of training and, if you've been working out consistently, every two to three months thereafter. A trainer who is really on the ball also reassesses your goals every few weeks to keep you motivated.

✔ **Listens to you:** If you mention that an exercise doesn't feel right, your trainer should figure out why and show you an alternative move for the same body part. There's no single exercise you absolutely must do. If you tell him you're feeling stagnant, overtrained, or underchallenged, he should alter your program.

✔ **Teaches you to be independent:** Ironically, good trainers train themselves out of a job by teaching you how to do everything on your own. After a few months, you should be able to set the correct amount of weight, adjust the machines, use proper form, and modify your routine as needed. Of course, if you'd never exercise by yourself, you're welcome to hire your trainer for life; she'll be glad to accommodate you. Regardless, you should know how to do everything on your own. This way, if you're out of town on business or vacation, you can keep up your workouts at a hotel or local gym. And if, heaven forbid, your trainer goes on vacation, you won't have an excuse to stop working out.

✔ **Speaks English, not jargon:** Some trainers say things like, "Your patella edema is a limiting factor in increasing your volume of oxygen uptake." Translation: "You can't run faster because you have bad knees." If you can't understand what your trainer is saying, find someone new. You shouldn't expend extra energy just trying to figure out what the heck you're being asked to do. Trainers with jargonitis tend to be really insecure. Occasionally, however, a small dose of fitness verbiage is good for you; a trainer may be trying to teach you something that you actually should know, like where your triceps are. (By the way, if you don't know where your triceps are, read Chapter 12.)

Getting the Most out of Your First Training Session

Even with the guidance of a trainer, your first session may be a little awkward. One friend of ours says she just had to swallow her pride while trying out the weight machines for the first time. "Here was this cute, young trainer helping me climb onto the hamstring machine," she remembers. "I felt like a 40-year-old woman trying to get on a horse for the first time. I'm lying on the bench with my butt in the air, and the trainer's saying, 'Keep your butt down.' And I'm saying, 'That's as far down as it goes. It's just big.'"

Having a good sense of humor can get you through a first workout session without any ego damage. So what if you sit backward on the shoulder machine? So what if you sink to the floor when you hop onto the stair-climber? Your trainer may as well earn his money showing you the right way to use the equipment.

Here are some tips to help ease your anxiety and make your first session a productive one:

✔ **Schedule the session at a time when the gym isn't busy (any time other than weekday mornings or evenings).** This way, you won't have 12 other members clamoring to use the arm-curl machine while the trainer teaches you to adjust the seat.

✔ **Take notes and draw pictures.** During the session, your trainer should fill out a card listing each exercise in your program, how much weight to lift, and how many sets and reps to do. But if you supplement this information with your own notes, you may find it easier to remember what to do when you work out alone. For example, if your trainer writes "lat pull-down," you can add, "pull bar down to chest; strengthens back muscles; adjust seat to second notch." You may even want to sketch some of the machines so that when you work out by yourself, you won't spend ten minutes searching for the right contraption. Some facilities number the machines to make them easier to remember and identify, too. Your trainer simply notes the machine number and the seat height.

✔ **Ask lots of questions.** Don't be too intimidated to ask the trainer why he picked a particular chest exercise or for a reminder of where your delts are. No question is too stupid (unless you're asking what time the 3 p.m. boxing class starts).

✔ **Don't expect to absorb everything your trainer tells you on the first day.** Every time you work out, you'll pick up more information, such as how to adjust each machine and how to stretch each muscle group. You can make things easier on yourself by scheduling a second training appointment to reinforce what you learned on the first go-around. Some gyms charge for a second appointment; some don't. If you bring up the issue when you join the gym, some clubs may throw in a few extra training sessions.

✔ **Don't try to impress the trainer by lifting too much.** The trainer doesn't expect you to be Arnold Schwarzenegger. One friend of ours lost any such illusions during his first session with a trainer. "I sat down on this machine and pulled the handles back, and the trainer said, 'Do you feel that?' I said, 'Yeah, it's really pulling on my muscles.' Then the trainer said, 'Oops, I forgot to put the weight on.'" When stuff like that happens, just laugh and realize that it doesn't take much time to get stronger.

Being the Best Client You Can Be

You have the right to demand a lot from your trainer, but your trainer can also expect a certain level of courtesy, attention, and effort from you. Keep in mind the following rules of client etiquette. Some of these tips apply just to home trainers; others apply to trainers at a gym.

✔ **Don't show up at the door in your pajamas.** Your trainer shouldn't have to serve as your alarm clock or wait a half-hour for you to get your act together. Like you, the trainer has a schedule, and time is money. If you're late getting started, the trainer has every right to cut your session short or charge you extra.

✔ **Don't answer your doorbell, phone, fax, pager, or e-mail.** This just wastes the trainer's time and distracts you from your workout. Also, if you have kids, make sure that someone is watching them. Your trainer won't be happy if your 5-year-old runs into the room screaming, "Mommy! Mommy! My Scene Barbie is sick!"

✔ **Don't whine.** Get yourself in a positive frame of mind before your training sessions.

Liz used to train a woman who wanted to tone her legs but who hated to do leg exercises. While working out, she used to curse at Liz very loudly, to the point where people would turn around and stare. The management eventually asked Liz and her client to go elsewhere, but Liz refused to work with the client any longer.

✔ **Schedule in advance.** You'll have a very happy trainer if you schedule a month in advance. (Just make sure that it's a schedule you can stick to.) At the very least, don't call in the morning and expect a session that afternoon.

If canceling or rescheduling, give your trainer as much time as possible. Many trainers have a 24-hour cancellation policy, which requires you to cancel or reschedule your session with at least 24 hours' notice. This allows your trainer time to adjust his schedule and possibly fit someone else into that spot. It also helps keep a positive rapport with your trainer.

✔ **Speak up.** Just because you've hired a trainer doesn't mean you've lost the power of speech. If something doesn't feel right, say so. Your trainer isn't a mind reader.

One woman we know severely pulled her inner-thigh muscles because a trainer went overboard on a stretch. Afterward, she said she felt pain for nearly a minute before she heard a loud pop. Why didn't she say anything? Because she didn't want to question the trainer. Granted, the trainer should have paid better attention, but he couldn't have been expected to know how the woman felt.

✔ **Keep the relationship professional.** Your trainer isn't your therapist. Inevitably, you'll get into personal stuff; after all, this is your personal trainer. But don't take your bad day out on your trainer, and don't expect your trainer to fix your life. And never make a pass at your trainer, just as he or she shouldn't be making a pass at you or making inappropriate comments.

Part II
Enjoying Total-Body Health: Eating Well and Staying Injury-Free

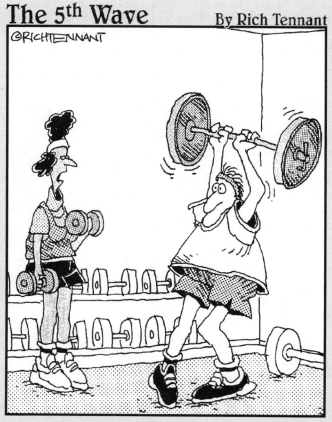

The 5th Wave   By Rich Tennant

@RICHTENNANT

"That's really great form — for someone taking his underwear off over his head."

In this part . . .

We tell you how to enjoy whole-body health, from injury prevention to stretching to eating well.

Chapter 5 helps you prevent and treat common exercise injuries — and discover the difference between a sprain and a strain.

We also introduce you to the most neglected — and, perhaps most important — component of fitness: flexibility. In Chapter 6, we make a darn good case for taking ten minutes out of each day to stretch. We also give you a rundown of the various stretching philosophies, cover the basic rules of stretching, and present a head-to-toe stretching workout that doesn't require the flexibility of a Cirque du Soleil troupe member.

Chapter 7 fills you in on nutrition basics: You get the skinny on low-carb diets, low-fat eating, food pyramids, vitamin supplements, and phytochemicals (an important group of substances with long and unpronounceable names).

Chapter 5

This Doesn't Have to Happen to You: Avoiding Common Injuries

. . . .

In This Chapter

▶ Differentiating between good pain and bad pain

▶ Recognizing and treating exercise injuries

. . . .

Sometimes, exercise hurts. If you never lift anything heavier than a tube of Pringles potato chips and then start lifting dumbbells, naturally you're going to feel some soreness. That type of pain is nothing to worry about. But, if you wake up the morning after a weight-lifting session and feel like your left arm has been shredded by a meat grinder, that's a different story. This chapter tells you how to differentiate the two, how to take care of an injury, and how to prevent injuries in the first place.

Taking Care of Common Injuries

Normal pain is achy, dull, and very general. Usually, you feel it throughout an entire muscle or over a large area of your body. Bad pain — the type that signals injury — tends to be sharp and specific. It usually hurts when you do certain movements, like bending your knee or lifting your arm overhead. It's important to recognize this type of pain and act accordingly. Not long ago, Suzanne ignored the shoulder pain that flared up after she performed certain chest exercises. Eventually, the pain got so bad — and her tendon so inflamed — that she couldn't lift a pitcher of water without wincing. Suzanne was forced to take off three entire months from upper-body weight training, which made her grouchy and a real annoyance to her friends and kept her from improving her fitness level.

You can avoid a scenario like that if you follow the advice in this chapter, which covers injuries common to people who exercise. We tell you how to recognize and treat them — and how to prevent them from happening in the first place.

Strains and sprains

First, we should clear up some terminology. One of your coworkers may hobble into the office announcing he has "strained" a muscle — or maybe he says he has "pulled" a muscle. These terms are interchangeable, but they're not synonymous with "sprain."

When you *strain* a muscle (commonly called a *pulled muscle*), you over-stretch or tear the *tendon* (the tough, cord-like end of the muscle that attaches to the bone). Strains happen when you push yourself harder than normal, like when you challenge your kid brother to a 100-yard dash. A *sprain* refers to a torn or overstretched *ligament* (the connective tissue that joins two bones together). You can sprain a joint — like when you turn your ankle while stepping off a curb — but you can't sprain a muscle.

Two of the most commonly strained muscles are the hamstrings (rear thigh muscles) and groin (inner-thigh) muscles. (See Chapter 12 for pictures of and more information about these muscles.) These muscles often pull because they're tight and because most people don't take five minutes to *warm up* (that is, to ease into a workout by starting slowly and gradually increasing the tempo — see Chapter 8) before working out. You know you've strained your hamstring if a sharp pain shoots up the back of your thigh when you straighten your leg. You have a groin pull if a stabbing pain prevents you from lifting your leg in toward your other leg or out to the side. In both cases, you may feel a lump or a knot where the muscle has tightened up. Stop the offending activity for a few days until the muscle repairs itself. Otherwise, you may be headed for a full-blown tear, in which case you could be sidelined for several months instead of being laid up for a few days. Light stretching may be beneficial (see Chapter 6).

To speed up the healing process for a strain, apply ice to the injured area for the first 24 to 48 hours. (See the "RICE, RICE Baby" section in this chapter for icing tips.) Gentle — emphasis on *gentle* — massage may help work out muscle kinks. To prevent future pulls, carefully stretch your muscles every day, always *after* a thorough warm-up, and increase your exercise program on a gradual basis. Check your shoes, too. Athletic shoes with *flared heels* — heels that are wider on the bottom than on the top — may restrain your foot and ankle from normal movement. That, in turn, may cause your thigh muscles to tighten up. Shoes that are too big cause the same type of problem.

Sprains occur most commonly at the ankle. If you sprain your ankle badly, you may hear a loud pop or tearing sound when the injury happens. Usually you're left with a bruise and swelling, and you can't place any of your weight on the injured foot without pain. The treatment for a sprain is to keep your shoe on for as long as possible (this keeps the ankle from swelling), and then following the RICE formula (see the "RICE, RICE, Baby" section later in this chapter).

Shin splints

Shin splints is a catch-all term for shin pain, usually caused by a slight separation between the shin muscle and the bone. You can develop shin splints from doing more exercise than your body is ready to handle or simply from introducing a new aspect to your training, such as wearing a new pair of shoes, running downhill, or running on the beach when you normally run on asphalt.

To cure shin splints, back off for a few days. When you're free of pain, start back up gradually. Don't increase your exercise time or distance by more than 10 percent a week (see Chapter 10). Ice helps by reducing inflammation and by dulling the pain. For shin splints, we recommend the ice massage method described in the "RICE, RICE, Baby" section. Also, gently but deeply massaging the area several times a day can help.

To prevent shin splints, strengthen your shin muscles so that they work more in harmony with your calves, the muscles that operate in opposition to them. Here's one simple exercise: Stand on the floor or with your heels on the edge of a stair, with your weight distributed evenly over the entire length of your foot, and lift and lower your toes and the balls of your feet 20 to 30 times, as shown in Chapter 14. Ask a trainer to show you some other shin exercises. Stretching the calf muscles (see Chapter 6) also helps prevent injury to the shin and ankle.

Also, be sure to replace your athletic shoes often so your shins don't take a pounding from lack of cushioning. We know one guy who solved his chronic shin splint problem overnight by buying a pair of shoes with a slightly wider heel. This seemed to suit his running style; a podiatrist or sports-medicine specialist (or even a well-informed running store associate) can help you find the solution that suits your style. If all else fails, your podiatrist may make a special pair of inserts, called *orthotics*, to properly position your feet in your shoes.

Achilles tendonitis

Achilles was the mighty Greek warrior whose mother had dipped him into the waters of the River Styx to make him invulnerable. The problem was, she missed a spot: the point on the back of his heel where she held him. This area, where the Achilles tendon connects to the heel, is a weak spot for just about anyone who happens to stand or move in an upright position, especially runners, walkers, in-line skaters, cyclists, and tennis players. When the Achilles tendon becomes swollen, sore, or inflamed, you have *Achilles tendonitis.*

The most common culprit is a calf muscle that's too short and tight. A regular stretching program that focuses on your foot, calf, and hamstring muscles (see Chapter 6) goes a long way toward preventing the problem. Your old friend ice also can reduce swelling and relieve pain (see the "RICE, RICE Baby" section for details). If you wear high heels, wean yourself from them and switch to flats; heels can contribute to Achilles tendonitis by keeping your calves in a contracted (shortened) position for hours on end.

For chronic Achilles inflammation, the remedy that works best is something many die-hard exercisers don't want to hear: Stop exercising. Give your Achilles tendon a few days off to rest and repair. Ice the spot, but don't do any stretching or strengthening exercises that put pressure on your heel. (You can swim, but only if you feel no pain.) If your Achilles problem persists, see an orthopedist or a podiatrist. You may need more-aggressive remedies.

Knee pain

On the surface, the knee seems to be a wonderfully uncomplicated mechanism with a pretty simple job description: to bend and straighten your leg. In reality, knee function is controlled by more muscles, tendons, ligaments, and cartilage than any other joint in your body. That's one reason why it's often the first joint to break down. The other is that the knees are involved in virtually every sport or activity, making it the most common joint to suffer injury.

Knee pain comes in more varieties than Baskin-Robbins ice cream. It can be caused by a tear in a ligament, a tendon, a muscle, or a piece of *cartilage,* the cushioning that prevents two bones from rubbing against each other. (See Chapter 12 for additional definitions of these high-tech terms.) We can't diagnose your specific ailment, but we can tell you this: Knee pain is often the result of doing the same movement over and over again. Typically, you can't trace it to a specific incident; it's more likely the result of one bike-a-thon or skate-a-thon too many. It's also affected or caused by a lack of stability and strength in the hips.

Cross training is a good way to avoid knee pain. By varying your exercise activities — running one day, cycling the next — you use different muscles, or at least you use the same muscles in different ways. You can still injure your knees with a cross-training regimen, so be careful not to overdo it. If you do feel knee pain coming on, cut back on your exercise routine or switch to an activity that doesn't aggravate the situation. Or, better yet, contact a qualified personal trainer to ensure that your form and technique are correct — improper technique is often the cause of joint problems. Some people with knee problems from running can bicycle with no pain whatsoever, and vice versa. Ice is always a good choice, too. But don't mess around here. If pain persists, recurs frequently, or is caused by a single incident, get thee to a doctor ASAP.

Stress fractures

The first large group of modern-day athletes to experience stress fractures were soldiers in World War II. The Army took out-of-shape civilians, placed heavy packs on their backs, and sent them off to march for miles in heavy combat boots. Soon the rookies complained about foot pain, but because nothing showed up on X-rays, doctors assumed they were faking it. Often, a second X-ray was taken several weeks later, revealing a fuzziness along the bone. *Bone callus* (a build-up of bone material) was forming; the healing process had started. Today, long-distance runners, hikers, backpackers, and in-line skaters are the most common sufferers of stress fractures.

Stress fractures are typically not one but a series of micro-fractures or hairline breaks that run along the bone. Typically, you don't have a telltale snap or pop that occurs in other breaks. More often, you wake up one day with pain radiating down the top of one or two of your toes to the center of your foot or along your shinbone. You may feel pain when you walk. You may even notice redness or swelling on top of your foot. When you press your finger on that spot, you feel a stabbing pain that immediately grabs your attention. The front of the shin is also a likely place for a fracture accompanied by the trademark pinpoint of pain.

Don't try to treat this kind of pain yourself. It definitely warrants a visit to your orthopedist or podiatrist, who will X-ray your foot to make sure that your injury is a stress fracture. The doctor will probably prescribe anti-inflammatory medication, ice, and elevation, and implore you to stay off your feet. In extreme cases, he may even put you in a soft or hard cast.

If you think you have a stress fracture, stop exercising immediately. We can't tell you how many times marathoners in agonizing foot pain at mile nine go on to finish the race anyway. When you continue to run on a stress fracture, you transform a minor injury into one that can take months to heal.

Lower-back pain

Nearly 80 percent of people utter the words "Oh, my aching back," at some point in their adult lives. You may be referring to a nagging stiffness that makes tying your shoes a difficult proposition, or you may be referring to chronic, debilitating pain that keeps you curled up in bed for weeks at a time. Although regular workouts (especially abdominal and back exercises) can do a lot to help prevent back pain, fitness activities can also cause back problems, particularly if you do a lot of pounding or use improper form when you run or cycle. You also can wrench your back by failing to bend your legs when you lift a weight off the rack.

Of course, you also can throw out your back by doing completely nonathletic activities, such as improperly lifting a child or a bag of groceries. Always use proper form (lifting and bending with your legs, not your back), when lifting and carrying anything.

In many instances of back pain, the worst thing you can do is just stay in bed. This weakens the very muscles that need to be loosened up and strengthened (and lack of activity may have led to the back pain in the first place). Another time-honored treatment, the heating pad, makes many back conditions worse by further inflaming the nerves.

So what helps back pain heal? Time, for one thing. Many cases of back pain disappear within four weeks without any treatment at all. If that doesn't work, you can see a variety of professionals. Most experts believe that the majority of back pain is muscular in nature and can be treated successfully with nonsurgical procedures, such as exercise, massage, physical therapy, and chiropractic. (To find a good chiropractor, get a recommendation from a friend, or better yet, from a medical doctor.) Swimming, walking, and yoga seem to be the best activities for limbering up tight back muscles. Back and abdominal strengthening exercises supervised by a physical therapist or trainer experienced in dealing with back pain can give you long-term immunity from further recurrence of back pain. For helpful back stretches, see Chapter 6.

For an episode you're having right now, ice and gentle movement are probably your best bet for relief. Some experts recommend seeing a *physiatrist,* a medical doctor who rehabilitates the disabled. Physiatrists are more likely to prescribe exercise than medication or surgery. If you experience severe back pain that prevents you from going about your normal activities, see your physician first to rule out any underlying medical causes, such as kidney infections or intestinal disorders.

Don't ignore the symptoms, like Liz's husband, Jay, once did. One night Jay woke up in the middle of the night to get some ice but got so dizzy from his back pain that he fainted. When he hit the floor, Liz woke up and found him lying in the hallway, blood dripping from his mouth. Liz thought he had been shot. For the next two days, Jay was confined to bed because he couldn't walk. His cut lip didn't feel too good, either.

Tennis elbow

You don't need to be a tennis player to experience a tenderness on the bony bump on the outside of your elbow or an aching sensation whenever you straighten your arm or pick up an object. In fact, *tennis elbow* (inflammation of the tendons in your elbow) can be caused by carrying a gym bag or briefcase with a straight arm or by lifting weights or any heavy object with improper form.

When you lift weights or use a stair-climber, take care not to lock your elbows. This is a very common mistake, and the people who do it often fail to make the connection between their elbow pain and their sloppy form.

If you feel pain in your elbow, stop the offending activity. Ice can help, and you can buy a brace or slip-on wrap at the drugstore to help support your elbow. Your doctor may even suggest that you wear the brace while you sleep, to keep up continuous compression on your elbow joint. To help prevent future episodes of tennis elbow, strengthen your wrists (forearms) and your triceps, the muscles at the back of your arm (see Chapter 12 for more information on tricep muscles; see Chapter 14 for a tricep-building exercise). Strong wrists are particularly important because most elbow pain is caused by swollen tendons that originate in the wrists and end in the elbow (see Chapter 14).

To prevent tennis elbow, lift objects with your palm facing your body. Also try doing strengthening exercises with hand weights: With your elbow cocked and your palm down, repeatedly bend your wrist, stopping if you feel any pain. Stretch the muscles in and around the elbow before beginning a potentially stressful activity by grasping the top part of your fingers and gently but firmly pulling them back toward your body, while keeping your arm fully extended and your palm facing outward.

Neck pain

You may not realize how useful your neck is until you can't move it, like when the guy standing next to you asks a question, and answering him requires a three-quarter turn of your body.

Just about anything can cause neck pain — you may sleep on your neck in a funny way or spend too much time cradling the phone on your shoulder. But neck pain is often caused by fitness activities. We're talking about poor weight-lifting technique, such as turning your head to the side while doing a shoulder press, and poor upper-body exercise posture, such as letting your head droop forward when you walk. If you experience neck pain after a traumatic incident, such as getting beaned on the head with a soccer ball, check with your doctor immediately. Also consult a physician if you have constant or recurring neck pain.

Neck pain of the non-traumatic kind usually signals tightness in the muscles of your neck, upper back, and/or shoulders. When you press a finger into the area between your shoulder and your neck and there's very little give or springiness, you have tight neck muscles. One remedy: Gently stretch your neck muscles; if you feel tightness on the right side of your neck, tip your head toward your left shoulder and stretch your right arm downward. See

Chapter 6 for details. Gentle massage is also useful for freeing up knotty neck muscles. You can give yourself a massage, but somehow that isn't as satisfying as enlisting a friend, significant other, or professional therapist.

Ice, usually an injury-friendly treatment, isn't always the best choice for neck pain. If you're stiff to begin with, applying ice may cause you to tense up even more. If your trouble is a stiff neck, moist heat in the form of a warm washcloth, shower massage, or whirlpool may be the way to go.

Rotator-cuff injuries

What's the capital of Belgium? If you can't raise your hand to answer that question, you may have a rotator-cuff tear. Throwing, catching, and lifting your arm to the side may also be painful. (By the way, the answer is Brussels.)

The *rotator cuff* is a group of four muscles that surround and protect your shoulder joint (see Chapter 12 for details about the muscles in your body, if you're interested). They're particularly delicate and susceptible to injury. They can tear if your arm is violently pulled or twisted or if you fall with your arm outstretched. But the most likely scenario is damage from repetitive movements such as throwing, catching, swimming, and lifting weights that are too heavy. Which movements cause pain depends on which rotator-cuff muscle you damage and how badly you injure it. Rotator-cuff tears are often the reason for the early retirement of baseball players and weekend softball players alike.

These injuries usually are treated with ice and compression (see the "RICE, RICE Baby" section later in this chapter), plus strength-training exercises using very light weights. Ease up on hard-core weight-training exercises, particularly heavy bench pressing, both on a flat and an incline bench, and ask a trainer to check your form. Reeducate yourself on throwing, catching, or swim stroke technique — make sure to involve your entire body rather than just your arm and shoulder. In some cases, the rotator cuff is too far gone to strengthen through exercise, and the damaged muscle needs surgical repair or, at the very least, physical therapy.

Chafing

Your legs feel great, and you've barely broken a sweat, yet you can't continue your bike ride because your butt is rubbed raw. You have what's essentially a case of adult diaper rash, an irritation that can crop up anywhere your clothing touches your skin and is known as *chafing*. It's particularly common in hot weather, when heavy sweating contributes to the problem. Every sport has special hot spots to look out for. The bra line, underarms, and sock line are the most common among runners. But you can also get chafed if your tights, shorts, or shirt rub against your skin as you move. Only streakers are immune.

You can also develop a similar condition, *blisters* (a small buildup of water or blood under your skin), when your feet rub against the seams in your shoes, slide around in too-loose shoes, or feel friction against too-tight or bunched-up socks. Small, deep blisters and large blisters are not only painful — they can keep you off your feet and knock you off your training routine for days at a time.

To prevent chafing, experiment with fabrics and cuts of clothing that don't irritate your skin. Softer fabrics that include at least some cotton tend to be the kindest to your skin, but it's a matter of personal preference. To prevent chafing or blisters, before your workout, try greasing up your hot spots with Vaseline or with a product like Sportslick or BodyGlide, all-purpose skin lubricants that lasts longer than Vaseline and won't come off until you wash with soap and water. (Check with your local running or walking store; some all-purpose sporting-goods stores also carry these products.) Long-distance cyclists also slather their butts with udder balm, an ointment made for cows but helpful for reducing chafing in humans. It feels kind of icky, but it usually does the trick.

We know one runner who used to get a severe case of irritation on his nipples. He solved this with the strategic placement of Band-Aids. Not very macho, but then, neither were the two spots of blood leaking through his shirt.

RICE, RICE Baby

If your doctor or trainer prescribes RICE for an injury, he isn't suggesting some New Age nutritional treatment. He's referring to the common way to treat sports injuries: Rest, Ice, Compression, and Elevation. Usually, this treatment is all you need to get back on your feet, particularly if you RICE diligently for the first 48 hours after an injury.

Rest

Stop doing activities that aggravate your injury. (If you sprain your ankle, don't try to "walk it off.") Rest can often mean the difference between an injury that heals right away and one that nags you for months. But don't use your injury as an excuse to quit exercising altogether. Simply choose an activity that doesn't hurt. If you pull a hamstring, you don't have to stop upper-body weight training. Swimming is also often a great activity when injured, unless, of course, your injury is swimming-related.

Ice

Ice reduces swelling and deadens pain by constricting blood flow into the injured area. Ice for 15 to 20 minutes three or four times a day for as long as you feel pain. Contrary to popular belief, ice is not useless after the first day. You can apply ice with a pack, a plastic bag full of cubes, or a package of frozen corn. Just don't allow the ice to rest directly on your skin; otherwise, you're inviting a whole new list of problems, such as ice burns. Instead, put a thin, damp washcloth between your skin and the ice.

One of our favorite icing techniques is ice massage. Fill a paper cup ¾ full of water and stick it in the freezer. When the water freezes, peel the cup down so you have what resembles an ice cream cone of ice. Use this to massage the injured area in a circular motion for as long as you can take it, usually four or five minutes. Ice massage penetrates deeper into your muscles than passively throwing an ice pack over the injured area. Be sure to keep the ice moving.

Compression

Put pressure on the injured area to keep the swelling down. Wrap a damp ACE Brand bandage around the injury, or buy a special knee, elbow, or wrist wrap or brace. Wrap tightly enough so that you feel some tension but not so firmly that you cut off your circulation or feel numbness.

Elevation

Elevating your injured body part reduces swelling by allowing fluids and waste products to drain from the area, much like water runs downstream. (Waste products are the bits of broken blood cells and other inflammatory agents hanging around the injury.) If your ankle is injured, you don't need to raise it so high that it's perpendicular to the ground. Propping it up on a couple of fluffy pillows will do. Elevation works best when used in conjunction with the rest of the RICE treatment.

Chapter 6

The Scoop on Stretching

*I*f you're like most people, stretching ranks right up there with flossing and oven cleaning on your list of least-favorite activities. Many of the most dedicated athletes we know hate to stretch. And prominent stretching researchers have admitted to us that they have trouble getting motivated to stretch — despite the fact that their own studies demonstrate the importance of flexibility training. The designer of a popular stretching device even admitted to Liz that he usually skips the stretching part of his workout. "Because stretching doesn't help you lose weight or make your muscles bigger, it's the first thing to go when you're short on time," he said.

True, stretching won't burn many calories or sculpt you a physique like Brad Pitt's, but a few minutes of daily stretching is a very wise investment. So, in this chapter, we explain what stretching can do for you, give you the lowdown on several different stretching methods — including the very-hot method called Active Isolated stretching — and show you some basic stretches that you can use right away.

Why You Need to Stretch

Stretching is the key to maintaining your flexibility — in other words, how far and how easily you can move your joints. As you get older, your tendons (the tissues that connect muscle to bone) begin to shorten and tighten, restricting your flexibility. Your movement becomes slower and less fluid. You don't stand up as straight. You walk more stiffly and with a shorter stride. You find it more difficult to step up to a curb or bend down to pick up the trash. Stretching your rear thigh, hip, and calf muscles can make a big difference.

Flexibility is one of the keys to good posture. When your front neck muscles are short and tight, your head angles forward. When your shoulders and chest are tight, your shoulders round inward. When your lower back, rear thigh, and hip muscles are tight, the curve of your back becomes exaggerated. A regular stretching routine also can reduce pain and discomfort, particularly in your lower back. In fact, the pain often disappears when you begin doing simple stretches for your lower-back and rear-thigh muscles.

What's more, flexibility exercises can correct muscle imbalances. Say that your front-thigh muscles are strong, but your rear thighs are tight and weak. (This is a common scenario.) As a result, you end up relying on your front thighs more than you should. Chances are, you won't even notice this, but it will throw off your movement in subtle ways — you may have a short walking stride or bounce too high off the ground. Muscle imbalances can eventually lead to injuries such as pulled muscles. They also contribute to clumsiness, which in itself can lead to injury. Finally, if you're any kind of a jock — even a bowler or a Saturday-afternoon softball player — stretching may help you perform better. The ability to move freely in a wide variety of directions makes you a better athlete.

Before, After, During? Knowing When to Stretch

Contrary to popular opinion, stretching is not the first thing you should do when you walk into the gym or arrive at the park for a jog. Don't stretch your muscles until you've at least warmed up thoroughly (see Chapter 8 for warm-up basics); we think stretching at the end of your workout, after you've finished your workout but before you shower, is even better. A post-workout stretch is a great way to relax and ease back into the rest of your day and has been shown to reduce injuries.

Can stretching prevent injury?

A recent study showing no link between stretching and injury rates has bolstered non-stretchers' self-confidence. Don't be too surprised if, while stretching at your gym, someone lectures you on how you're wasting your time.

But before you throw stretching out the window altogether, consider that what this study showed was that *warming up* with stretching does not reduce injuries. As we clearly recommend in this chapter, you don't want to stretch *before* you work out, but *after*. (Although you want to ease into any workout by doing a full warm-up — see Chapter 8.) Research actually shows that, although runners who stretch before they work out have higher injury rates compared to runners who don't stretch at all, those who stretch *after* workouts have lower rates of injury.

Don't stretch before you cool down (see Chapter 8 for more on cooldowns). Putting your head below your heart right after a workout can cause fainting and nausea. Wait until your heart rate dips below 100 or you aren't feeling breathless before you lie down to stretch.

Following a Few Rules of Stretching

Watch runners at the park or weight lifters at the gym. Chances are, they have the wrong idea about stretching. Maybe they'll grab their heel for a split second to stretch their front thigh, or bend over for a moment to touch their toes. Liz recently saw a very short woman wind up and throw her leg onto the hood of a very tall car. The sight made Liz cringe with fear for the woman's hamstring. That sort of "stretching" isn't going to make you more flexible, and it may even injure you.

Here are the basic rules for a useful and safe flexibility workout:

- ✔ **Stretch as often as you can — daily, if possible.** Always stretch after every workout, both cardiovascular and strength training. When you stretch on days you don't work out, be sure to warm up with a few minutes of easy movement like shoulder rolls, gentle waist twists, or light cardio activity.

- ✔ **Move into each stretching position slowly.** Never force yourself into a stretch by jerking or snapping into position.

- ✔ **Notice how much tension you feel.** A stretch should rate anywhere from mild tension to the edge of discomfort on your pain meter. It should never cause severe or sharp pain anywhere else in your body. Focus on the area you're stretching, and notice the stretch spread through these muscles.

- ✔ **Never bounce.** No matter which type of stretching you choose (traditional, PNF, or AI — see the "Finding Alternative Ways to Stretch" section) after you find the most comfortable stretch position, stay there or gradually deepen the stretch. Bouncing only tightens your muscle — it doesn't loosen it. Forceful bouncing increases the risk of tearing a muscle.

- ✔ **As you hold each position, take at least two deep breaths.** Deep breathing promotes relaxation.

A Simple Stretching Routine

In the following sections, we show you a thorough, basic stretching routine to get you started. If you consider stretching too boring, too painful, or too complicated, you'll like this section. It features a no-brainer stretching routine that won't pull your hamstrings like a rope in a tug of war. Although we like alternative stretching techniques such as AI and PNF (described in the following section), in this section, we demonstrate classic stretches because they're the type most fitness experts recommend. After you master these moves, the workout should take about five minutes.

Keep in mind that this is just a starting point. We think it's a great idea to learn additional stretches; there are literally hundreds to choose from. Varying your flexibility routine allows you to stretch your muscles at a number of angles. Plus, you'll be able to give the necessary extra attention to the muscles you use most in your particular workout. For example, if you're a tennis player or rower, you may want to do a few extra upper-body stretches. If you're a runner, do a few additional hamstring and lower-back stretches. If you're a cyclist, emphasize your quadriceps and glutes.

Neck stretch

This stretch is designed to loosen and relax the muscles in your neck.

Stand or sit comfortably. Drop your left ear toward your left shoulder, and gently stretch your right arm down and a few inches out to the side (see Figure 6-1), using your opposite hand to assist the stretch by gently pulling on the side of your head. Repeat the stretch on your right side.

Keep these tips in mind as you perform the neck stretch:

- Keep your shoulders down and relaxed.
- Your ear may or may not touch your shoulder, depending on how stiff you are.

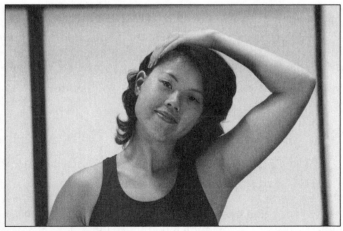

Figure 6-1:
The neck stretch loosens and relaxes the muscles in your neck.

Photograph by Sunstreak Productions, Inc.

Chest expansion

This stretch targets your shoulders, chest, and arms and helps promote good posture.

Sit or stand up tall and bring your arms behind you, clasping one hand inside the other (see Figure 6-2). Lift your chest and raise your arms slightly. You should feel a mild stretch spread across your chest.

Keep in mind the following tips as you perform the chest expansion:

✔ Resist arching your lower back as you pull your arms upward.

✔ Try to keep your shoulders relaxed and down.

✔ Don't force your arms up higher than is comfortable.

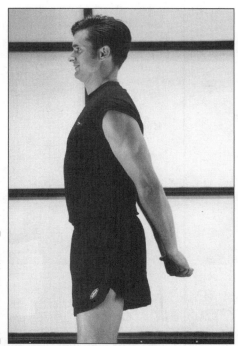

Figure 6-2:
The chest expansion promotes good posture.

Photograph by Sunstreak Productions, Inc.

Back expansion

This move stretches and loosens your shoulders, arms, upper-back, and lower-back muscles.

Standing tall with your knees slightly bent and feet hip-width apart, lift your arms in front of you to shoulder height. Clasp one hand in the other. Drop your head toward your chest, pull your abdominals inward, round your lower back, and tuck your hips forward so that you create a C shape with your torso. Stretch your arms forward so that you feel your shoulder blades moving apart and you create an "opposition" to your rounded back. You should feel a mild stretch slowly spread through your back and shoulders. (See Figure 6-3.)

Keep in mind the following tips as you perform the back expansion:

✔ Keep your abdominal muscles pulled inward to protect your lower back.

✔ Lean only as far forward as you feel comfortable and balanced.

✔ Keep your shoulders down and relaxed.

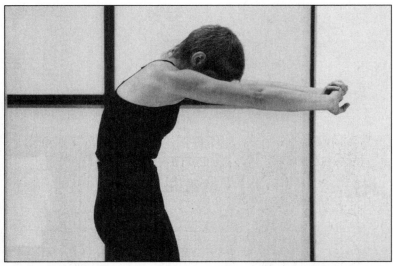

Figure 6-3:
The back expansion stretches your shoulders, arms, and back.

Photograph by Sunstreak Productions, Inc.

Standing hamstring stretch

This is a great stretch for your hamstrings (rear-thigh muscles) and your lower back. If you have lower-back problems, do the same exercise while lying on your back on the floor and extending your leg upward.

Stand tall with your left foot a few inches in front of your right foot and your left toes lifted. Bend your right knee slightly and pull your abdominals gently inward. Lean forward from your hips, and rest both palms on top of your right thigh for balance and support (see Figure 6-4). Keep your shoulders down and relaxed; don't round your lower back. You should feel a mild pull gradually spread through the back of your leg. Repeat the stretch with your right leg forward.

Keep in mind the following tips as you perform the standing hamstring stretch:

✔ Keep your back straight and your abs pulled inward to make the stretch more effective and to protect your lower back.

✔ Don't lean so far forward that you lose your balance or feel strain in your lower back.

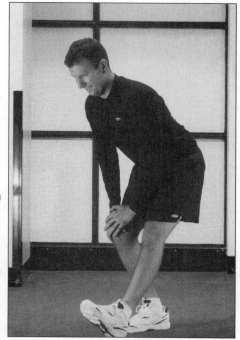

Figure 6-4:
The standing hamstring stretch targets your rear-thigh muscles.

Photograph by Sunstreak Productions, Inc.

Standing quad stretch

This stretch focuses on the quadriceps (front-thigh muscles). Be extra gentle with this stretch if you're prone to knee or lower-back pain. If back pain is an issue for you, you can do a similar stretch while lying on your side, bending your top knee, and bringing your heel toward your buttocks.

Stand tall with your feet hip-width apart, pull your abdominals in, and relax your shoulders. Bend your left leg, bringing your heel toward your butt, and grasp your left foot with your right hand (see Figure 6-5) or with your left hand, if the opposite hand is too uncomfortable. You should feel a mild pull gradually spread through the front of your left leg. Then switch legs.

Keep these tips in mind as you perform the standing quad stretch:

- ✔ Hold onto a chair or the wall if you have trouble balancing.
- ✔ Don't lock the knee of your base leg.

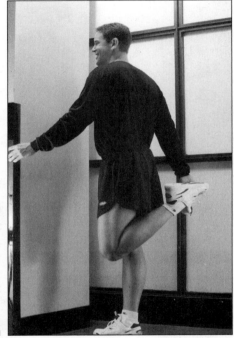

Figure 6-5:
The standing quad stretch targets your front-thigh muscles.

Photograph by Sunstreak Productions, Inc.

Double calf stretch

This stretch offers some relief for the calf muscles, which tend to be tight and bunched up from daily activities such as walking and standing.

Stand with your feet together about 2 feet from a wall that you're facing. Pull your abdominals gently inward and don't round your lower back. With straight arms, press your palms into the wall and lean forward from your ankles, keeping your heels pressed as close to the floor as possible (see Figure 6-6). You should feel a mild stretch spread through your calf muscles.

Keep in mind the following tips as you perform the double calf stretch:

✔ Keep both heels flat on the floor or as close to the floor as your flexibility allows.

✔ Keep your abs pulled in to prevent your lower back from sagging or arching.

✔ To increase the stretch, bend your elbows, leaning your chest toward the wall.

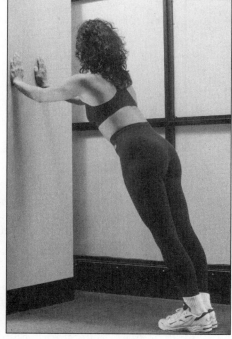

Figure 6-6:
The double calf stretch helps relieve tightness in your calf muscles.

Photograph by Sunstreak Productions, Inc.

Horse biting tail

This movement stretches your abdominals, sides, and lower back. Take care not to force this stretch, especially if you have lower-back problems.

Kneel on your hands and knees so that your palms are directly beneath your shoulders and your knees are directly below your hips. Pull your abdominals gently inward so that your back neither sags nor arches. Slowly twist your spine to the left as much as your flexibility allows, so that you're looking back over your shoulder toward your left buttock, and your left buttock moves slightly forward (see Figure 6-7). You should feel a mild stretch spread through your spine. Slowly move back to center and repeat to the right.

Keep in mind the following tips as you perform this stretch:

- ✔ Keep your abs pulled in to prevent your lower back from sagging.
- ✔ Don't force the stretch.

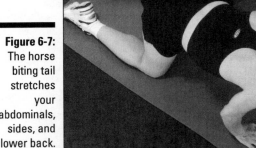

Figure 6-7:
The horse biting tail stretches your abdominals, sides, and lower back.

Photograph by Sunstreak Productions, Inc.

Butterfly stretch

This exercise stretches your inner thighs, groin, hips, and lower back. If you are prone to lower-back discomfort, take extra care to lean forward from your hips rather than rounding your lower back. This exercise may also cause some knee discomfort.

Sit up tall with the soles of your feet pressed together and your knees dropped to the sides as far as they will comfortably go. Pull your abdominals gently inward and lean forward from your hips. Grasp your feet with your hands and carefully pull yourself a small way farther forward (see Figure 6-8). You should feel the stretch spread throughout your inner thighs, the outermost part of your hips, and lower back.

Keep in mind these tips as you perform the butterfly:

- ✔ Increase the stretch by carefully pressing your thighs toward the floor as you hold the position.
- ✔ Don't hunch your shoulders up toward your ears or round your back.
- ✔ To reduce stress on your knees, move your feet away from your body. To increase the stretch, move your feet toward your body.

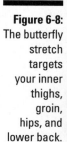 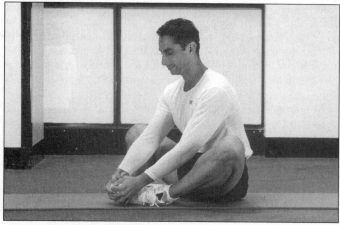

Figure 6-8:
The butterfly stretch targets your inner thighs, groin, hips, and lower back.

Photograph by Sunstreak Productions, Inc.

Finding Alternative Ways to Stretch

Traditional stretching — holding a position for 10 to 30 seconds — isn't the only way to make your muscles more flexible. Here's a look at a few other popular methods.

Active Isolated stretching

Some exercise experts theorize that conventional stretching techniques can damage muscles by pulling on them too hard, too far, and for too long, causing muscles to tighten up and spring back to prevent ripping and tearing. This automatic defense mechanism has many technical names too long to pronounce, but in laymen's terms, it's referred to as the *rebound reflex.*

Active Isolated stretching, or AI, is a method designed to avoid the rebound reflex. To do an AI stretch, using a rope or stretch band, you tighten the muscle opposite the muscle you're targeting for a stretch and then move the targeted muscle into a stretched position and hold it for about two seconds — that's right, two seconds — just long enough to elongate the muscle without triggering the rebound reflex. The theory is that when you *contract,* or shorten, a muscle, the opposite muscle has no recourse but to relax and lengthen. You repeat the process 8 to 12 times in each position before moving on to the next stretch.

Little research has been conducted yet on AI, but we think this method works, and we particularly like it for people who don't exactly have the flexibility of a ballerina. When you're very inflexible, holding a stretch for even ten seconds can seem like a lifetime. We also like the fact that there is a reliable certification program for AI, offered by New York City exercise physiologists Jim and Phil Wharton and their company, Maximum Performance. Maximum Performance has certified thousands of trainers nationwide. Look for these trainers, who can either teach group classes or do one-on-one instruction. Also pick up *The Whartons' Stretch Book,* which takes you step-by-step through an Active Isolated stretching routine.

To use the AI method, lie on your back and bend your right leg so that you can wrap a towel or rope around the instep of your right foot. (Buy boating rope at your local hardware store and have them seal the ends; buy a length that's about twice your height.) Then proceed with the instructions in this section; at the end of the movement, while your leg is still straight, use the rope to actively pull your leg toward your torso into a stretch, holding for about two seconds before releasing.

Hamstring stretch

To stretch your hamstrings (rear thigh muscles), with your rope around your right foot, lie on your back, keeping your left leg straight or slightly bent, and follow these steps:

1. **Straighten your right leg, lock your right knee, and using your rope, pull your right leg up toward your chest (see Figure 6-9).**

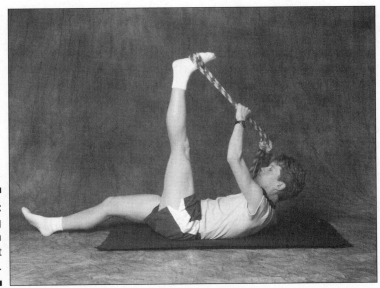

Figure 6-9: Hamstring stretch (straight knee).

Photograph by C.D. Stouffer, Detroit

2. **Hold for two seconds, and then release, allowing your right leg to relax for a few seconds.**

3. **Repeat Steps 1 and 2 for a total of eight to ten counts.**

   If necessary, do an additional set of eight to ten repetitions.

Quadriceps stretch

You may not even know your quads (thigh muscles) are tight, but as soon as you do this stretch, you'll know. Although you may feel like a contortionist, work through the following steps to get a fantastic stretch in your quads:

1. **With your rope wrapped around your right foot, lie on your left side.**

2. **Bend your left leg and pull it up toward your chest and chin.**

   The quadriceps of your left leg should be parallel to the top of your head.

3. **Bend your right leg and pull your right foot toward your butt.**

4. **Pull the rope over your head and hold for two seconds (see Figure 6-10).**

5. **Release, allowing your right leg to relax for a few seconds.**

6. **Repeat Steps 2 through 5 for a total of eight to ten counts.**

   If necessary, do an additional set of eight to ten repetitions.

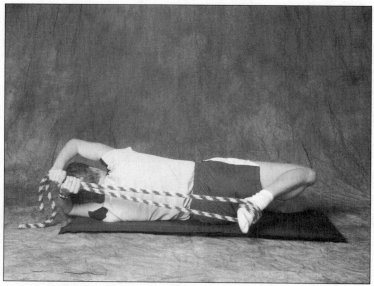

Figure 6-10:
Quadriceps
stretch.

Photograph by C.D. Stouffer, Detroit

Calf stretch

To keep your calves loose and supple, sit up and wrap the rope around your right foot (left foot bent or straight — makes no difference), and then follow these steps:

1. **Lock your right knee and pull your right foot straight back toward your chest.**

2. **Lean your upper body forward (toward your lower leg) about 10 degrees and hold for two seconds (see Figure 6-11).**

   This leaning-forward part is critical. If you simply pull your foot toward your chest without the forward lean, you won't get much of a stretch.

3. **Release, allowing your right leg to relax for a few seconds.**

4. **Repeat Steps 1 through 3 for a total of eight to ten counts.**

   If necessary, do an additional set of eight to ten repetitions.

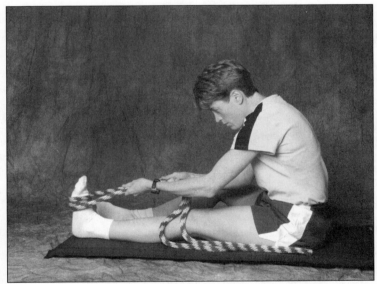

Figure 6-11:
Calf stretch.

Photograph by C.D. Stouffer, Detroit

PNF

If you have a trainer or go to a gym, you may come across a stretching technique with a name that, in our opinion, sets a new standard for fitness jargon: *proprioceptive neuromuscular facilitation* — PNF for short.

PNF involves tightening a muscle as hard as you can right before you stretch it. PNF is most often used for stretching the hamstrings. You lie on your back with your heel resting on your trainer's shoulder and your leg almost straight. To exhaust your hamstrings, you press your heel into the trainer's shoulder, while he pushes his shoulder into your heel. You hold this position for five to ten seconds. Then, you relax and hold the stretch for about 15 seconds. You may repeat the whole push/relax scenario three or four times.

You can do a PNF hamstring stretch yourself by lying in the same position and wrapping a towel around your ankle and holding an end in each hand. The theory behind PNF is that the act of tightening, or squeezing, causes a reflex in the muscle so that it becomes relaxed and more "receptive" to the stretch. So, after you tighten your hamstring for a few seconds, you're able to stretch it a little bit further than usual immediately after you release the tension. Many experts also feel that having someone push the stretch just a little bit further than you're likely to do yourself gets better results.

Does PNF work? Research does look promising. We know many trainers — and clients — who swear by PNF. Some gyms offer 45-minute private training sessions entirely devoted to this type of stretching.

Chapter 7

Nutrition Basics

*N*ot long ago, we came across a fitness book that proclaimed, "A great exercise program can make up for lack of a great diet." Unfortunately, that just isn't so.

But wait — if you scarf an extra donut at the office, can't you just burn off the calories on the treadmill? Sure, except that it takes an entire hour of brisk walking to burn off that single honey-dipped cruller. On a daily basis, exercise isn't a realistic way to make up for overeating. Besides, weight control isn't the only reason you should watch what you eat. If you make consistently poor choices, you deprive your body of nutrients that fight cancer and heart disease, prevent your bones from becoming brittle, fuel you through your kickboxing class, and give you the energy to keep reading this book (not that this book isn't a real page turner, of course).

So what's the right way to eat? Americans seem to be obsessed with finding the answer. The bestseller lists are always filled with diet books, whether it's *The South Beach Diet, The Abs Diet, Superfoods,* or *Dr. Atkins' New Diet Revolution,* and many contain specific rules about how to eat.

We say: Forget about all these rules and gimmicks. No single eating plan works for everyone. How much, how often, and what time of day you should eat depends on so many factors, including your body size, how much you exercise, your daily schedule, and your personal preferences. What appears to work for Dr. Atkins may not work for you — and may not be nutritionally sound, anyway. Plus, figuring out what to eat shouldn't be so complicated!

You shouldn't have to carry around a diet book and constantly glance at your watch. A better plan is to know nutrition basics, listen to your body's own signals for hunger and food preferences, and develop eating habits that you can sustain for life — not just for five days.

In this chapter, we present sensible, basic guidelines for nutritious eating. Adopting these common-sense rules will help you maintain your weight and your health yet, at the same time, keep your taste buds interested. If you're interested in a more in-depth discussion of nutrition, visit www.dummies.com for a wealth of health and nutrition books that answer your every question.

Control Your Calories

As a country, we eat less fat than we used to, but we're more overweight than ever. How come? Because people don't pay enough attention to calories. The reality is, if you eat more calories than your body consumes, you're going to gain weight. If your nutrition analysis — or simply the fit of your jeans — indicates that you're eating too much, use the strategies in this section to keep your calories under control. Just make sure you don't drop your calorie intake too low, especially if you exercise regularly. If you drastically cut calories — particularly if you drop below 1,200 — your body will think it's being starved and will compensate by hanging on to the few calories that you do eat.

- **Start with small portions.** You don't need to model your dinner plate after the Eiffel Tower. You can always go back for more. Also, buy single-serving packages of snack foods. You're less likely to keep eating if you have to rip open a whole new bag of chips than if you have your hand buried in a bargain-sized package.

- **Don't confuse fat-free with calorie-free.** Many fat-free foods are plenty high in calories because they make up for the lost fat by adding sugar. One Reduced-Fat Chips Ahoy! cookie has 50 calories, while a regular Chips Ahoy! has 53. Not exactly major savings.

- **Don't deprive yourself.** If you lust after a slice of chocolate cake, eat a small piece; otherwise you'll end up inhaling an entire cake tomorrow.

- **Eat slowly.** Utter at least one complete sentence between bites or chew 32 times before taking another spoonful. Many people eat so fast that they don't taste anything and then rush back for seconds. Give your body a chance to feel full.

- **Go easy on the booze.** Alcohol stimulates your appetite and weakens your reserve. This combination can lead to some serious overeating. Instead of drinking before a meal, drink while you eat.

> ✔ **Stop when you're satisfied.** Eat half of what's on your plate and then take a ten-minute break and assess whether you're still hungry. People often eat for reasons other than hunger, such as depression and exhaustion. Make sure that you're eating for the right reasons.
>
> ✔ **Eat regular meals.** Skipping meals sets you up for losing control and overeating. You're less likely to pig out if you avoid becoming a ravenous monster in the first place.

Get the Skinny on Fat

For years we've heard a single message about fat: It's bad for you. There's just one problem with this message: It's not true. In reality, only certain types of fat are harmful to your health. Others may actually help prevent heart disease. And we all need some fat to absorb certain vitamins and maintain a healthy immune system; fat also provides the material for hormone production, such as testosterone.

Distinguish between healthful and unhealthful fats

In the following sections, we take a look at the different types of fat.

Saturated fat

Saturated fat is the really bad stuff. In excess quantities, saturated fat raises your levels of blood cholesterol and clogs your arteries. It's found mostly in animal products, such as beef, pork, chicken, milk, ice cream, and cheese. But the amount of saturated fat in these foods varies greatly. For instance, 4 ounces of roasted pork tenderloin contain only about 2 grams of saturated fat, compared to 12 grams of saturated fat in 4 ounces of beef ribs.

How much saturated fat is too much? The major health organizations recommend keeping saturated fat to less than 10 percent of your total calories. If you eat 2,000 calories per day, that means you can get 200 of those calories from saturated fat. Because 1 gram of saturated fat (or fat of any kind) contains 9 calories, you can eat about 22 grams of saturated fat per day. (By the way, that's four *fewer* saturated fat grams than the amount in one Burger King Double Whopper with cheese.)

Trans fats

These artery-clogging fats may be just as harmful as saturated fats; they're created through *hydrogenation,* a process that turns liquid oils into solids like margarine and shortening. Hydrogenation makes pie crusts flakier and french fries crispier. (Thanks to their trans fat, McDonald's french fries have roughly as much artery-clogging fat as if they were fried in lard.)

Chips, crackers, cookies (yes, even low-fat cookies), granola bars, pastries, microwave popcorn, many types of bread, many cereals, and many peanut butters often contain trans fats. Look for the words *hydrogenated* or *partially hydrogenated* on labels and avoid those products that use hydrogenated oils, especially when near the top of the list. Keep reading labels and don't give up: For every ten cereals or microwave popcorn products that have trans fat, you can find one that doesn't.

Unsaturated fat

All right, now we're getting to the fats that may actually be good for your health. Unsaturated fat is the kind found in foods such as:

- Avocados
- Canola and flaxseed oils
- Fatty fish, such as salmon and mackerel
- Nuts and seeds
- Peanuts and "natural" peanut butter (the kind made only from peanuts and salt, as opposed to the processed kinds, like Jif and Skippy, which have hydrogenated fats, mentioned in the preceding section)
- Olives and olive oil

Unsaturated fats fall into two categories: mono and poly. Olive and canola oils are predominantly monounsaturated, as are peanut butter and avocado. Corn, soybean, safflower, and sunflower oils are mainly polyunsaturated.

The evidence is strong that monounsaturated fats may help protect against heart disease by reducing levels of LDL cholesterol (the artery-clogging kind) without affecting HDL cholesterol (the kind that acts as a vacuum cleaner within your bloodstream). There's less of a consensus about polyunsaturated fats, but you want to eat a balance of both.

So how much fat is it okay to eat?

That's debatable. Most major health organizations recommend keeping your total fat intake to less than 30 percent of your total calories (about 66 fat grams per day if you eat 2,000 calories). However, the 30 percent figure is not backed by solid evidence. Certain Greek populations of the 1960s ate as much as 40 percent fat — primarily from olive oil — and their heart disease rates were a remarkable 90 percent lower than those of Americans. There may be a range of acceptable fat intake levels. Keeping your saturated fat to less than 10 percent of total calories appears to be the more important figure.

Choose Your Carbs Carefully

Read some of the most popular low-carb diet books and you get the impression that carbohydrates are the root of all evil. Many of these books claim that pasta, bagels, fruit, sweet potatoes, and other high-carbohydrate foods trigger the body to store excess fat. But, as with many wacky diet theories, this one takes a scientific theory and distorts it beyond recognition.

In reality, carbohydrates are your body's main source of fuel, and exercisers need plenty of them. Sports nutritionists recommend that between 50 percent and 70 percent of calories should come from carbohydrates.

Choosing the best carbs

The key is to favor complex carbohydrates and natural simple sugars over processed and nutritionally-void simple sugars. Complex carbohydrates have sugar molecules strung together in long chemically bonded chains. These carbs are found in beans, whole-wheat pasta, grains, veggies, and the like. Most complex carbs are low in calories, low in fat, and high in fiber. The sugar in complex carbohydrates is absorbed relatively slowly into your bloodstream so that your blood-sugar level and energy level remain fairly constant, and you feel full for a good while.

Getting enough fiber

Although most Americans eat just 12 to 17 grams of fiber per day, the federal government recommends 20 to 35 — nearly double. Fiber comes from whole-grain products (veggies, fruits, oats, whole-wheat bread), plus in dry beans, peas, nuts, and seed. Check labels, of course, and you'll find very little fiber in processed foods. To get the most fiber, eat whole-grain flour-based products and the skin on vegetables and fruits.

Perhaps the most well-known benefit of fiber is to keep your colon healthy and keep your bowel movements regular. Fiber also plays a role in reducing cholesterol. But the most tangible benefit? Fiber keeps you feeling full longer throughout the day.

If you just don't eat a lot of fiber in your diet and can't seem to change that pattern, try using a fiber supplement such as Metamucil. Although you want to get your fiber from the foods you eat, a supplement is a good idea if you don't.

Avoiding processed carbs

Simple carbohydrates, on the other hand, are single or double sugar molecules. They're found in table sugar and processed foods like Pepsi and Twinkies, but they also occur naturally, like in fruit. Simple carbs, whether they're found in a papaya or a Pop Tart, are absorbed quickly, causing the amount of sugar in your blood to skyrocket and then plunge soon after, leaving you feeling tired and hungry. But there's a difference between the natural simple sugars found in fruit and the refined simple sugars found in candy. When you eat that papaya, the sugar comes packaged with vitamins, minerals, water, and fiber. Also, the sweetness in fruit comes from fructose (as opposed to sucrose or glucose in other simple sugars), and fructose doesn't cause the sort of sharp insulin spike that other simple sugars do.

In general, eat foods that are processed as little as possible. Choose an apple over apple juice, and whole-wheat bread over white bread. Be sure to buy bread that is actually labeled "whole wheat." Many wheat and grain breads are mostly refined white bread colored with molasses, despite the brown wrapping that depicts wheat fields waving in the wind and names like "12-grain health nut bread."

Read food labels carefully and find out where you're getting most of your refined sugar. Breakfast cereals such as Kellogg's Raisin Bran and Frosted Flakes are more than 42 percent sugar. Flavored yogurts are loaded with sugar, too. Be aware that sugar goes by other aliases, including corn syrup, honey, maple syrup, maltodextrin, sucrose, and other words that end in -*ose*. Sugar is sugar.

Going low-carb — with modifications

If you've been bitten by the low-carb craze, don't fret. Low-carb eating could be an ideal way to eat with the following simple modifications:

- ✔ Consume an unlimited variety of vegetables.
- ✔ Choose dense, whole grains and avoid processed carbs.
- ✔ Eat two to four half-cup servings of unsweetened fruit each day. (Most low-carb diets eliminate fruit, but fruit contains many vitamins and minerals that are important to consume.)
- ✔ Substantially reduce your intake of saturated fat and trans fats, which many popular low-carb diets don't limit.

Eating a wide variety of foods

Ever notice that you stroll down the same aisles of the grocery store every week and fill your basket with almost the exact same items? People who have researched these things have found that most of us are in a serious rut, eating only 20 to 25 different foods on a regular basis. Not only does this repetition take a lot of the adventure out of eating, but eating the same foods over and over again limits the nutrients you get.

Even if you consume adequate amounts of vitamins and minerals, you may be missing out on thousands of *phytochemicals,* substances in fruits and vegetables that appear to help fight heart disease and cancer, strengthen the immune system, and slow the aging process. These substances have catchy names like quercetin, genistein, ferulic acid, and inositol hexaphosphate. Research into phytochemicals is relatively new, so nutrition experts don't yet know how much of them we need or which ones are most important. The best strategy is to eat as wide a variety of foods as possible. If you're a big fan of broccoli and eat it several times a week, the next time you're in the grocery store, instead of choosing only broccoli (high in organosulfides, flavonoids, and indoles — to name a few), go for asparagus, too (high in lutein, zeaxanthin, and glutathione).

Get Enough Protein, but Don't Fall for High-Protein Propaganda

Protein is crucial because it's made up of amino acids, which your body uses to build and repair your muscles, red blood cells, enzymes, and other tissues. Are you a protein overeater or undereater? Or are you right on target? The general rule of thumb for inactive people is to eat 0.4 grams per 1 pound of body weight. For example, a 180-pound couch potato multiplies 180 by 0.4. He needs about 72 grams of protein a day; a 130-pound person needs about 52.

Exercisers need a bit more protein, although not nearly as much as many protein advertisements would lead you to believe. A recreational exerciser should aim for 0.5 to 0.75 grams of protein per pound of body weight. A competitive athlete may need as much as 0.9.

To get an idea of how easy it is to rack up protein, consider that a Philly Cheese steak (36 grams), a side of fries (6 grams), and an 8-ounce glass of chocolate milk (8 grams) provide 50 grams of protein. In general, about 15 to 20 percent of your total calories should come from protein.

You can assess your protein needs by following the tips in the "Analyze Your Eating Habits" section later in this chapter. If you find that you're overshooting the mark on protein, cut back by using high-protein foods as a side-dish rather than as your main course. Sprinkle meat on your spaghetti or top your salad with strips of grilled chicken rather than planning your entire meal around a slab of steak. If you find that you're not getting enough protein because you fear the fat, focus on the plant sources, such as dried peas and beans, lentils, soybeans, and black beans. Also, turn to dairy foods like fat-free cottage cheese and fat-free plain yogurt. If you're a vegetarian, even a vegan, you have plenty of protein-rich choices.

Analyze Your Eating Habits

Do you have any idea whether you're even in the ballpark for how much saturated fat, protein, and other nutrients you need each day? Do you know whether you're consuming enough fiber or calcium or carbohydrates? One of the best ways to enlighten yourself about your diet is to track it for a while. Now, we're not suggesting that you write down every morsel you eat on a daily basis for the rest of your life. But we do recommend that you keep a food and beverage diary for a few days every now and then to get a handle on where your eating habits need improvement.

The simplest, low-tech way is to buy books that list how many calories and how much fat, saturated fat, protein, fiber, and other nutrients are contained in pretty much every food or drink you can think of, from Brussels sprouts to Japanese fish paste cake — whatever that is. (You can also find several online sources, but their locations change frequently. Search on "calorie counter" and see what pops up.)

If you want to compare the number of calories you're eating with the number of calories your body burns each day, you can use the following formula. In general, the number of calories you need to eat each day depends on how big your body is and how active you are.

We carry through the math for a man who's 5'10" and weights 180 pounds and is trying to maintain his current weight, not lose anything:

1. **Change your weight to kilograms by dividing your weight in pounds by 2.2.**

   For our sample man, we divide 180 by 2.2 and get 82.

2. **If you're a man, don't do anything. If you're a woman, multiply the result of Step 1 by 0.9.**

3. **Multiply the result of Step 2 by 24.**

   This calculation estimates your resting metabolic rate, the number of calories you'd need to consume if you did absolutely nothing but lie motionless in bed 24 hours a day.

   For our sample man, we multiply 82 by 24 and get 1,968.

4. **Add a percentage of Step 3 to account for your activity.**

   For a relatively sedentary day — say, a day lying around the pool — tack on 20 percent of your Step 3 result. For our sample man at the pool, we perform this calculation: $1,968 \times 0.20 = 394$; $394 + 1,968 = 2,362$ calories.

   On days when you exercise, you may need to add 30 to 50 percent of your resting metabolic rate, depending on how long and how hard you work out.

You may also want to make an appointment with a registered dietitian every so often. A visit with an R.D. can be very enlightening. He can not only tell you where you're falling short but also offer concrete suggestions on how to boost your iron intake, reduce your calorie consumption, or sneak more fiber into your diet.

Follow a Food Pyramid

Back in the days of Wonder Bread and Bosco, you and your fellow fourth-graders probably were treated to an educational film about the basic four food groups: meat, dairy, fruits and vegetables, and cereals and grains (in case you forgot). The idea was that if you got enough servings from each group, you'd cover all your nutritional bases.

In 1992, the federal government exiled the four food groups and unveiled the food guide pyramid (see the following section). Nutrition experts applauded the basic concept — that plant foods should form the base of our diet while animal products, perched near the top of the pyramid, should be eaten less often. But to many nutritionists, the pyramid does not reflect the latest nutrition research and may, inadvertently, promote a diet linked to heart disease and cancer. In the last several years, experts have erected more than a dozen competing nutritional structures, including various vegetarian pyramids, a Latin American pyramid, an Indian pyramid, and several Asian pyramids. There's even a vegan trapezoid. (A geometry refresher course, anyone?)

We're not going to analyze each and every pyramid in existence, but here's a brief look at the government's pyramid, the Mediterranean Diet Pyramid, and a newer pyramid from Harvard University. You can take the best of these structures and create a model of nutritious eating that works for you.

The USDA Food Guide Pyramid

Does three glasses of whole milk and a half-pound of hamburger per day sound like a healthy eating plan? Of course not. But that scenario is technically permitted under the USDA Food Guide Pyramid (shown in Figure 7-1), and it illustrates one of the pyramid's main flaws: failure to distinguish healthful fats from disease-causing fats. The pyramid lumps together meat, poultry, fish, dry beans, eggs, and nuts, and recommends two to three daily servings from this group of protein-rich foods. (One meat serving is 3 ounces, thereby allowing for the 8-ounce burger.) But these foods aren't equally healthful. Some cuts of red meat are loaded with saturated fat, while nuts, which contain vitamin E and heart-healthy (monounsaturated) fat, are very nutritious.

As for that whole milk: The pyramid recommends two to three daily servings of milk, yogurt, or cheese but doesn't specifically recommend low-fat or nonfat versions of these high-calcium foods. (Full-fat varieties are loaded with saturated fat.) At the same time, the pyramid groups fats, oils, and sweets at the top of the pyramid, with the admonition to "use sparingly." Yet research clearly shows that the fats found in olive oil and canola oil may protect against disease.

One benefit of the USDA Food Guide Pyramid is that it specifies a range of daily servings for each food category. Still, the numbers can be confusing. The pyramid recommends two to four fruit servings a day, but this is intended as a minimum. On the other hand, two to three servings from the protein-rich group is intended as a maximum.

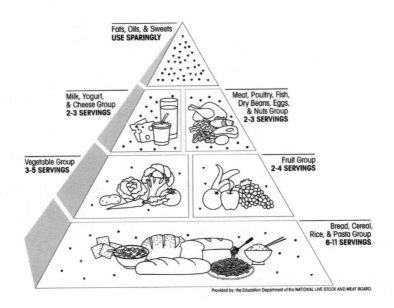

Figure 7-1:
The USDA
Food Guide
Pyramid.

A final gripe: The base of the pyramid — which includes bread, cereal, rice, and pasta — fails to distinguish between whole grains (thought to decrease risk of heart disease, diabetes, and some cancers) and refined grains (which are essentially stripped of vitamins, minerals, and fiber). For this reason, the federal government is now putting together panels to update its pyramid. As we went to print, the new pyramid wasn't ready, but check the Internet to see whether the USDA has made the radical revisions to the food pyramid that they've proposed.

The Mediterranean Diet Pyramid

Many of the USDA pyramid's problems are addressed by the Mediterranean Diet Pyramid (shown in Figure 7-2). Although refined in light of current nutrition research, the Mediterranean diet pyramid essentially reflects the eating habits of certain Greek and Italian populations around 1960, when their chronic disease rates were among the world's lowest and adult life expectancy was the highest despite limited medical services.

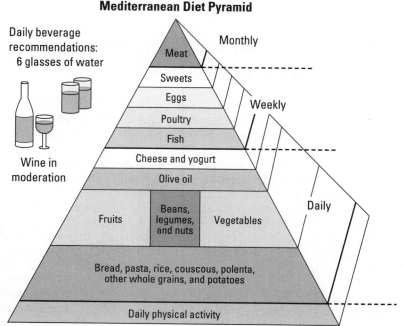

Mediterranean Diet Pyramid

Daily beverage recommendations: 6 glasses of water

Wine in moderation

Monthly

Meat

Sweets

Eggs

Weekly

Poultry

Fish

Cheese and yogurt

Olive oil

Fruits | Beans, legumes, and nuts | Vegetables

Daily

Bread, pasta, rice, couscous, polenta, other whole grains, and potatoes

Daily physical activity

Figure 7-2: The Mediterranean Diet Pyramid.

The Mediterranean Diet Pyramid prioritizes the high-protein foods that are lumped together in the USDA model. Beans and nuts sit near the base of the pyramid, recommended daily. Fish, poultry, and eggs are permitted a few times per week, but fish is given more emphasis than poultry, which is favored over eggs. That's because fish, high in omega-3 fatty acids, may protect against heart disease, whereas the skinless white meat of poultry appears to be neutral, neither increasing nor decreasing disease risk. Eggs may raise cholesterol levels but don't appear to be a problem (for non-diabetics) if no more than seven eggs are consumed per week. Red meat is relegated to the tip-top of the pyramid, recommended only a few times per month. (Although red meat consumption is clearly linked to deadly disease, there's no evidence that eating 12 to 16 ounces a month is actually more harmful than eating none at all.)

The Mediterranean Diet Pyramid also scores points for highlighting legumes, a term that doesn't roll off the tongue of most Americans. *Legumes* — basically edible seed pods — include chick peas, lentils, garbanzo beans, and soybeans. They're not only high in protein but also free of saturated fat and crammed with disease-protective nutrients.

Is the Mediterranean Diet Pyramid perfect? No. Like the USDA version, it doesn't distinguish between whole grains and refined grains.

Harvard School of Public Health's Healthy Eating Pyramid

When the folks at Harvard's School of Public Health decided to build their own food pyramid (shown in Figure 7-3), they came up with one that addressed the deficiencies of the USDA and Mediterranean Diet models.

Specifically, the Harvard model specifies whole grains at the base of the pyramid, with plant oils sharing the stage. Plant oils? Sure. Healthy, unsaturated oils like olive, canola, soy, and so on can lower cholesterol levels and protect the heart. The Harvard pyramid then stresses vegetables in whatever quantity is desired and some fruits. Going up the pyramid, you find a recommendation for nuts, fish, poultry, and eggs, but in moderation. Also recommended is a daily supplement, one specifically providing calcium. The top of the pyramid includes refined grains, sweets, red meat, and butter.

This pyramid does address many of the weaknesses of the other two pyramids. Its deficiency is in calcium intake, which is relegated to a supplement. Low-fat and nonfat dairy products, especially those low in sugar, are a good source of calcium. Supplements are a potential substitute for food sources (see the "Don't Waste Money on Useless Supplements" section for details), but getting your vitamins and minerals from food is always a better goal than relying on supplements.

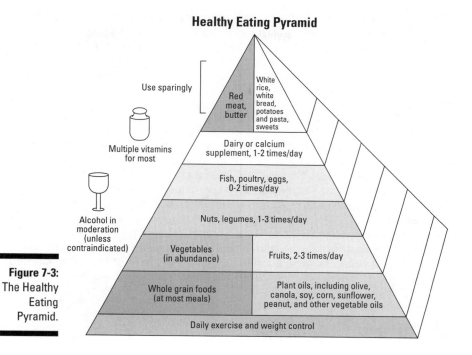

Healthy Eating Pyramid

Use sparingly

Red meat, butter

White rice, white bread, potatoes and pasta, sweets

Multiple vitamins for most

Dairy or calcium supplement, 1-2 times/day

Fish, poultry, eggs, 0-2 times/day

Alcohol in moderation (unless contraindicated)

Nuts, legumes, 1-3 times/day

Vegetables (in abundance)

Fruits, 2-3 times/day

Whole grain foods (at most meals)

Plant oils, including olive, canola, soy, corn, sunflower, peanut, and other vegetable oils

Daily exercise and weight control

Figure 7-3:
The Healthy Eating Pyramid.

Fuel Up for Your Workouts

ANECDOTE

Don't underestimate the power of food to get you through a workout and beyond. This goes for novices and athletes alike. Several years ago, professional triathlete Brad Kearns went on a wacky diet that had one rule: Eat nothing but fruit until noon. "I'd have a melon, a banana, and some berries, then I'd go ride my bike for three hours and swim for an hour and a half," Brad told us. Three months later, he hadn't lost any weight and was struggling to finish his races. "I was so starved that I was eating peanut butter straight from the jar," he recalls. "It made me realize that your body doesn't like your messing with it. You have to eat." You also need to drink — before, during, and after your workout. (See the "Drink Lots and Lots of Fluids" section later in this chapter for more about staying hydrated.) Here are some strategies for maintaining the energy to perform your best.

Before you work out

Your mom may have told you not to go swimming until at least an hour after you eat, but we tell you the opposite: If your stomach can handle it, eat within an hour of your workout. (For some activities, such as running, you may need two or three hours between eating and working out.) We recommend a couple hundred calories of (primarily) complex carbohydrates, such as a bagel or a couple pieces of fruit. A little protein may help if you're going for a long workout lasting a few hours or more.

During your workout

During most workouts, you don't need to eat anything unless you feel a major dip in energy. But if you're going for a three-hour bike ride or an afternoon hike, bring along snacks. Energy bars like PowerBars and Clif Bars or frosting-like gels such as GU or Power Gel are convenient choices. They easily slip into your pocket or fanny pack and don't get smashed like Fig Newtons or bananas.

For workouts that last longer than about an hour, sports drinks such as Gatorade and Cytomax are a good idea. They provide fluid as well as sodium and easily-digestible energy. Water is preferred for shorter workouts.

After your workout

Some people are under the impression that if they eat right after exercise, they somehow negate the benefits of their hard work. Just the opposite is true. If you eat within an hour of your workout, your body is more receptive to replenishing your energy stores. A post-workout snack that combines lots of carbs and some protein is ideal.

Don't go too long without eating

At one of the gyms that Liz used to manage, the staff members witness at least one fainting a month. Usually it's someone who shows up for a lunchtime workout without having eaten anything since an English muffin at 6 a.m. To maintain a consistent energy level throughout the day — and to prevent fainting episodes — make an effort to eat small, frequent meals.

Even on days when you don't exercise, eating frequently throughout the day is important. Waiting long periods between meals can cause wide swings in your blood sugar levels, which in turn can zap your energy, disturb your concentration, and turn you into a crankpot. Plus, if you let yourself become ravenous, you're likely to overeat at your next meal, a pattern that can lead to weight gain.

So, start your engines in the morning with a good breakfast — plenty of complex carbohydrates with an accent of protein and a dash of fat. A good example: hot oatmeal with skim milk, half a banana, walnuts, and a glass of orange juice. Then graze through the day, eating up to six small meals, aiming for a mix of carbs and protein each time — the combination will keep you satisfied longer than carbs alone. Eating breakfast can boost your metabolism 25 percent for the day!

Drink Lots and Lots of Fluids

Staying hydrated isn't just important for when you work out. More than 75 percent of your body is made up of water — even bone is more than 20 percent water. When you don't drink enough water, your blood doesn't flow properly, and your digestive track doesn't run smoothly. New research even suggests that drinking plenty of water can reduce the risk of breast, colon, and urinary tract cancers.

You've probably heard that you need to drink 8 glasses of water a day — 9 to 13 if you exercise. Here's where that number comes from: You typically lose about 10 cups of water per day — 2 cups to sweating and evaporation, 2 cups to breathing, and 6 cups to waste removal. You can replace up to 2 cups through the water in the foods you eat, but you have to make up the remaining 8 cups by drinking fluids, water being the best choice.

Recent research suggests that you need a much higher fluid intake, from 3 to 6 *quarts* per day (and because there are 4 cups in a quart, that's 12 to 24 cups per day). The low end is if you're eating lots of fruits and vegetables (and you are, aren't you?), because those foods are high in fluids. The high end is if you're working out for many hours per day, in hot weather (which we, incidentally, don't recommend). Your fluid intake can come from many sources, as outlined in the following list:

✔ **Water:** Good old-fashioned water is far and away the best way to get your fluids. Water is critical for proper functioning of your organs, so you want to get the majority of your fluids by drinking water. Keep a water bottle with you at all times: on your desk, in your purse, and in your car.

If you don't like the taste of water, you may have substances in your water that create an off-taste. Note, however, that most bottled water is just a bottled version of whatever's in your tap, so you need to decide whether it's worth the extra expense. You can try filtering your water: Brita and other companies make low-cost filter systems that attach to your kitchen or bathroom faucet. If you're still not thrilled with the taste of water, trying squeezing a slice of lemon into each glass.

✔ **Sports beverages:** Sports beverages include Gatorade, Powerade, Accelerade, and so on, and if you've never tried them, they're actually quite palatable — most taste just like Kool-Aid. The advantage of a sports beverage over water is that it includes *electrolytes* like potassium, magnesium, calcium, and sodium that you lose as you sweat. Sports beverages can also keep you from getting a stomachache after exercising.

The disadvantage is that sports beverages are pretty high in calories, and if you get in the habit of thinking of sports beverages like water, you can easily gain weight. If you really feel you need to include a sports beverage after workouts, try to limit your daily intake of sports beverages to 12 ounces, just after you finish exercising.

Sports drinks are expensive if you buy them in individual bottles. To save money, buy the powdered version at your local grocery store. You simply mix the powder with water, and you pay less than one-tenth the price with the exact same flavor. You can dilute sports beverages in extra water to reduce calories and sugar content.

✔ **Carbonated sodas and carbonated sports drinks:** Carbonated beverages, including sugary sodas, add calories to your diet without adding any vitamins or other nutrients, and they don't contain the electrolytes that sports beverages offer. One alternative is the new variety of carbonated flavored water. However, all carbonated beverages, even carbonated water, also contain phosphates, which can interfere with calcium absorption and may lead to bone-density problems. A treat now and then isn't going to hurt you, though.

✔ **Juice:** One-hundred-percent orange juice is rich in potassium, vitamin C, and other important vitamins. However, it's high in calories and doesn't really fill you up, so go easy on it. One small glass per day (6 to 8 ounces) is about all you need. You get a better bang for the buck by eating the whole fruit, so if you're choosing between the fruit and the juice, go with the fruit — it's more filling than juice and provides additional nutrients.

✔ **Low-fat or nonfat milk:** Two or three 8- to 12-ounce glasses of low-fat or fat-free milk are an excellent source of calcium, but you may not be able to stomach a glass of milk right after working out. If not, try drinking a glass of skim milk just before bed (warm it up in the microwave, if you like). In addition to helping you get much-needed calcium, milk has protein, which may help you fall asleep quickly.

✔ **Coffee and tea:** Coffee and tea are hot, tasty beverages, but a better choice is water. However, coffee and tea are fluids that count in your daily total of 8 cups, and if you look forward to your mug(s) of coffee or tea everyday, you don't need to stop drinking it completely. Just limit the total number of mugs, because caffeine can have a dehydrating effect, negating some of the benefits of drinking the fluids in the first place.

Don't rely on thirst to tell you when to drink. By the time your mouth feels parched, you're already mildly dehydrated. Prevent dehydration by drinking all day long. Keep a water bottle at your desk, and always carry a bottle when you work out. See Chapter 26 for some innovative products that make drinking water more convenient. You know that you're not drinking enough if your urine is dark and scanty rather than clear and plentiful. Keep in mind that vitamin supplements can make your urine dark or fluorescent yellow; in this case, volume is a better indicator.

Don't Waste Money on Useless Supplements

Supplements are promoted everywhere these days — on infomercials, in health-food stores, and at health clubs. Whether they claim to build muscle, burn fat, or boost your metabolism, the vast majority of supplements — including pyruvate and chitin — aren't worth the cost of the plastic bottles they come in. That's why we include them in our list of fitness rip-offs in Chapter 27.

Are any supplements worth taking? Actually, yes. A multivitamin/mineral supplement isn't a necessity, but for many people, it may be a good idea. According to the United States Department of Agriculture, about 90 percent of us fail to get enough magnesium, chromium, vitamin A, B vitamins, vitamin E, zinc, and many other nutrients. The typical woman gets less than two-thirds the calcium she needs to help prevent osteoporosis. In a typical four-day period, nearly half of all women fail to eat a single piece of fresh fruit, and the vast majority fail to eat even one dark green leafy vegetable. This explains why women are so deficient in vitamin C, folic acid, and other vital nutrients.

The second reason we recommend supplements is that even if you make all the right food choices, getting optimal amounts of a few particular vitamins and minerals is tough. For instance, research suggests that vitamin E may lower your risk of cancer and heart disease, but only when you consume at least 100 IU (international units, a way of measuring tiny amounts). To get this much vitamin E from your diet, you'd have to eat 25 cups of cooked spinach or drink 1¼ cups of vegetable oil (not recommended, by the way). Unlike with vitamin C, there's no easy way to get vitamin E from food.

However, none of this means that you should rely on supplements for your vitamins and minerals. Scientists are learning that the vitamins or minerals alone may not prevent certain diseases; instead the benefit may come from the way these nutrients mingle with other components in food. Aim to get the vast majority of your vitamins and minerals from food and take the word *supplement* literally. No pill will compensate for a diet of Doritos and Budweiser. When you eat healthy foods, you not only get vitamins and minerals, but you also get protein, carbohydrates, fiber, and other nutrients.

Choose a multivitamin (rather than individual pills) with doses that don't go much beyond 100 percent of the U.S. RDA (Recommended Dietary Allowance). Don't bother with super potency megavitamins, which often contain more than ten times the U.S. RDA (and cost you bundles). Your body can absorb only so much of each nutrient; if you go overboard, most of the excess is just excreted when you go to the bathroom. As one doctor told us, "You'll have very expensive urine." Also, some vitamins are stored in your body, so megadoses can lead to dangerous outcomes.

Also, forget those designer vitamins hawked infomercial-style by has-been celebrities and former athletes. Generic drugstore brands are identical. Manufacturers have yet to come up with the magical combination of dosages to banish wrinkles or to make you live to 196, although a telemarketer once called to inform Liz that every single Olympic athlete today swears by her particular brand of supplements. "Really, every single one?" she asked. Yes, she said. She was quite sure — every single one.

Part III
Getting to the Heart of the Matter

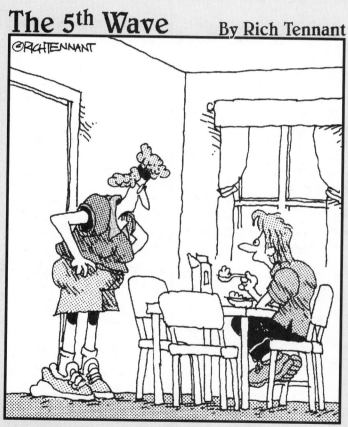

The 5th Wave   By Rich Tennant

"I know I walk regularly and I do it on the
street, but if anyone asks, I'm a fitness-
walker, or a power-walker, NOT a street-walker."

In this part . . .

We explain what the heck *aerobic* and *cardiovascular* mean and tell you everything you need to know about this type of exercise, also known as *cardio* exercise. In Chapter 8, we give you a crash course on cardio basics, explaining terms such as *target heart rate* and *anaerobic threshold.* We also help you design a cardio workout program suited to your goals and fitness level. In Chapter 9, we explain how to use indoor cardio equipment such as elliptical trainers, stair-climbers, treadmills, and other machines. Chapter 10 covers tips and equipment for popular outdoor cardio activities — such as walking, running, in-line skating, cycling, and swimming — along with up-and-coming activities such as snowshoeing.

Chapter 8

Cardio Crash Course

*I*f you hang around people who exercise, you're going to hear the word *cardio* pretty often. Someone may say, "I prefer to do cardio after I lift weights" or "My gym has awesome cardio equipment." *Cardio* — which means "for your heart" in medical jargon — is short for cardiovascular exercise, the kind that strengthens your heart and lungs and burns lots of calories.

In Chapter 24, we list all kinds of reasons to pursue this sort of exercise — everything from lowering your blood pressure to sleeping more soundly to trimming that spare tire. This chapter explains how exactly to get those benefits — in other words, what type of exercise counts as cardio. We introduce you to terms such as *aerobic, anaerobic,* and *target heart rate zone,* which, in case you were wondering, has nothing to do with what happens to your heart when there's a sale at Target. After you understand the basic concepts involved in cardio exercise, use the cardio plans near the end of this chapter to design a cardio workout program based on your goals.

Two Cardio Rules That You Can't Break

You wouldn't try to sell someone a stereo without a few pleasant introductory words to your potential customer, right? You need to ease her into things with a couple of jokes or at least a "Good morning. How can I help you?" And certainly you wouldn't turn your back on her the minute she handed over her credit card; you'd congratulate her on the purchase and wish her a nice day. Well, the same principles apply to exercise. No matter what type of cardio workout you do — whether it's walking, playing basketball, or cross-country skiing — you need to ease into it with a warm-up and ease out of it with a cooldown. (Weight-training workouts also require a warm-up, as we explain in Chapter 14, although they typically don't require a cardio cooldown.)

Warming up

A *warm-up* simply means 5 to 15 minutes of aerobic exercise at a very easy pace. For example, runners may start out with a brisk walk or a slow run. If you're going on a hilly bike ride, start with at least a few miles on flat terrain. Be aware that stretching is not a good warm-up activity (see Chapter 6).

What does *aerobic* mean, anyway?

The term *cardio* is often used interchangeably with *aerobic.* Aerobic exercise is any repetitive activity that you do long enough and hard enough to challenge your heart and lungs. To get this effect, you generally need to use your large muscles, including your butt, legs, back, and chest. Brisk walking, bicycling, swimming, and stair climbing count as aerobic exercise.

Movements that use your smaller muscles, like those leading into your wrists and hands, don't cut it. Channel surfing with your remote control can certainly be repetitive, sustained, and intense — particularly when performed by certain husbands and boyfriends we know — but it's not aerobic.

Aerobic means with air, and *cardio* was coined in the late 1960s by fitness pioneer Dr. Kenneth Cooper, and it means heart. When you exercise aerobically, your body needs an extra supply of oxygen, which your lungs extract from the air. Think of oxygen as the gas in your car: When

you're idling at a stoplight, you don't need as much fuel as when you're zooming across Montana on Interstate 90. During your aerobic workouts, your body continuously delivers oxygen to your muscles.

However, if you push yourself hard enough, eventually you switch gears into using less oxygen: Your lungs can no longer suck in enough oxygen to keep up with your muscles' demand for it. But you won't collapse, at least right away. Instead, you begin to rely on your body's limited capacity to keep going without oxygen. During this time, you're exercising *anaerobically,* or without air.

Anaerobic exercise refers to high-intensity exercise like all-out sprinting or very heavy weight lifting. After about 90 seconds, you begin gasping for air and you feel a burning sensation in your legs. That's when your body forces you to stop.

People who are out of shape need to warm up the longest. Their bodies take longer to get into the exercise groove because their muscles aren't used to working hard. If you're a beginner, any exercise is high-intensity exercise. As you get more fit, your body adapts and becomes more efficient, thereby warming up more quickly.

Many people skip their warm-up because they're in a hurry. Cranking up the LifeCycle or hitting the weight room right away seems like a more efficient use of time. Bad idea. Skimp on your warm-up, and you're a lot more likely to injure yourself. Besides, when you ease into your workout, you enjoy it a lot more. A trainer we know says, "If you don't have time to warm up, you don't have time to work out!"

What exactly does warming up do for you? Well, for one thing, a warm-up warms you up — literally. It increases the temperature in your muscles and in the tissues that connect muscle to bone (tendons) and bone to bone (ligaments). Warmer muscles and joints are more pliable and, therefore, less likely to tear. Warming up also helps redirect your blood flow from places such as your stomach and spleen to the muscles that you're using to exercise. This blood flow gives you more stamina by providing your muscles with more nutrients and oxygen. In other words, you tire more quickly if you don't warm up.

Finally, warming up allows your heart rate to increase at a safe, gradual pace. If you don't warm up, your heart rate will shoot up too quickly, and you'll feel like you're walking through a knee-high snowdrift.

Cooling down

After your workout, don't stop suddenly and make a dash for the shower or plop on the couch. Ease out of your workout just as you eased into it, by walking, jogging, or cycling lightly. If you've been using a stair-climber at Level 5 for 20 minutes, you could cool down by dropping to Level 4 for a couple minutes, then to Level 3, and so on. This *cooldown* should last five to ten minutes — longer if you've done an especially hard workout.

The purpose of the cooldown is the reverse of the warm-up. At this point, your heart is jumping, and blood is pumping furiously through your muscles. You want your body to redirect the blood flow back to normal before you rush back to the office. You also want your body temperature to decrease before you hop into a hot or cold shower; otherwise, you risk fainting. Cooling down prevents your blood from pooling in one place, such as your legs. When you suddenly stop exercising, your blood can quickly collect, which can lead to dizziness, nausea, and fainting. If you're really out of shape or at high risk for heart disease, skipping a cooldown can place undue stress on your heart.

How Hard Do You Need to Push?

To reap the benefits of cardio exercise, how much huffing and puffing do you need to do? Not as much as you probably think. Sure, you won't benefit much from walking on the treadmill at the same pace you stroll down the grocery store aisles; they don't call it working out for nothing. On the other hand, exercising too hard can lead to injury and make you more susceptible to colds and infections; plus, you may get so burned out that you want to set fire to your stationary bike. Also, the faster you go, the less time you can keep up the exercise. Depending on what you're trying to accomplish, you may gain just as much, if not more, from slowing things down and going farther.

To get fit and stay healthy, you need to find the middle ground: a moderate, or aerobic, pace. You can find this middle ground in a number of different ways. Some methods of gauging your intensity are extremely simple, and some require a foray into arithmetic. This section looks at three popular ways to monitor your intensity.

The talk test

The simplest way to monitor how hard you're working is to talk. You should be able to carry on a conversation while you're exercising. If you're so out of breath that you can't even string together the words "Help me, Mommy!" you need to slow down. On the other hand, if you're able to belt out "Livin' La Vida Loca" at the top of your lungs, that's a pretty big clue you need to pick up the pace. Basically, you should feel like you're working, but not so hard that you feel like your lungs are about to explode.

Perceived exertion

If you're the type of person who needs more precision in life than the talk test offers, you may like the so-called *perceived exertion* method of gauging intensity. This method uses a numerical scale, typically from 1 to 10, that corresponds to how hard you feel you're working — the rate at which you perceive that you're exerting yourself.

An activity rated 1 on a perceived exertion scale would be something that you feel you could do forever, like sit in bed and watch *Chariots of Fire*. A 10 represents all-out effort, like the last few feet of an uphill sprint, about 20 seconds before your legs buckle. Your typical workout intensity should fall somewhere between 5 and 8. To decide on a number, pay attention to how hard you're breathing, how fast your heart is beating, how much you're sweating, and how tired your legs feel — anything that contributes to the effort of sustaining the exercise.

The purpose of putting a numerical value on exercise is not to make your life more complicated but rather to help you maintain a proper workout intensity. For example, suppose you run 2 miles around your neighborhood, and it feels like an 8. If after a few weeks running those 2 miles feels like a 4, you know it's time to pick up the pace. Initially, you may want to have a perceived exertion chart in front of you. Many gyms post these charts on the walls, and you can easily create one at home. After a few workouts you can use a mental chart. Table 8-1 shows a sample perceived exertion chart.

Table 8-1	Perceived Exertion Chart	
Numerical Rating	**Subjective Rating**	**Sample Activities**
0	Nothing at all	Sitting still, reading
1	Very light	Standing in line
2	Light	Taking a leisurely stroll
3		
4	Light/moderate	
5	Moderate	Walking at a moderate pace, gardening
6		
7	Hard	Jogging briskly, cycling over rolling hills
8	Very hard	Running
9		
10	Extremely hard	Sprinting up a steep hill

Measuring your heart rate

The talk test and the perceived exertion chart are both valid ways to make sure that you're exercising at the right pace. But there's a more precise way: measuring your *heart rate,* the number of times that your heart beats per minute. (Your heart rate is also called your *pulse*.) You can determine this number either by counting the beats at your wrist or neck or by wearing a gadget called a heart-rate monitor. This section discusses both and also lets you know why you want to measure your heart rate and how you can determine your own target heart-rate zone.

Why monitor your heart rate?

Keeping track of your heart rate, by whatever method, sounds like an incredibly advanced thing to do — something way beyond a beginner's needs. But even if you're just starting out, heart-rate monitoring is abundantly effective.

When you're just starting to work out, you may not have a good sense of how hard to push yourself. And with all that "no pain, no gain" propaganda, you may be working harder than you really need to. Actually, this happens to advanced exercisers and athletes all the time. Left to their own devices, they try to outdo themselves every day. The smart ones use a heart-rate monitor to remind them to slow down. However, for most people, the problem is getting into a higher gear.

Knowing how hard you're working during a workout is far more helpful than simply knowing how fast you're going. For example, running nine-minute miles on a hot, humid afternoon takes a lot more effort than running at the same pace on a cool, overcast morning. If you rely only on your stopwatch, you may push yourself to run nine-minute miles in the heat, when that pace may put excess stress on your body. If you pace yourself according to your heart rate instead, you know when you need to back off.

The same goes for when you're tired. If you've had a particularly hard week at work, your body may not be up to your usual workout. Without checking your heart rate, you may force yourself to do Level 4 on the stair-climber, when, in fact, your body isn't up to the task. If you monitor your pulse, you may find that, in order to keep up with Level 4, you have to exceed the high end of your training zone — a signal to drop down a notch or two.

By keeping track of your heart rate over a long period of time, you discover some interesting things about your progress. When you're a beginner, your heart has to work a lot harder to keep up with your body's demands for blood and oxygen. If you work out on a regular basis, your aerobic system gradually becomes more efficient. Suppose when you started, Level 1 on the exercise bike used to get your heart up to about 140 beats per minute; now, two months later, your heart rate is 125 beats per minute. This drop means that you need to step up the difficulty of your workout. You can see why keeping good records of your workouts is a good idea.

To find out how much your fitness level is improving, watch how fast your heart rate drops after a workout. Measure your heart rate immediately upon finishing your exercise session and then one minute later. The better shape you're in, the faster your heart rate drops. Ideally, your heart rate should plunge at least 20 beats in the first minute. People in really good shape drop 40 beats or more. Keep track of this measure. You'll see a gradual improvement over a period of weeks and months. (Taking prescription or over-the-counter medication may affect the way your heart and blood pressure respond to exercise. Check with your doctor about this.)

As we mention in Chapter 2, monitoring your resting heart rate is also a good idea. Your *resting heart rate* is the number of times your heart beats per minute when you're just sitting around. When you start exercising, your resting heart rate may be as high as 90. But after a few months of exercising, your resting heart rate may drop 10 or 20 beats. Some top athletes in endurance sports have resting heart rates as low as 30 beats per minute. However, don't compare your heart rate to anyone else's. Your resting heart rate is partly determined by heredity.

Your resting heart rate also can tell you a lot about your recovery from day to day. Keep your monitor by your bed and strap it on first thing in the morning, on a daily basis. Or, take your pulse manually. If your heart rate is ten beats higher than usual, you probably haven't recovered from yesterday's workout.

Your target heart-rate zone

Your heart rate can tell you so much about your body — how fit you are, how much you've improved, and whether you've recovered from yesterday's workout. But how do you know what heart rate to aim for? There's no magic number. Rather, there's a whole range of acceptable numbers, commonly called your *target heart-rate zone.* This range is the middle ground between slacking off and knocking yourself out. Typically, your *target zone* (as it's called for short) is between 50 percent and 85 percent of your *maximum heart rate,* the maximum number of times your heart should beat in a minute without dangerously overexerting yourself.

The point at which your body switches from using oxygen as its primary source of energy to using stored sugar is referred to as your *anaerobic threshold.* (You may also hear this referred to as the point at which *lactic acid* builds up.) When you're in poor physical shape, your body isn't very efficient at taking in oxygen, and you hit your anaerobic threshold while exercising at relatively low levels of exercise. As you become more fit, you're able to go farther and faster, yet still supply oxygen to your muscles. If a couch potato tries to run an eight-minute-mile pace, he's going to go anaerobic pretty darned fast. An elite runner can run an entire marathon at about a five-minute-mile pace and still stay primarily aerobic.

At the low end of your zone, you're barely breaking a sweat; at the high end, you're dripping like a Kentucky Derby winner. If you're a beginner, stick to the lower end so you can move along comfortably for longer periods of time and

The Karvonen method for target heart rate

One of the problems with the standard formula for finding your target heart rate is that it takes only your age into consideration. This is a valid consideration because your recommended maximum heart rate declines as you age. However, the following formula, called the Karvonen method, is somewhat more accurate because it also factors in your *resting heart rate*, the number of times your heart beats when you're sitting still. Typically, as you become more fit, your heart rate drops.

The Karvonen method requires a bit more math, but don't let that intimidate you. In this example, we use the case of a 40-year-old man who has a resting heart rate of 60 beats per minute and wants to work at between 50 percent and 85 percent of his maximum heart rate. Grab your calculator and follow these step-by-step instructions:

1. **Subtract your age from 220.**

   Using our example, $220 - 40 = 180$.

   This is our subject's estimated maximum.

2. **Subtract your resting heart rate from your estimated maximum.**

   $180 - 60 = 120$.

3. **Multiply the number you arrived at in Step 2 by 50 percent. Then add your resting heart rate back in.**

   $120 \times 0.50 = 60$

   $60 + 60 = 120$

   120 is the low end of the man's target zone.

4. **Multiply the Step 2 result by 85 percent. Then add your resting heart rate back in.**

   $120 \times 0.85 = 102$

   $102 + 60 = 162$

   162 is the high end of the man's target zone.

Okay, now that you feel like you've earned your Ph.D. in calculus, you can compare the results of this formula with those of the traditional formula. Using the age-related formula, this 40-year-old's target zone is 90 to 153 beats. But when you factor in his resting heart rate, this allows him to work up to 162 beats per minute. And he knows that if he drops below 102 beats, he probably needs to pick up the pace.

with less chance of injury. As you get more fit, you may want to do some of your training in the middle and upper end of your zone. In Chapter 7, we offer examples of ways to mix up your training.

So how do you know what your maximum heart rate is? Well, we don't recommend running as hard as you can until you keel over, and then counting your heartbeats for one minute. A safer and more accurate way is to have your max measured by a professional such as a physician or exercise specialist. (See Chapter 2 for details on exercise testing.) You can also use a number of mathematical formulas to estimate your max.

The most time-honored method for determining maximum heart rate is for men to subtract their age from 220 and for women to subtract their age from 226. Keep in mind that this formula gives you only an estimate. Your true max may be as many as 15 beats higher or lower. Also, this formula is generally used for activities during which your feet hit the ground. (To estimate your max for bicycling, subtract about five beats from the final result; for swimming, subtract about ten beats.)

Using that easy formula to find your max, find your target heart-rate zone by calculating 50 percent and 85 percent of your maximum. Here's the math for a 40-year-old man:

$$220 - 40 = 180$$

This is his estimated maximum heart rate.

$$180 \times 0.50 = 90$$

This is the low end of his target zone. If his heart beats less than 90 times per minute, he knows that he's not pushing hard enough.

$$180 \times 0.85 = 153$$

This is the high end of his target zone. If his heart beats faster than 153 beats per minute, he needs to slow down.

Okay, so now you know how to figure out your target heart-rate zone. But how do you know if you're in the zone? In other words, how do you know how fast your heart is beating at any given moment? As we mention earlier in this chapter, you can check your heart rate in two ways: taking your pulse manually or using a heart-rate monitor.

Taking your pulse manually

Watch any quality aerobics video or take any decent cardio class at the gym, and you hear the instructor yell out, "Okay, everybody, time for a heart-rate check." On this cue, the participants place their fingers on their necks or on their wrists. Taking your pulse manually can be wildly inaccurate, so concentrate when you do it.

To use the neck method, place your index and middle fingers (not your thumb) in the groove on either side of your throat pipe. When you feel a beat, you've found your carotid artery. The neck method isn't our favorite because your heart rate is harder to find on your neck and because some experts feel that the act of pressing against this artery may actually shut off blood and oxygen supply to the brain, causing you to faint. If you use this method, be careful not to push too hard. We prefer the wrist method, which we explain in Chapter 2.

Whichever method you choose, you don't need to keep your fingers on your neck or wrist for an entire minute while you count the beats. Feel the steady pounding of blood flowing through your arteries. When you're fairly comfortable with the rhythm, count how many beats you feel in 15 seconds. Then multiply this number by four — voilá, your heart rate.

If you flunked Mr. Dyshuck's fifth-grade math class and multiplying by four proves to be out of your range of talents, that's okay. Just take your pulse for 6 seconds and add a zero onto the number of beats you count; this, in effect, is multiplying by 10. For example: You take your pulse for 6 seconds and count 14 beats. Add a zero and you get 140 — that's approximately how many times per minute your heart is beating. Just know that this shortcut method can be extremely inaccurate. If you miss a single beat, you miscalculate your heart rate by 10 beats per minute. We mention this method only because it's commonly used in health clubs.

During your workout, take your pulse about every 15 minutes and be sure to concentrate. Otherwise, you may end up counting the number of steps you take on the stair-climber rather than the number of pulses in your wrist. You may want to slow down or even stop while you take your pulse. True, this is disruptive to your workout, but it's not nearly as disruptive as getting launched off the treadmill.

Using a heart-rate monitor

You can eliminate the inaccuracy and inconvenience of taking your heart rate by wearing a heart-rate monitor. With a monitor, you don't need to stop exercising or take the time to count anything. At any given moment you can find out your heart rate by glancing at your wrist. A good monitor can cost less than $60. The really fancy ones cost up to $400. They offer features such as a clock, a timer, and an alarm that you can set to beep when you wander out of your target zone.

Most of the cardio equipment in gyms is now "heart-rate-monitor compatible." The machines pick up the signal from the monitor, and your heart rate pops up on the display console, so you don't have to wear the wrist watch. This saves you the trouble of bringing your wrist up to your eyeball while you're moving.

The most accurate type of monitor is the *chest-strap variety,* which operates on the same principle as a medical electrocardiogram (ECG). You hook an inch-wide strap around your chest. This strap acts as an electrode to measure the electrical activity of your heart. This information is then translated into a number, which is transmitted via radio signals to a wrist receiver that looks like a watch with a large face. All you have to do is look at your wrist, and you instantly know how many times your heart is beating that moment, whether it's 92 or 164. Turn to Chapter 25 for more details on purchasing a monitor.

Chest monitors are very accurate, but some are subject to interference from electromagnetic waves like those given off by some treadmills and stair-climbers. (Better, newer models come equipped with coded signals that prevent this interference.) Exercising next to someone else who's wearing a monitor may also scramble signals, a sort of electronic equivalent of getting your braces locked with someone else's when you're kissing. You may need at least 4 feet between users for monitors to function properly, although several companies now offer models with a special device to eliminate interference.

Less accurate than chest monitors are *photo-optic models,* often sold with home equipment. These clip onto your earlobe or fingertip and detect the heartbeat there. Your heart rate shows up on a handheld or clip-on digital screen or special wristwatch. Those models cost only about $30, but any movement of your wrist, hand, or fingers can cause highly erratic or false readings. Daylight, poor circulation, and high-intensity exercise may also skew the results.

How Much Do You Need to Do?

Unless you're a professional athlete or wealthier than the average Third World dictator, you probably don't have unlimited time to work out. So you may be wondering: Just how much cardio exercise does it really take to get fit?

The answer depends on your goals. Exercise is not an all-or-nothing proposition. You can be fit to live a long life, fit to bicycle 30 miles, fit to run the Mount Everest Marathon (there really is such a thing) — or anywhere in between. In the cardio plans near the end of this chapter, we discuss how long, how often, and how hard you need to exercise in order to achieve three general goals: good health, fat loss, and maximum fitness. We also explain how you can cut back on your workouts during a serious time crunch without losing your fitness.

That said, recent research published in the *Archives of Internal Medicine* attempted to answer the question of how much exercise is needed to maintain body weight by placing subjects into four categories:

- No exercise at all
- Low amount of exercise (12 miles per week of walking or running) with moderate intensity (equivalent to 4 to 5.5 in Table 8-1)
- Low amount of exercise (12 miles per week of walking or running) with vigorous intensity (also 6.5 to 8 in Table 8-1)
- High amount of exercise (20 miles per week of walking or running) with vigorous intensity (6.5 to 8 in Table 8-1)

The subjects did not change their total caloric intake or alter the makeup of their diets. Researchers discovered that 73 percent of subjects in the control group (who didn't exercise at all) gained weight during the study, indicating that some exercise is absolutely essential for maintaining weight. Perhaps not surprisingly, 75 percent of the other three groups lost weight and decreased in size. But here's the best news: The high-amount/vigorous-intensity subjects lost far more weight and body fat and had the largest reductions in size (namely, waist circumference) of the four groups. Although the issue of how much exercise is enough won't be resolved anytime soon, this study suggests that the most benefits are gained from combining a high amount of exercise with vigorous intensity.

Following a Cardio Plan for Good Health

If your goal is to feel better and live longer, a little aerobic exercise goes a remarkably long way. Research shows that the people who gain the most from aerobic exercise are those who go from being completely slothful to only marginally slothful — not the ones who go from being fit to super fit. The people in the bottom 20 percent of the population, fitness-wise, are 65 percent more likely to die from heart attack, stroke, diabetes, or cancer than the highly fit people in the top 20 percent. However, when those couch potatoes move up just one notch on the fitness scale, by simply adding a daily 30-minute walk, they're only 10 percent more likely to die from these causes than super-fit people.

If you have no designs on hiking the Appalachian Trail or losing 50 pounds, you may want to know the minimum amount of exercise that can make a difference in your health. Here are some answers.

How often you need to do cardio for good health

Research suggests that you can lower your risk of heart disease just by walking for 20 minutes three times a week. This typically is enough exercise to increase your energy level and stamina, too, although not enough to cause much in the way of fat loss. If you're a beginner, we recommend working out five or six days rather than three days a week (keeping the workouts short) simply so you get in the habit of exercising.

How long your workouts should last for good health

If your goal is to improve your health, you do not need to do all your exercise in big chunks. Nowhere is it written — in the U.S. Constitution, the Talmud, or the California Penal Code — that in order to benefit from aerobic exercise, you need to do it for 30 consecutive minutes. Studies show that doing three ten-minute bouts of aerobic exercise has nearly the same health benefits as doing one half-hour session.

How hard you need to push for good health

If you're simply looking to feel better and improve the quality of your every-day life, being active is the key, even if you don't always reach your target zone (see the "Your target heart-rate zone" section earlier in this chapter). However, to realize the maximum health benefits — significantly lowering your heart-disease risk, for example — it's wise to work out in your target zone the majority of the time. Plus, even if you have modest goals, you may want to crank up your intensity just to keep things interesting.

Realize that, when you're a beginner, any exercise you do is high-intensity exercise. As you get more fit, you need to adapt your routine to match your increasing strength and lung power. When Liz's mom started working out, she couldn't complete 10 minutes on the treadmill at 2 mph. After three months, she was able to do 20 minutes at 4 mph — an improvement that in the beginning would have seemed inconceivable.

Following a Cardio Plan for Weight Loss

If your goal is permanent fat loss, the "cardio plan for good health" isn't going to cut it. You simply won't burn enough calories to make a significant impact. Here's why: In order to lose a pound in one week, you need to create a 3,500-calorie deficit; in other words, you need to burn off 3,500 more calories than you eat. A 30-minute power walk on flat ground burns about 120 calories. (See the "Which activities burn the most calories" section later in this chapter.) So, to burn off 1 pound of fat by walking, you'd have to hoof it for more than 2 hours a day.

Don't worry — we're not suggesting that you exercise two hours every day! In fact, we think the best way to lose fat is to create a calorie deficit by burning calories through exercise and cutting calories you eat. For example, over the course of a week, you may cut 250 calories per day by switching from mayo to mustard on your sandwich at lunch and snacking on Yoplait Lite yogurt instead of Columbo Fruit-on-the-Bottom. Meanwhile, you could burn an extra 250 calories a day by taking a one-hour walk or a half-hour jog.

Cardio exercise is only one part of a weight-loss plan. You also need to revamp your eating habits (see Chapter 7 for tips) and embark on a weight-training program (see Chapter 11 to find out why). Also, keep in mind that losing weight is not as easy as it sounds on TV diet commercials. It takes a lot more commitment than just drinking that delicious shake for breakfast. And it takes time. Don't try to lose more than ½ pound to 1 pound each week, and don't eat fewer than 1,200 calories per day (preferably more). On a super-low-calorie diet, you deprive your body of essential nutrients, and you have a tougher time keeping the weight off because your metabolism slows down. Realize, too, that genetics plays a large role in weight loss. It's easier for some people to lose weight than it is for others.

Here are some general cardio guidelines for weight loss. We suggest that you consult a registered dietitian and certified fitness trainer to come up with a plan best suited to your specific goals and schedule.

How often you need to do cardio for weight loss

Here's the cold, hard truth: You probably need to do five or six workouts a week.

How long your workouts should last for weight loss

Here's another dose of reality: You should aim for at least 45 minutes of exercise, a mix of cardio and strength training, six days per week. Again, you don't need to do all this sweating at once, but for the pounds to come off, the calories you burn need to add up.

How hard you need to push for weight loss

To make a serious dent in your fat-loss program, we suggest that you work out in your target zone most of the time. But keep in mind: If you're pretty darned "deconditioned," as the politically correct like to say, even exercising at 50 percent of your maximum heart rate can help build up your fitness level.

You may have heard that exercising at a slow pace is more effective for weight loss than working out more intensely. In fact, many cardio machines have "fat burning" programs that keep you at a slow pace. But this is misleading. As it turns out, the concept of a fat-burning zone is no more real than the *Twilight Zone*.

During low-intensity aerobic exercise, your body does use fat as its primary fuel source. As you get closer to your breaking point, your body starts using a smaller percentage of fat and a larger percentage of carbohydrates, another fuel source. However, picking up the pace allows you to burn more total calories, as well as more fat calories.

Here's how: If you go in-line skating for 30 minutes at a leisurely roll, you might burn about 100 calories — about 80 percent of them from fat (so that's 80 fat calories). But if you spend the same amount of time skating with a vengeance over a hilly course, you might burn 300 calories — 30 percent of them from fat (that's 90 fat calories). So at the fast pace, you burn more than double the calories and 10 more fat calories.

Of course, going faster and harder is not always better. If you're just starting out, you probably can't sustain a faster pace long enough to make it worth your while. If you go slower, you may be able to exercise a lot longer, so you'll end up burning more calories and fat that way.

Which activities burn the most calories

"Maximize your workout and burn over 1,000 calories per hour!" That's a claim you may see in advertisements for treadmills, stair-climbers, and other cardio machines. And it's true. You can burn 1,000 calories per hour doing those activities — if you crank up the machine to the highest level and if you happen to have bionic legs. If you're a beginner, you'll last about 30 seconds at that pace, at which point you will have burned 8.3 calories, and the paramedics will be scooping you off the floor and hauling your wilted body away on a stretcher.

There's a better approach to calorie burning: Choose an activity that you can sustain for a good while — say, at least 10 or 15 minutes. Sure, running burns more calories than walking, but if running wipes you out after a half mile or bothers your knees, you're better off walking.

Table 8-2 gives calorie estimates for a number of popular aerobic activities. The number of calories you actually burn depends on the intensity of your workout, your weight, your muscle mass, and your metabolism. In general, a beginner is capable of burning 4 or 5 calories per minute of exercise, while a very fit person can burn 10 to 12 calories per minute.

The table includes a few stop-and-go sports such as tennis and basketball. Activities like these are not aerobic in the truest sense, but they can still give you a great workout and contribute to good health and weight loss. The numbers in this chart apply to a 150-pound person. (If you weigh less, you'll burn a little less; if you weigh more, you'll burn a little more.)

Table 8-2	Calories Burned during Popular Activities			
Activity	*15 min.*	*30 min.*	*45 min.*	*60 min.*
Aerobic dance	171	342	513	684
Basketball	141	282	432	564
Bicycling at 12 mph	142	283	425	566
Bicycling at 15 mph	177	354	531	708
Bicycling at 18 mph	213	425	638	850
Boxing	165	330	495	660
Circuit weight training	189	378	576	756
Cross-country skiing	146	291	437	583
Downhill skiing	105	210	315	420
Golf (carrying clubs)	87	174	261	348
In-line skating	150	300	450	600
Jumping rope, 60–80 skips/min.	143	286	429	572
Karate, tae kwon do	192	834	576	768
Kayaking	75	150	225	300
Racquetball	114	228	342	456
Rowing machine	104	208	310	415
Running 10-minute miles	183	365	548	731
Running 8-minute miles	223	446	670	893
Ski machine	141	282	423	564
Slide	152	304	456	608
Swimming freestyle, 35 yds/min.	124	248	371	497
Swimming freestyle, 50 yds/min.	131	261	392	523

Activity	15 min.	30 min.	45 min.	60 min.
Tennis, singles	116	232	348	464
Tennis, doubles	43	85	128	170
VersaClimber, 100 ft./min.	188	375	563	750
Walking, 20-minute miles, flat	60	120	180	240
Walking, 20-minute miles, hills	81	162	243	324
Walking, 15-minute miles, flat	73	146	219	292
Walking, 15-minute miles, hills	102	206	279	412
Water aerobics	70	140	210	280

Following a Cardio Plan to Maximize Your Fitness

When you get the hang of this exercise thing, you may find that you want more of a challenge. Instead of being satisfied with a boost in energy and a decrease in heart-disease risk, you may want to test yourself in a 5K run or a weeklong hiking tour of Canada.

Bernie Kalkbrenner, a funeral director we know from Duluth, Minnesota, smoked 2½ packs of cigarettes a day for 25 years. One day, Bernie realized that if he didn't get his act together, he was going to become one of his own customers. So he quit smoking and took up bicycling. At age 51, he cycled 3,230 miles across the United States in less than seven weeks. "I've never felt this good in my life," Bernie said upon finishing. "To be able to pedal my butt up a hill without any shortness of breath — that's exhilarating."

How can you get in shape like Bernie? In Chapter 10, we offer specific tips on how to train for several outdoor sports, including cycling. The following sections also give you some general tips for getting in really good cardio shape. Be sure to increase your training gradually; don't go longer, more often, and harder all at once. Otherwise, you really increase your chances of injuring yourself. In other words, it's not a great idea to do three 20-minute workouts one week and then jump to three 45-minute workouts the next. It's more sensible to increase the time of just one of your workouts to 25 minutes and keep the others at 20.

The best approach is to increase no more than 10 percent each week. So, if you walk 150 minutes one week, walk no more than 165 minutes the next.

Treat getting into good cardiovascular shape like a really important ongoing project. You may struggle through the first session, maybe even the first five to ten. But if you stick with it three times a week for at least six weeks, you'll start to notice dramatic changes. At that point, you'll recover much more quickly from your workouts. Instead of going home and crashing on the couch, you may feel ready to go bowling or out for a walk.

How often you need to do cardio for maximum fitness

Five days a week is a good goal to shoot for. Most people feel best with two days off a week; everyone should take at least one day of complete rest. In the "Giving It a Rest" section later in this chapter, we explain how to tell whether you need more rest.

How long your workouts should last for maximum fitness

Depending on your sport and your goal, you probably need to mix in at least a couple long workouts — an hour or more — per week. Just make sure you don't increase the length of your workouts by more than 10 percent a week; otherwise, your risk of injury shoots pretty high.

How hard you need to push for maximum fitness

Even when you're training to get in your best shape ever, you don't want to go all-out every day. (In fact, only serious athletes peaking for an event should ever go all-out — and even then, only once or twice a week.) Your target zone includes a large range of intensity levels. On some days, stay near the bottom of the range and go for a longer workout; on other days, push harder and go for a shorter workout. Try any or all of the training techniques described in the next section.

Four ways to boost your fitness

You can play plenty of games to challenge your body. This section discusses four training techniques that you can try after about a month or two of training at 50 to 60 percent of your maximum heart rate. The less conditioning you start with, the more cautious you should be.

✔ **Interval training:** With *interval training,* you alternate short, fairly intense spurts of exercise with periods of relatively easy exercise. For example, say you're out bicycling. After warming up for 15 minutes or so, you may try cycling all-out for 30 seconds and follow this with a few minutes of easy pedaling until your heart rate slows down a little, to about 120 or fewer beats per minute. Then you do another tough 30-second interval, and so on. In essence, you're switching between the low and high ends of your target zone.

When you first try interval training, keep the high-intensity periods short — 15 to 30 seconds. Follow these periods with at least three times as much active rest (so, 45 to 90 seconds). *Active rest* means that you keep moving between intervals instead of stopping dead. So after you do that 30-second bike sprint, pedal slowly for about 90 seconds. You may need even more recovery than that, especially if you're a beginner. As you become more accustomed to higher levels, you can increase the length of the high-intensity intervals as you decrease the length of the low-intensity intervals. Eventually, you can aim for a 1:1 hard-to-easy ratio, measuring intervals in terms of time or distance.

✔ **Fartlek:** This charming word means "speed play" in Swedish. *Fartlek* is basically interval training without an exact measure of time or distance. You just do your intervals whenever you feel like it. You may try sprinting to every other telephone pole. Or set your sights on that horse standing in the field down the road and pick up your pace until you reach him.

✔ **Uphill battles:** You can add hills to walking, biking, running, or skating workouts. You have to work harder when you come to a hill, but ultimately you're rewarded with extra strength and stamina. As a bonus, going uphill can burn twice as many calories as exercising on flat land. One fun drill is to do hill repeats. Find a long, fairly steep hill and then sprint up it and jog down it, repeating this sequence four to eight times.

Here's a trick to make hill workouts seem easier: Pick a landmark that's partway up the hill, such as a bush or mailbox. Pretend that you have a rope in your hands and cast it over your landmark. Now pull yourself up the hill with your imaginary rope. When you reach your landmark, cast your rope on something farther up the hill and keep doing this until you reach the top.

✔ **Tempo workouts:** *Tempo workouts* help you learn to move faster. During a tempo drill, you move at a pace that you consider challenging but not brutal, keeping that pace for four to ten minutes. Do that a couple of times each workout. In between, exercise at your normal pace. If you're new to tempo training, begin with short tempos and gradually increase their length. Anyone training for a local road race or a bike-a-thon will find tempo work helpful.

Training for a specific event

Thinking of training for a 5K or 10K race, half-marathon, century bike ride, or triathlon? Ideally, you want to spend at least 16 weeks (about 4 months) preparing for your event. Take the first six to ten weeks just getting used to running, cycling, swimming, and so on, slowly building your weekly mileage at 10 percent each week. Starting at about 9 to 11 weeks, begin using the techniques listed in the "Four ways to boost your fitness" section earlier, mixing them into your routine. For example, one week, you might do uphill training one day; the next week, you might try a tempo workout on a Monday and a fartlek on a Thursday. In between, you run, cycle, or swim at a more moderate pace or take a day off, allowing your body time to recover before your next workout. By 16 weeks, you should be ready for the big day.

For more specific information about training for a running event, check out Wiley Publishing's *Running For Dummies,* by Florence Griffith-Joyner and Jon Hanc, or *Marathon Training For Dummies,* by Tere Stouffer Drenth, which includes information on racing at distances from 5K to marathons.

Giving It a Rest

For most people, exercising too much is about as big a problem as saving too much money. However, some beginners — in their zeal to make up for 20 years of neglecting their bodies — vow to exercise every day for the next 20 years. This is not a good idea. If you're trying to get fit, your workouts are only part of the equation; rest is just as important.

Aim for a balance between hard days and easy days. If you do an intense interval day on Monday, do an easy workout Tuesday. If you do two tough days in a row, your legs may feel like someone inserted lead pipes in them while you were sleeping. Everyone should rest at least one day a week. (Just don't let that one day off slip into three years.) And when we say take a rest day, we mean no exercise. Nada. Zippo. An easy day does not count as a rest day. In addition to taking a day or two off each week, you may also want to take an easy week every month or two. So if you usually jog 15 miles a week, cut back to 7 just for the week. Drastic cutbacks can help remotivate you and give your body the vacation it may need.

There's no magic formula to determine exactly how much rest is best for your goals and fitness level. But here's a good rule: If you're doing everything right, you should be able to wake up in the morning and say, "I know my workout's going to be really good," rather than, "How the heck am I gonna drag my butt to the gym?"

What happens if you stop exercising?

Aerobic conditioning is a use-it-or-lose-it proposition. A couple of days of inactivity won't set you back, but if you continue to slack off, your improvements fade in a matter of weeks. Research indicates that most of the benefits from aerobic training are lost within two weeks to three months.

But there's good news, too. You can preserve your hard-earned fitness even if you go through a period when you don't exercise as much as usual. Suppose you're a CPA. You get into a really good routine of jogging on the treadmill four days a week for a half-hour, and you keep up the routine for four straight months. Then, suddenly, tax time arrives, and for two months you're buried in 1099s, IRS long forms, and 401(k) plans. Well, instead of abandoning exercise altogether, which would practically guarantee that you lose all your conditioning, you can cut back and still maintain your fitness for up to 12 weeks.

Instead of running 30 minutes 4 days a week, you could get by with 30 minutes twice a week or 15 minutes 4 times a week. The only requirement is that you keep up your usual pace. When you get back to your regular routine after tax time, you may find that you've lost no fitness at all — or maybe just a tiny bit.

Exercisers of all levels are susceptible to overtraining. For an elite athlete, overtraining might be running 80 miles in a week; for a beginner, running 8 miles might be too much. Here are some signs that you've overdone it:

- ✔ **Your resting heart rate sounds like a jackhammer drilling through concrete.** In other words, if your heart rate is way above what it normally is — say, about 10 beats — take it very easy or take a day or two off. (For details about your resting heart rate, see Chapter 2.)

- ✔ **You feel chronically sore or weak.** If you lift a ketchup bottle and it feels like a 10-pound dumbbell, stay home.

- ✔ **You get chronic colds and infections.**

- ✔ **You're not sleeping well.**

- ✔ **You're irritable, anxious, or depressed.** It's not a good sign if you lock your keys in your car and smash the window to retrieve them instead of calling the auto club.

- ✔ **You can't concentrate or you feel disoriented.** If you make a left-hand turn signal while you're on a stationary bike, it's time for a rest.

Chapter 9

Using Cardio Machines

*W*alk into a health club or fitness-equipment store and you're likely to encounter rows of high-tech contraptions that appear to be part video game, part escalator, and part lawn mower. Don't be alarmed. The consoles of these machines may resemble the control panel of Apollo 13, but with a little help, even a rookie can understand all the flashing red dots and beeping green arrows. Be thankful for all this technology because it makes indoor aerobic exercise a lot more fun than it used to be. For all your sweat, the screen offers you instant gratification — the number of miles that you walk, steps that you climb, minutes that you cycle, and calories that you burn.

Cardiovascular machines tend to come and go. Since the first edition of this book, we've seen the rise and fall of various riders, gliders, and skaters. So we're not going to give you a rundown of every crazy invention that's made its way onto an infomercial. Instead, this chapter covers the solid, proven machines, such as treadmills, rowers, bikes, and stair-climbers, as well as a relative newcomer that we believe is here to stay: the elliptical trainer. We tell you how to take the drudgery out of exercising in place and how to position your body on each machine so that you burn the most calories and avoid injury.

Can You Trust Those Calorie Counters?

At the gym one day, Suzanne was pumping away on the stair-climber next to a very fit woman. For a brief moment, the woman looked away from her machine to say hello to a friend. When she looked back, her 45-minute workout had ended, and she had missed the final calorie readout. Horrified, the woman uttered several curse words and then stormed into the locker room — as if not knowing her exact calorie burn negated the entire 45 minutes of effort.

That may be an extreme case, but most of us do get a psychological boost from knowing how many calories we just burned. There's just one problem: The information may not be accurate.

For the most part, the formulas used to calculate calories burned are derived from tests done on healthy young males — and in some cases, elite athletes working near their maximum effort. This does not always translate accurately for the rest of us. For instance, a recent study conducted found that fitness equipment readouts may overestimate calorie count for obese women by as much as 80 calories for 30 minutes of moderate intensity walking.

Other research has found that calorie predictions are skewed even further if you lean your body weight against the handrails, grip tightly, or otherwise position your body on a machine in a way that makes the exercise less strenuous. Some studies have shown that calculations can be off by as much as 50 percent.

Sometimes it's not the formulas or your technique that skew the calorie count; it's the deceptive marketing strategy of the machine's manufacturer. A researcher for one cardio-equipment manufacturer admitted to us that his company intentionally boosts the calorie information by as much as 30 percent so that people may, subconsciously, prefer their machines over other brands.

We suspect that elliptical machines (described in the "Elliptical trainer" section later in this chapter) have particularly generous calorie readouts. Case in point: When Liz does a fairly easy elliptical workout, the machine tells her that she burns 12 calories per minute — a number that seems suspiciously high. In fact, in order to achieve the same calorie burn on the treadmill (known to be an accurate machine), she needs to run at a brisk 8 mph, a pace that shoots her heart rate way up into the huff-and-puff zone. We're skeptical that these two workouts are equivalent.

The most accurate machines tend to be the treadmill and the stationary bike because the contraptions have been so well studied. In recent years, stair-climbers have adjusted calorie estimates drastically downward to better reflect reality.

The bottom line: Realize that the calorie figures are simply estimates.

Use the calorie information to motivate you, but don't be a slave to it, and don't rely on the numbers to validate your efforts.

Combating Boredom on Aerobic Machines

It's no coincidence that "treadmill" is listed under "tedium" in *Roget's Thesaurus;* imitating a laboratory rodent is not among life's thrills. No matter what type of exercise machine you use and no matter how many flashing dots you're rewarded with, boredom is bound to hit you at some point. In this section, we suggest ways to divert your attention so that your 20, 30, or 40 minutes pass before you know it. Eventually, you may actually begin to enjoy the sensations of sweat and fatigue, and using these machines won't seem like a chore.

Take a cardio-machine class

It used to be that if you wanted a cardio workout in the company of a perky instructor and enthusiastic classmates, you had to take step aerobics or some type of dance class. But now the group-exercise concept includes machines, too. The trend started with indoor cycling classes known as spinning or studio cycling and has since expanded to treadmills, stair-climbers, and rowing machines. Group cycling has become so popular that most new clubs now build separate rooms for these classes. (See Chapter 4 for more details about group cycling.) Treadmill classes that go by the name of Treading and Trekking are also catching on. Concept II, a top rowing machine brand, has developed a half-hour group class called Boathouse, and StairMaster has introduced a 20-minute climbing class called Stomp.

Instructors of these cardio classes guide you through a workout as if you're running, climbing, or rowing outdoors. You imagine bounding up pristine mountain hills, sprinting through meadows, or finishing the Tour de France. A good instructor can make the experience so much fun that you almost forget you're in a room with a dozen other stinky, sweaty people going absolutely nowhere.

Vary your workouts

If you don't want to take a class or you work out at home, you can make your workouts more entertaining simply by varying your pace. Most machines have a manual mode that allows you to control the intensity of the workout.

You push one arrow to speed up the pace, another to slow it down. Use the manual mode to design your own workouts, incorporating the training techniques that we describe in Chapter 8.

You should also experiment with the various programs already entered in the computer's memory. These programs are great because you don't have to decide what to do next. Most programs have built-in warm-up and cooldown periods; in between, you vary your pace. For instance, many machines offer a random program; every 10 to 30 seconds, the machine surprises you by changing the tension. Most treadmills offer programs like "A Romp in the Park," which may be a 3-mile walk or jog over rolling hills. The treadmill automatically inclines and declines during these workouts.

Listen to music or a book on tape

Rock, rap, pop, or country — go with whatever gets your adrenaline pumping. If Shania Twain works for you, so be it. A tape that mixes fast and slow songs can add variety to your workout, because your pace tends to be in sync with the music. One study showed that women who exercised to music lasted 25 percent longer than those who worked out in silence. At some gyms you can plug your headphones into a system that offers dozens of CD selections and audio channels.

Or try listening to a book on tape. You may prefer to get wrapped up in a good story or learn how to manage your love life. If you rely on a tape or CD player to keep you going, make sure that you keep a load of extra batteries in your gym bag. We can't count the times we've shown up at the gym with our tape players only to find that the batteries are dead — along with our motivation.

At some gyms, you can listen to music without the need for batteries, or even a tape or CD player. At these clubs, the cardio machines are equipped with high-tech systems: Attached to each treadmill, bike, or other machine is a tape and CD player, along with a small TV screen that even offers Internet access. The only catch is you have to buy special wireless headphones that cost up to $100. These systems require you to bring your own headphones and plug them into a small box attached to the machine. Or, you need your own personal stereo and must tune into an FM frequency to pick up the various TV stations.

Watch TV or a video

Park your stationary bike in front of your TV and tune in to whatever you consider entertaining, whether it's Truckin' USA on Country Music Television or British Parliament debates on C-SPAN. You can also pop in a video designed for indoor exercise workouts. For example, you can buy videos that simulate a group cycling class, including hill sprints and interval drills. Other videos, designed for bikes, treadmills, and stair-climbers, transport you to the Grand Canyon, a Hawaiian rain forest, or the Swiss Alps. You can find a selection of these videos in the resources we describe in Chapter 19.

If you work out at a gym, plug into the TVs that are either suspended in front of the cardio machines or attached to each individual contraption. (We're fond of all this new technology; gone are the days when you had to negotiate with your fellow gym members to find a mutually agreeable show. Suzanne once had to miss a crucial episode of *Melrose Place* because two guys on the bikes next to her insisted on watching a basketball game. The nerve. . . .)

Read a magazine

Kill two birds with one stone: Burn calories while you catch up on your reading. Suzanne is a much more informed citizen during the winter, when she spends a fair amount of time on the stair-climber, than she is during the summer, when she's outside on her road bike.

This is a good time to read the fitness magazines we talk about in the Appendix. Exercise magazines offer lots of encouragement and tend to contain easy-to-skim lists. When you're drenched in sweat on the elliptical trainer, taking in "Ten Ways to Boost Energy and Get Stronger" is a lot easier than concentrating on an essay about Indonesian politics. ***Note:*** As we explain in the "Treadmill" section later in this chapter, don't read while you're walking or running on the treadmill.

Exercise in short spurts

To break up the monotony, do ten minutes on the treadmill, followed by ten minutes on the bike, and then ten minutes on the rowing machine. Or try short bouts on a cardio machine with five minutes of weight lifting. As we explain in Chapter 8, it's a myth that you must exercise for 20 or 30 consecutive minutes. Breaking up your workout into small chunks isn't a good strategy to use every day if you're training for a marathon, but if your goal is simply to burn calories and improve your health, the total time you spend exercising is what matters most.

Think, but not too hard

People tend to have their most creative ideas when they're doing something repetitive that doesn't involve their mind completely. But don't set out to solve the U.S. health-care crisis during your workout. Instead, use your time to ponder more solvable dilemmas, like how you can get your boss off your back. You may even want to keep a tape recorder handy, in case a flash of brilliance comes along.

Monitor your heart rate

To keep yourself occupied, use a heart-rate monitor to create an interval program. For instance, after warming up, alternate five minutes at the low end of your target zone with five minutes at the high end. (If all this talk about monitors, intervals, and target zones is complete gibberish to you, read Chapter 8.)

Many machines have heart-rate monitors built into them. Your heart rate registers when you grasp the handles. Or, you can wear a strap around your chest; the machine picks up the signal from the strap and beams it to the console so that your heart rate is displayed right alongside your speed and distance. The strap is more accurate than the handles, but you do have to bring your own heart-rate-monitor chest strap from home, if your gym doesn't provide them. Chapter 8 includes tips on buying a heart-rate monitor.

Talk to a friend

Some people think that if they're able to speak while exercising, they must not be working hard enough to do their body any good. As we explain in Chapter 8, that's not true. In general, your breathing should be light enough so that you can hold up your end of a conversation.

One health club in L.A. has started a book club. Members of the "Brains and Brawn" workout group do their reading at home and then convene on the treadmills and stair-climbers to discuss the latest murder mystery or popular novel. (Tolstoy and Dickens aren't popular in this book club.)

Exercising in the Great Indoors

Most exercisers have a favorite cardio machine and one that they probably can't stand. Some people find the treadmill invigorating; others consider it more tedious than peeling potatoes. We suggest you try all the machines at your gym or at an equipment store before you buy one. No single cardio machine is better than the rest. What matters most is how often you use the thing.

No matter what machine you use, always keep a water bottle and a towel within reach. Many gym machines have water bottle holders, and you can buy them cheaply for your home equipment. Also, stay tuned to how your body feels. If your knee hurts or you start to feel faint, don't ignore the pain or try to drown it out by cranking up the volume on your stereo headphones. You may be damaging muscles or joints.

That said, here's a look at the most popular cardiovascular machines.

Treadmill

Treadmills are the motorized equivalent of walking or running in place. You simply keep up with a belt that's moving under your feet. Treadmill workouts burn about the same number of calories as walking or running outdoors. The only exception seems to be running uphill. When you incline the treadmill to simulate running uphill, it's somewhat easier than running up real-life hills of the same grade. But walking uphill on a treadmill is virtually the same as walking uphill outdoors.

Who will like it

Treadmills are especially popular in crowded cities, where you need to be part cutting horse, part smog filter to run or walk through the streets. Treadmills are great for beginners because they require little coordination to use. Plus, treadmills can move at a slow enough pace to accommodate even the most out-of-shape exercisers. People with back pain, bad knees, or weak ankles often find treadmills kinder to their joints than concrete or cement. Today's treadmills are springier and more shock-absorbing than ever. Many have added flashy new features, such as Internet hookups so that you can run and walk with other treadmillers from all over the globe. Some treadmills can store up to 100 personal programs.

Who will hate it

You need a very strong or very blank mind to do long workouts on a treadmill. Most people find more than a half-hour on this machine mind-numbing, even with entertainment. If you crave the wind whipping through your hair and scenery flashing by, reserve the treadmills for emergency aerobic situations only. Running also places more impact on your joints than most other exercises and may not be a favorite if you have a bad lower back, achy knees, or weak ankles.

Treadmill user tips

Treadmills are among the easiest cardio machines to use. Still, treadmill users are not immune to poor posture. And if you're not paying attention, you can stumble. On occasion you may see someone slide off the treadmill like a can of beans on a supermarket conveyor belt. Here are some tips to make sure this doesn't happen to you:

✓ **Start slowly.** Most treadmills have safety features that prevent them from starting out at breakneck speeds, but don't take any chances. Always place one foot on either side of the belt as you turn on the machine, and step on the belt only after you determine that it's moving at the slow set-up speed, usually between 1 and 2 miles per hour.

✓ **Don't rely on the handrails.** Holding on for balance when you learn how to use the machine is okay, but let go as soon as you feel comfortable. You move more naturally if you swing your arms freely. You're working at too high a level if you have to imitate a water-skier — in other words, if you hold onto the front rails and lean back. This is a common phenomenon among people who incline the treadmill, and this position is bad news for your elbows and for the machine. Plus, you're not fooling anyone; you're burning far fewer calories than the readout indicates. However, if you have balance issues, go ahead and grasp the handrails lightly so that you feel steady and secure.

✓ **Look straight ahead.** Your feet tend to follow your eyes, so if you focus on what's in front of you, you usually walk straight ahead instead of veering off to the side. When you're in the middle of a workout and someone calls your name, don't turn around to answer. This piece of advice may seem obvious now, but wait until it happens to you.

✓ **Expect to feel disoriented.** The first few times you use a treadmill, you may feel dizzy when you step off. Your body is just wondering why the ground suddenly stopped moving. Don't worry. Most people only experience this vertigo once or twice.

✓ **Never go barefoot.** Always wear a good pair of walking or running shoes for your treadmill workout.

✓ **Don't read on the treadmill.** You risk losing your balance and stumbling off the side or back.

Elliptical trainer

Just when we thought that all good cardio machines had been invented, along came the elliptical trainer. Ellipticals have two large, fat foot pedals. Your feet follow a path that's sort of a stretched-out oval known as an ellipse (hence, the name elliptical trainer) — see Figure 9-1. The motion feels like a mix between fast walking, stair-climbing, and cross-country skiing. Precor, Reebok CCS, Life Fitness, StairMaster, and Startrac make the most popular models. The popularity of this machine has exploded in the past two years, rivaling that of the treadmill. Newer models allow you to work your arms in an opposite motion to your feet, which can get confusing if you think too much about it while exercising! Working your arms allows you to burn additional calories, though.

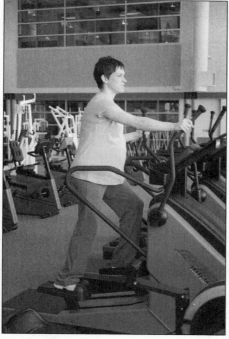

Figure 9-1:
Elliptical
trainers are
gentle
enough for
prenatal
workouts.

Photograph by John Urban

Who will like it

Runners who need a day off from the pounding gravitate toward this machine like moviegoers to the concession stand. It's also popular with walkers looking for a more spirited workout and people who once used the cross-country skier but can't find one because NordicTrack has gone out of business. The elliptical trainer is also popular among people who are bored with stair-climbing or find stair-climbing hard on their knees.

Who will hate it

Suzanne! She finds the elliptical motion unnatural. She feels that if your feet are going to be moving in a circular-type motion, you should be sitting down, like on a bike; and if you're going to be standing, your feet should be going up and down or back and forth. But then again, Suzanne may be a poor judge of this machine — she can't pat her head while rubbing her tummy in circles. Also, Suzanne finds it tough to read while using the elliptical trainer, and because she uses her machine cardio time to peruse the TV section of *USA Today,* this is a problem.

Elliptical-trainer user tips

Elliptical trainers can take a bit of getting used to, but they don't require great skill. You'll be up and running in no time by following these tips:

- ✔ **Limit backward pedaling.** Contrary to popular belief, pedaling backward does *not* work your buttocks more than pedaling forward (and it may even be hard on your knees). Both motions emphasize the front thigh muscles, so do it once in a while, but not for any prolonged amount of time.

- ✔ **Use the machine's versatile features.** To adjust the intensity of your workout, you can pedal faster, raise the incline, increase the resistance, or any combination.

- ✔ **Don't lock your knees.** Keep a slight bend in your knees, keeping the motion smooth.

- ✔ **Remind yourself to stand up straight.** Although the elliptical trainer lends itself to better technique than the stair-climber, you can still commit postural violations such as leaning too far forward and hugging the console.

Stationary bicycle

Bikes come in two varieties: upright and recumbent. Upright bikes simulate a regular bike, only you don't go anywhere (see Figure 9-2). Recumbent bikes, have bucket seats so you pedal out in front of you. Neither type is superior; it's a matter of preference. The recumbent does offer more back support and may be more comfortable for people with lower-back pain. If you're new to exercise or heavyset, you may also find a recumbent bike more comfortable.

Who will like it

Bikes are great for toning your thighs (and recumbents are especially good for your butt), and they give your knees a break while offering a terrific aerobic workout. Bikes also suit anyone who wants to read while working out. Holding a book or magazine in place on a stair-climber or treadmill is much tougher — and it's impossible on a skier or rowing machine.

Who will hate it

Hard-core cyclists complain that most stationary bicycles don't have the same feel as outdoor bikes. They're right: The pedal positions usually are different, and the seats on a stationary bike usually are wider. Also, most indoor bikes force you to sit upright rather than allow you to lean forward, like you do on a regular bike. The exceptions are bikes specially designed for spinning and other versions of group indoor cycling; these contraptions are designed more like road bikes, although they lack the high-tech computer programs that keep many people motivated. Different bike brands offer very different positioning. You may like some bike brands more than others.

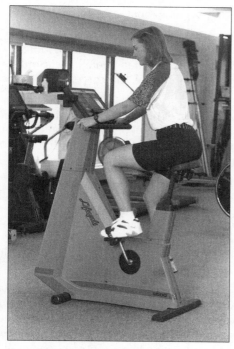

Figure 9-2:
An upright stationary bike.

Photograph by Sunstreak Productions, Inc.

Bikes give you less opportunity to use atrocious form than do most other machines. Still, there's room for injury or discomfort. Here are some tips to help you avoid both:

- ✔ **Adjust the seat.** When the pedal is at the lowest position, your leg should be almost, but not quite, straight. You shouldn't have to strain or rock your hips to pedal. Your knees shouldn't feel crunched when they're at the top of the pedal stroke. With a recumbent bike, you adjust the seat forward and back, rather than up and down, but the principles are the same.

- ✔ **Set the handlebars correctly (if your bike allows adjustments).** You should be able to hold the bar so that your arms extend out at shoulder level. You shouldn't have to squirm around to get comfortable. Handlebar adjustment is especially important if you're very tall or very short.

✔ **Get to know the display panel.** For instance, notice how many levels the bike has. Some bikes feature 12 levels; others have 40. So if you just hop on and press Level 6, you'll get two very different workouts. Also, pay attention to your *cadence* — that is, how many revolutions per minute (rpm) you're cycling. Varying your cadence is a good idea. You may want to hum along at 80 rpm for 5 minutes and then do 30-second intervals at 100 rpm using the same tension level.

✔ **Adjust the pedal straps so that your feet feel snug — but don't let the straps cut off your circulation.** Riding a bike with the foot straps is much more comfortable and efficient than pedaling without them. Don't remove the pedal straps from your bike; this forces the next person to waste time putting them back on.

✔ **Don't pedal with just your toes.** Otherwise you may bring on foot and calf cramps. Instead, press from the ball of your foot and through your heel as you pump downward on the pedal, and pull up with the top of your foot on the upstroke.

✔ **Don't hunch over.** Rounding your back is the way to develop back and neck pain. Don't get your upper body into the effort, either. Instead, keep your chest up, shoulders back and down, ears in line with your shoulders, and belly button drawn in. Unlike some other machines, riding a stationary bike is not a total-body workout; don't try to make it one. If you have to rock wildly from side to side, grit your teeth, or clench the handlebars, you need to lighten your load.

✔ **Make sure the bike is sturdy.** At one New York City gym, a guy was pedaling furiously when the frame collapsed and the bike shot forward and out the second story window — with the guy still seated. Ironically, he landed on a bike rack below. This being New York, the doorman said, "Hey buddy, you can't park that thing here." Actually, we made the last part up, but the rest of the story was reported on the news. Although the guy was hospitalized, he walked away more or less unscathed.

We're not thrilled about the trend of attaching arm handles to treadmills, but we do like the so-called *dual-action bikes,* at least the brands that you find in health clubs. On a good bike, it's easy to keep upper- and lower-body movements coordinated while still getting a smooth ride. Operating one of these bikes looks complicated, but it's not nearly as difficult as, say, rubbing circles on your stomach while patting your head. We especially like the new recumbent bikes with arm handles, particularly a brand called Cycle Plus, the only such bike that allows you to adjust the arm and leg tension separately (see Figure 9-3). We're also fond of the upright Schwinn AirDyne; the flywheel fan generates a cool, gentle breeze as you pedal your legs and pump your arms.

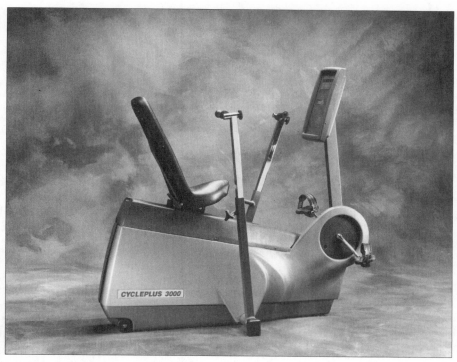

Photograph by Sunstreak Productions, Inc.

Figure 9-3: A recumbent bike with arm handles.

For bikes with arm handles, adjust the seat height as you would with a regular bike, and set the arm handles at shoulder height. Coordinating upper- and lower-body motions can take some getting used to. Start by focusing on your legs and then gradually add in more arm resistance. If you find that exercising your arms and your legs at the same time is too tiring, alternate arm and leg movements until you build more stamina. As long as you keep moving, you're still getting an aerobic workout. (For a definition of aerobic, see Chapter 8.) Keep in mind that even if you use a dual-action bike regularly, you still need to do upper-body strength training. The resistance on the bike is too low to build significant strength in your upper body.

Stair-climber

The most common type of stair-climber is the pedal stepper, which many exercisers refer to as the StairMaster. In fact, StairMaster is a specific brand — just one of many excellent makes that you find in health clubs and home equipment stores. Stair-climbing on a machine is a big improvement over jogging up and down the bleachers at your local high school football stadium. The machine eliminates most of the wear and tear on your joints.

Who will like it

Women in particular love stair-climbers because these machines do a good job of toning the butt and thighs. People who want to get in shape for skiing, climbing, hiking, and running also love steppers, as they're often called.

This is a good time to clear up the myth that stair-climbing builds big, bulky muscles in your legs. The truth is, virtually any type of activity will increase the size of your muscles if you work very slowly against a lot of tension. And if you have a genetic predisposition toward building muscular thighs, you're pretty much going to fight against that no matter what you do. But for most people, this isn't an issue. The fact is stair-climbing is a terrific way to burn calories and tone your legs.

Who will hate it

Beginners may get frustrated because stair-climbing is no vacation in Maui. If you're a complete novice, you may not last five minutes even on the lowest level. In this case, use other machines, such as the treadmill or stationary bike, until you build up some stamina and strength. Also, stair-climbing can be tough to get the hang of; novices sometimes find themselves sinking to the floor before they're able to get into the rhythm of stepping. Finally, stair-climbing bothers some people's knees. If you're one of those people but have your heart set on stair-climbing, you may be able to eliminate the pain with a solid weight-lifting program. Do exercises that strengthen your thighs, both front and back, because those are the muscles that hold your knees together.

Stair-climber user tips

Proper form is butchered on the stair-climber more than on any other single piece of machinery. We've seen people clutch the railings so tightly their knuckles turn white — or hug the console like it's a long-lost relative. Some less-informed exercisers think it's really cool to be able to climb at the machine's highest level, regardless of their form. It's not. When you clutch the rails (or lean forward), you transfer your weight from your legs to your arms or the machine, which drastically reduces the number of calories you burn.

Fortunately, many stair-climber manufacturers have rectified this problem by designing handles that point straight up. This makes cheating more difficult. Still, we see people hanging on these newer handles. Here's how to use this machine the right way:

✔ **Rest your hands — or better yet, your fingertips — lightly on the bar in front of you or on the side rails.** Don't grip the rails any tighter than you'd grip a paper cup. And never reverse your wrists so that your fingertips are pointing toward the floor and your elbows are turned up to the ceiling. You really should be able to use the stair-climber without holding on to the railing at all, but using the railing for balance (within reason) is okay. If you must hang on in order to keep up with the machine, you're going too fast. Believe us, nobody will think less of you if you drop down a few notches. In fact, you'll probably impress people with your stellar posture and noncompetitive attitude.

✔ **Stand upright with a slight forward lean at the hips (see Figure 9-4).** Don't overcorrect your form by standing upright like a Marine at inspection. A slight — and we mean slight — forward lean helps keep your knees from locking and protects your lower back from overarching.

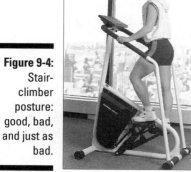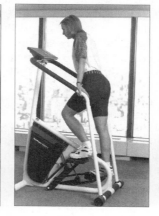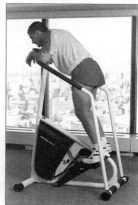

Figure 9-4:
Stair-climber posture: good, bad, and just as bad.

Photograph by Sunstreak Productions, Inc.

✔ **Take even, moderately deep steps.** Don't take short, quick hopping steps, a technique known as *shaking the machine*. This technique is hard on your calf muscles and cuts down on the number of calories you burn.

✔ **Keep your entire foot on the pedal.** This helps your rear end and thighs get a full workout and prevents you from overburdening your calf muscles.

Rolling stair-climber

This machine looks like a section of a department-store escalator (only it's hardly a free ride). A set of stairs rotates in a circle so that you climb continuously, like Sisyphus up the mountain, ever upward, but never getting anywhere. You look straight ahead into the console, which allows you to adjust the speed.

Rolling staircases have been around a lot longer than steppers. At the turn of the century, federal prisoners were forced to climb on them to provide electrical power to the prison facility. When modern rolling staircases first came out, there were a few kinks to work out, like the fact that they had a habit of collapsing when in use. Liz had a client who came in for a workout on her wedding day. The stairs folded underneath her and she slid to the ground, breaking an arm and a leg in the process. We're happy to report that this defect has been fixed, and rolling staircases are as safe as any other piece of equipment in the gym, as long as you use them correctly.

Who will like it

In many ways, the rolling stair-climber is a better workout than a regular stair-climber. It's harder to cheat, because you're forced to take a fairly deep stride to place your foot onto the next step. (However, you can still cheat by clenching the side rails.) This machine gives you a tremendous butt and thigh workout, and you work up one helluva sweat. Start at a very slow speed until you can confidently navigate the height of the step.

Who will hate it

If you're used to the stepper-type climbers, the rolling stair-climber takes some getting used to. Also, if you're just getting into shape, this contraption may be a bit much for you. At some health clubs, this workout is referred to as "climbing the stairway from hell." If you have knee or back problems, this form of exercise may not agree with you.

Rolling-stair-climber user tips

The rolling stair-climber is a good machine to try when you're looking to make stair-climbing even more challenging. We know one woman who used this machine to train for a race up the Empire State Building — 102 flights of stairs. She came in second place. Here are some tips to keep in mind (whether or not you plan to climb tall buildings):

- **Start at a very slow speed.** This is one machine you can definitely slide off of if you can't maintain the pace.

- **Start with just five or ten minutes.** Even if you're in great shape on the traditional stair-climber, treadmill, or other machine, you may find this contraption startlingly tough.

- **Try climbing every other step.** This technique gives you a killer butt workout and a good stretch in your legs — but this technique is *not* for beginners.

VersaClimber

In this case, we're using a brand name to refer to a whole class of machines, the ladder-climbing simulator. The VersaClimber is by far the best ladder climber, and the one that you're likely to encounter at gyms (see Figure 9-5). The VersaClimber is a stick of metal or wood that's about 8-feet high and leans slightly forward. You step onto the foot pedals, grip the handles, and do the vertical equivalent of crawling in place. Some models have handrails so that you can omit the upper-body motion and simply move your legs in an action similar to stair-climbing. Other models have detachable seats so that you can do the upper-body motion by itself. Many VersaClimbers also have a built-in heart-rate monitor.

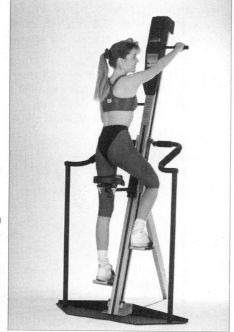

Figure 9-5:
This machine simulates climbing a ladder.

Photograph by Sunstreak Productions, Inc.

Who will like it

The VersaClimber has a reputation for being the exclusive domain of aerobic animals, but actually, it's ideal for beginners, too. You can easily adjust the variables — step height, arm motion, speed, and tension — to customize the workout for any level. People with bad knees who like to climb may have an easier time on this machine than any other type of climber. Many athletes use this total-body trainer, and in case you care, Madonna has one.

Who will hate it

We have a theory about why the VersaClimber isn't more popular: People don't like to be up high with their butts on display for the rest of the world. Some gyms put their VersaClimber off in a corner where exercisers tend to forget about it. That's a shame because the VersaClimber is a great piece of equipment. Vanity aside, there are some good reasons to avoid it, like if you have a bad back or poor circulation in your feet.

VersaClimber user tips

Don't be scared off by this admittedly scary-looking contraption. The VersaClimber is not as tough to operate as you think. Here's how to look like a pro:

- **Always warm up with small, quick strides for three to five minutes.** Then experiment with different speeds, stride lengths, and tension levels. If you get tired, you can eliminate the arm movement by holding onto the handrails, or eliminate the leg movements by sitting on the seat, if there is one.

- **Practice good climbing posture.** Keep your back straight and keep your torso parallel to the machine. Don't round your back or lean back away from the machine. Even if you take long strides, don't stretch out your body so far that your foot hits the floor, your knees and elbows lock, or you're forced to overarch your back.

- **Don't get fixated on the mileage.** A vertical mile is not the same as a mile on the treadmill or the road. A mile may still be 5,280 feet (1,609 meters), but we're talking straight uphill.

Rowing machines

Good rowers consist of a flywheel, a fan, and a cable with a handle attached to one end (see Figure 9-6). You pull the handle toward you as you slide the seat backward. The fan creates air resistance, which makes the movement feel pretty close to skimming across the water.

Who will like it

Anyone looking for a great total-body workout will love rowing. If you're trying to get in shape for a rowing or paddling sport, this is the way to go. Contrary to popular belief, rowing isn't bad for your back. If you row correctly, you initiate the movement from your legs and buttocks, which eliminates excess stress on your back muscles.

Figure 9-6:
Although rowing is a demanding activity, its low-impact nature makes it a good fit for prenatal exercise.

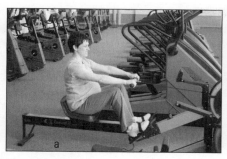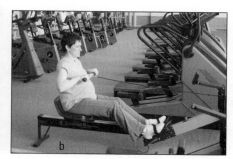

Photograph by John Urban

Who will hate it

Some people get bored with rowing in a matter of seconds. Others are intimidated because rowing is not as natural as walking, running, or biking. We know one guy who smacked the handle into his forehead over and over again until some kind soul in the gym showed him the proper form.

Rowing-machine user tips

Experienced rowers make rowing look easy, but when you actually sit down at the machine, you may find that it takes a fair amount of coordination. Here are some tips to fine-tune the motion:

- **Think legs, legs, legs.** Concentrate on initiating the movement with your buttocks rather than your lower back. Don't fully straighten your knees. Even when you're completely extended, your knees should be a little soft.

- **Don't round your back.** Hunching over is the way to give yourself back pain. Don't lean all the way back at the end of the stroke, either. You're in proper position when your upper body is leaning backward about 45 degrees.

- **Pull the handle in a smooth, continuous stroke.** Don't stop at the most stretched-out and bent positions.

Chapter 10

Exercising Outdoors

*F*resh air: What a concept. With all the hoopla these days about space-age, indoor exercise contraptions, it's easy to forget you can get a great workout in the great outdoors. You may even get a better workout — burning more calories per minute — because outdoor activities sometimes involve more muscles than their indoor counterparts. For example, when you park yourself on a stationary bicycle, your upper-body muscles basically get a free ride — you can easily read a magazine as you pedal away. But when you take your bike out for a spin, your chest, arm, abdominal, and back muscles are all called up for active duty.

In this chapter, we cover some of the most popular and invigorating outdoor aerobic activities. We discuss what gear you need and how much it costs, and we offer training strategies and safety tips for rookies and klutzes alike.

Walking

Can you really get fit by walking? Absolutely — as long as you walk long enough, hard enough, and often enough. (If you're asking, "How long?", "How hard?", and "How often?", check out Chapter 8.) A recent study found that, among people who are successful in maintaining long-term weight loss, nearly 80 percent walk as their main physical activity.

The beauty of walking is, it's simply a matter of putting one foot in front of the other. Sure, walking burns fewer calories per minute than jogging, but most people last longer on a walk than a run, so you can make up for the deficit. Plus, compared to runners, walkers enjoy a relatively low injury rate.

However, we're not going to sugar-coat this: Some exercisers find walking to be a big, fat bore. Suzanne hates walking so much that she'll spend 15 minutes searching for a good parking space at her gym before a one-hour workout on the stationary bike. (She can't help it; she grew up in Los Angeles, where you drive to visit your next-door neighbor.)

Essential walking gear

Although the rest of the animal kingdom does fine without the benefit of special equipment, human feet don't have adequate padding to meet the demands of walking in the modern world. You need a good pair of walking shoes to avoid foot, ankle, knee, hip, and lower-back problems. Expect to spend at least $50 for good walking shoes, which should hold up for 1,000 to 1,500 miles. (Running shoes usually have to be tossed after 400 to 500 miles.) Replace your shoes when the tread begins to wear thin or when the sides start to cave inward or outward.

Walking shoes may sound like a marketing conspiracy hatched by shoe-industry executives. After all, it's only walking — won't any pair of sneakers suffice? Actually, the concept of a walking shoe is a valid one. Walking shoes need to be more flexible than running shoes because you bend your feet more when you walk, and you push off from your toes with more oomph. Also, because your heels bear most of your weight when you walk, you need a firm, stable *heel counter,* the part of the shoe that wraps around your heel to keep your foot in place.

If you plan to hike or walk over rugged terrain, look for a walking shoe with treaded soles and added heel and ankle support. If you're focusing on speed walking or high mileage, go for a little more cushioning in the *midsole,* the area between the tread and the inside of the shoe.

Walking the right way

Okay, we lied to you: There actually is more to walking than simply putting one foot in front of the other. The biggest mistake walkers make is bending forward, a sure way to develop problems in your lower back, neck, and hips. Your posture should be naturally tall. You needn't force yourself to be ramrod straight, but neither should you slouch, overarch your back, or lean too far forward from your hips. Relax your shoulders, widen your chest, and pull your abdominals gently inward. Keep your head and chin up and focus straight ahead.

Meanwhile, keep your hands relaxed and cupped gently, and swing your arms so that they brush past your body. On the upswing, your hand should be level with your breast bone; on the downswing, your hand should brush against your hip. Keep your hips loose and relaxed. Your feet should land firmly, heel first. Roll through your heel to your arch, then to the ball of your foot, and then to your toes. Push off from your toes and the ball of your foot.

Run through a mental head-to-toe checklist every so often to see how you're doing. To find out more about fitness walking (yep, there's plenty more to tell), read Liz's book *Fitness Walking For Dummies* (published by Wiley).

Walking tips for rookies

Although walking is the most basic of all fitness activities, novice fitness walkers can still benefit from the following pointers:

- ✔ **Increase your workout time gradually.** Most people can start off with five 10- to 20-minute walking sessions a week; after about a month, they can increase each workout by 2 or 3 minutes per week until walking 30 to 45 minutes is comfortable. (Five days a week may sound like a lot, but an almost-daily walk makes it easier to get in the habit.)

- ✔ **Walk as fast as you comfortably can.** If you walk very fast — at a 12-minute-mile to 15-minute-mile pace — you can burn twice as many calories as when you walk at a 20-minute-mile pace. You may not be able to move at such supersonic speeds in the beginning, but as you get fit, you can mix in some fast-paced intervals. (For details about interval training, see Chapter 8.)

- ✔ **If you're walking on the shoulder of a road, walk against traffic so you can watch cars approach.** On sidewalks or trails, walk any old way you want.

- ✔ **Add some hills.** Walking over hilly terrain shapes your butt and thighs and burns extra calories (about 30 percent more calories than walking on flat terrain, depending, of course, on the grade of the hills).

- ✔ **Sneak in a walk whenever you can.** Leave your car at home and hoof it to the train station. Take a 15-minute walk during your lunch break. Traverse the airport on foot rather than on that automatic walking belt. It all adds up.

Running

Like walking, running is a workout that you can take with you anywhere. You don't need a rack on your car or a suitcase full of equipment; you just open the door and go. Plus, as any pathological runner will tell you, nothing is quite as satisfying as getting a good run under your belt. You work up a great sweat, you burn lots of calories, and your muscles feel pleasantly invigorated after you finish.

[handwritten annotations in margin:]

min mcH
12   5
15   4
20   3

No single type of exercise is better than all the rest. It's merely a question of what's best for you. Many runners develop frequent, chronic injuries. Many people have joints that simply will not tolerate all that pounding. If you're not built to run, don't argue with your body. You can get in great condition in other ways. And if you're a beginner, hold off on running until you've built up stamina and strength.

Essential running gear

Although you can spend hundreds of dollars on spiffy warm-ups, tights, and tops, the only equipment that's truly essential for running is a good pair of shoes (although women will want a supportive jogging bra, too). Be prepared to spend at least $50 to $60 a pair, but know that a hefty price tag doesn't always correspond to the best shoe.

The shoe that's best for you depends on your weight, the shape of your foot, your running style, and any special problems you may have, such as weak ankles or bad knees. Try on several models at the store, and take each one for a test drive around the mall or at least run a couple laps around the store.

Your running shoes should be fairly flexible, especially across the ball of the foot. Hold the shoe at both ends and bend it; it should break right at the ball of the foot. You want cushioning, but not so much that you can't feel your foot hitting the ground. Look for a stable *heel counter* (the part of the shoe that wraps around your heel to keep your foot in place). If your foot slides around a lot, that can mean trouble down the road.

Running the right way

Runners have a habit of looking directly at the ground, almost as if they can't bear to see what's coming next. Keeping your head down throws your upper-body posture off-kilter and can lead to upper-back and neck pain. Lift your head and focus your eyes straight ahead.

Relax your shoulders, keep your chest lifted, and pull your abdominal muscles in tightly. Don't overarch your back and stick your butt out; that's one of the main reasons runners get back and hip pain.

Keep your arms close to your body, and swing them forward and back rather than across your body. Don't clench your fists. Pretend you're holding a butterfly in each hand; you don't want your butterflies to escape, but you don't want to crush them, either.

Lift your front knee and extend your back leg. Don't shuffle along like you're wearing cement boots. Land heel first and roll through the entire length of your foot. Push off from the balls of your feet instead of running flat-footed and pounding off your heels. Otherwise, your feet and legs are going to cry uncle long before your cardiovascular system does.

If you experience pain in your ankles, knees, or lower back, stop running for a while. If you don't, you could end up having to sit on the sidelines for months.

Running tips for rookies

These tips help you get fit and avoid injury.

✔ **Start by alternating periods of walking with periods of running.** For example, try two minutes of walking and one minute of running. Gradually decrease your walking intervals until you can run continuously for 20 minutes. If you have the inclination, you can build from there. Of course, sticking with a walk-run routine is fine; you're less likely to injure yourself that way.

✔ **Vary your pace.** Different paces work your heart, lungs, and legs in different ways. Experiment with the techniques described in Chapter 8.

✔ **Always run against traffic when running on the shoulder of a road.** This allows you to see oncoming cars and dive for the side of the road, if necessary. If you're running on steeply *banked* (angled away from the center line) country roads and the road is flat, you can run in the middle of the road to save wear and tear on your legs. But as you head up or down hills, get as far over on the shoulder (that is, away from the road) as possible to avoid speeding cars mowing you down. Consider carrying a lightweight cell phone for emergencies.

✔ **Don't increase your mileage by more than 10 percent a week.** If you run 5 miles a week and want to increase, aim to do 5½ miles the following week. Jumping from 5 miles to 6 miles doesn't sound like a big deal, but studies show that if you increase your mileage more than 10 percent, you set yourself up for injury.

Bicycling: Road and Mountain

Talk to a group of cyclists and, chances are, you're talking to a group of ex-runners. Cycling is perfect for people who can't take the relentless pounding of running or find the slow pace a real drag. Cycling is the best way to cover a lot of ground quickly. Even a novice can easily build up to a 20-mile ride.

Cycling can be a hassle. You can't just grab your shoes and head out the door. You need your helmet, water bottle, gloves, sunscreen, and glasses. And even with all your protective gear, you can never be too cautious. Cycling is a low-impact sport — unless you happen to impact the ground, a car, a tree, a rut, or another cyclist.

Essential cycling gear

If you haven't owned a bike since grammar school, prepare yourself for sticker shock. *Mountain bikes,* the fat-tire bikes with upright handlebars, are somewhat less expensive than comparable *road bikes,* the kind with the curved handlebars. In both categories, you won't find many decent bikes under $500; many cost more than $2,000. Don't take out a second mortgage to buy a fancy bike, but if you have any inkling that you may like this sport, don't skimp, either. You'll just end up buying a more expensive bike later.

What distinguishes a $500 bike from a $2,000 steed? Generally, the more expensive the bike, the stronger and lighter its frame. A heavy bike can slow you down, but unless you plan to enter the Tour de France, don't get hung up on a matter of ounces. Cheaper bikes are made from different grades of steel; as you climb the price ladder, you find materials such as aluminum, carbon fiber, and titanium. The price of a bike also depends on the quality of the *components* — the mechanics that enable your bike to move, shift, and brake.

Cheaper bikes come with *toe clips* (pedal straps) that enable you to pull up on the pedal as well as push down. But you can pull up even more efficiently with clipless pedals, which lock into cleats affixed to the bottom of your cycling shoes. These pedal systems are like ski bindings: You're locked in, but your feet pop out easily when you fall. To clip out, you simply twist your foot to the side.

Beginners usually have an accident or two with clipless pedals because they haven't developed the instinct to twist sideways. Suzanne once tipped over with both feet clicked into her pedals. We'll spare you the details of her injury, but let's just say that she ended up at the gynecologist.

Find a bike dealer you trust and know that bike prices are negotiable. Ask the salesman to throw in a few free extras, like a bike computer to measure your speed and distance or a seat bag to carry food and tools.

Don't even think about pedaling down your driveway without a helmet snug atop your noggin. Cycling gloves make your ride more comfortable and protect your hands when you crash. Glasses are important to protect your eyes from the dust, dirt, and gravel.

Buy a pair of padded cycling shorts and a brightly colored cycling jersey so that you can easily be seen. Unlike cotton t-shirts, jerseys wick away sweat so that you won't freeze on a downhill after you worked up a big sweat climbing up. Plus, jerseys have pockets in the back deep enough to hold half a grocery store worth of snacks. Always carry a water bottle or wear a hydration pack, a clever backpack-like water pouch that we describe in Chapter 25.

Finally, carry gear to change a flat tire, and learn how to use it. There's no cycling equivalent of the auto club to come save you.

Cycling the right way

To protect your knees from injury, position your seat correctly (ask your salesperson for advice) and pedal at an easy cadence. *Cadence* refers to the number of revolutions per minute that you pedal. Inexperienced cyclists tend to use a higher gear than they can handle, which forces them to turn the pedals in slow motion; their legs tire prematurely, their knees ache, and they cheat themselves out of a good workout. Set your bike's gear so you're pedaling at a comfortable cadence.

Road cycling can wreak havoc on your lower back because you're in a crouched position for so long. Relax your upper body and keep your arms loose. Grasp your handlebars with the same tension that you'd hold a child's hand when you cross the street. Pedal in smooth circles rather than simply mashing the pedals downward. Imagine that you have a bed of nails in your shoes, and you have to pedal without stomping on the nails.

Cycling tips for rookies

You can learn a lot about cycling — and get faster in a jif — by riding with a club or friends who have more experience. Here are some pointers to start your cycling career:

- ✔ **Remember that you are a vehicle and are required to follow the rules of the road.** Ride with traffic, not against it.

- ✔ **Stop at all signs and lights, and use those hand signals you learned in driver's ed.** Don't trust a single car, ever. Assume that the driver doesn't see you, even if he happens to be staring you in the face.

- ✔ **When you go off-road, start on wide fire roads rather than narrow "single-track" trails that require technical skills.** And don't think that you're immune to injury because there are no cars. More crashes happen on mountain trails than on the road because there are more obstacles and riders get careless and cocky.

- ✔ **Head into a turn at a slow enough pace that you maintain control, and never let your eyes wander from the road or trail.** Never squeeze the brakes — particularly the front brake — with a lot of pressure. You'll go flying over the handlebars, a maneuver known as an *endo,* and go right into a *face plant,* a maneuver that we think is self-explanatory.

In-Line Skating

In 1980, Rollerblade introduced a new kind of skate: Instead of two wheels at the toe and two wheels at the heel, the four wheels were positioned in a single-file line. This was the biggest innovation in skating since a 16th-century Dutchman patterned the first pair of roller skates after ice skates. Now in-line skating — often called *Rollerblading* — is the skate of choice for more than 15 million people.

Skating is fun because it isn't as linear as running, walking, and cycling. You can curve, turn, glide, sprint, and spin. Skating is also a terrific tush toner because you push your legs out to the side, which works several seldom-used hip muscles. Skating is a good calorie burner, too.

But in-line skating is also dangerous. About 270,000 skaters per year wind up at the doctor or emergency room with injuries. Liz got a first-hand look at one of these injuries not long ago. While running over the 59th Street Bridge in New York City, Liz spotted a woman walking in bare feet and sobbing. The woman's entire left side was so bloody that she appeared to have been mauled by a tiger. It turns out the woman had attempted to skate over sharp metal teeth on the road — teeth designed to provide traction for cars during icy conditions in winter.

Most skaters use more common sense than that, but injuries are still common because the sport requires so much balance and concentration. Plus, stopping on in-line skates is darn tough. (See "Skating the right way," later in this chapter, for stopping tips.)

Essential skating gear

Skating equipment isn't cheap — a good pair of skates costs between $150 and $500. (We suggest you rent several times before you buy.) Try on several pairs at the store and wear each for at least ten minutes, until your feet start to get hot. Tilt your feet to the inside and the outside, putting plenty of pressure on your feet to make sure nothing hurts. Otherwise, you're asking for blisters. The boots should feel snug in the toe and heel. If your heel is loose, you won't have enough control when you skate.

In-line skates have more on conventional roller skates than just wheel placement. The wheels are faster, smoother, and more durable. Most skates have a plastic shell and foam-lined bootie, so they breathe more easily and conform to your feet much better than leather skates. You typically can get a more comfortable fit with skates that buckle rather than lace. Be sure to wear synthetic socks; cotton fibers retain moisture, which can irritate your feet. (See Chapter 25 for details about sports socks.)

By the way, we don't recommend that novices try off-road skates, which have fat, nubby wheels similar to mountain-bike tires. Skating is dangerous enough; we can't see a reason to do it over gravel and tree roots. We do, however, like skates with wheels that pop off, leaving you with decent walking boots. Because many buildings ban skates, removable wheels are a nice convenience.

A helmet is as essential for skating as it is for biking. A cycling helmet will suffice, but you can buy special in-line helmets with more protection at the rear of the head. Also crucial: wrist guards, knee guards, and elbow guards. Purchase safety equipment before you buy your skates so you won't be tempted to take a quick spin before suiting up.

Skating the right way

Keep your hands in front of your body at all times with your elbows in, your forearms straight ahead, and your palms down, as if you're placing your hands on a table. If you move your hands off center, your body is likely to follow. Keep your arms as still as possible — don't pump them back and forth.

Travel in a modified squat position, bending at the knees as if you're about to sit down. Keep your weight on your back wheel and push off straight with your heel. Pull your abdominal muscles inward and don't round your back. If you start to lose your balance, crouch lower — don't stand up straighter. If you veer off the pavement and onto mud or grass, run on your skates instead of stopping cold.

Skating tips for rookies

To find out whether skating is the sport for you, take a few lessons. (You can find an instructor through a skate shop, or call the International In-Line Skating Association for a referral.) In the meantime, here are some suggestions to get started:

- ✔ **Practice balancing by walking on the skates on your living-room carpet or your lawn.** Head to a parking lot to practice skating, turning, and stopping. Stick to bike paths until you're quite comfortable skating, and when you do head for the open road, always skate with — not against — traffic. *Remember:* You're responsible for abiding by the same rules as motorists.

- ✔ **Don't expect brakes to bring you to a complete halt.** The best a novice can hope to do is slow down. To do this, simultaneously lean forward from your waist, tilt the braking skate up, and exert pressure on the heel pad while maintaining your balance. Skip hills until you master stopping, and always skate slowly enough that you feel as though you could stop at any time.

✔ **Don't skate on the side of a busy road, where a cyclist might ride.**
Stick to bike trails, sidewalks, and other smooth, well-maintained, no-traffic areas.

✔ **Don't skate while holding anything in your hand, even a can of soda.**
When you fall, your reflex is to save what you're holding, not to protect your body.

Swimming

Swimming is truly a zero-impact sport. Although you can strain your shoulders if you overdo it, there's absolutely no pounding on your joints, and the only thing you're in danger of crashing into is the wall of the pool. You can get a great aerobic workout that uses your whole body. Plus, water has a gentle, soothing effect on the body, so swimming is helpful for those with arthritis or other joint diseases.

Swimming is great for people who want to keep exercising when they're injured and for people who are pregnant or overweight. That extra body fat helps you glide along near the surface of the water, so you don't expend energy trying to keep yourself from sinking like a stone.

Lap swimming has the reputation of being drudgery — after all, the scenery doesn't change a whole lot from one end of the pool to the other. The trick is to use an array of gadgets that elevate swim workouts from forced labor to bona fide fun. You can even buy an underwater tape player with pretty decent sound.

Essential swimming gear

Obviously, a body of water is helpful — preferably one manned by a lifeguard. And in most instances, you must wear a swimsuit. By the way, we said *swimsuit,* not bathing suit. You don't want a suit that looks good while you're sunbathing but creeps up your butt when you get in the water.

If you swim in a chlorinated pool, goggles are a must to prevent eye irritation and to help you see better in the water. Buy goggles from a store that lets you try them on. You should feel some suction around your eyes, but not so much that you feel like your eyeballs are going to pop out. You also need a cap so that your hair doesn't get plastered on your face as you swim or turn to straw from the chemicals.

As for the fun swimming gadgets: Many pools let you borrow equipment, but you can buy a whole set for less than $75. We especially like rubber swimming fins which give you a lot more speed and power in the water and give your legs a better workout. If you're a beginning swimmer, you may feel like you're going nowhere, and you may have trouble moving fast enough to get your heart rate up.

You can use fins when you kick with a *kickboard,* a foam board that helps you stay afloat. But don't use fins so much that they become a crutch. As you get in better shape, you may want to switch from long swim fins to short fins, which make you work a lot harder. Don't swim with scuba fins; they're too big and too stiff.

Swimming with plastic paddles on your hands gives your upper body an extra challenge. Some paddles are flat and rectangular; others are shaped more like your hand, with a comfortable contour in the palm area. With both styles, you place your hand on top of the paddles and slip your fingers through a thick rubber band that secures your hand to the paddles. Paddles can help you perfect your stroke technique and increase the intensity of your workout, but use them sparingly; overuse can lead to shoulder injuries. When you swim with paddles, put a *pull-buoy* (a foam gadget) between your thighs. This keeps your legs buoyant so that you can concentrate on paddling rather than kicking.

Swimming the right way

You'll probably spend the bulk of your workouts doing the front crawl, also called *freestyle.* It's generally faster than the other strokes, so you can cover more distance. Don't cut your strokes short; reach out as far as you can, have your hand enter thumb-first so it slices the water like a knife, and pull all the way through the water so your hand brushes your thigh. Use an S-shaped sculling movement, where you hand moves out, then in, then out again across your body/thigh and out of the water. Elongate your stroke so that you take fewer than 25 strokes in a 25-yard pool. The fewer strokes, the better. Top swimmers get so much power from each stroke that they take just 11 to 14 strokes per length of a 25-yard pool.

Kick up and down from your hips, not your knees. Don't kick too deeply or allow your feet to break the water's surface. Proper kicking causes the water to "boil" rather than splash.

Breathe through your mouth every two strokes, or every three strokes if you want to alternate the side that you breathe on. You need as much oxygen as you can get. Beginners sometimes make the mistake of taking six or eight strokes before breathing, which wears them out quickly. To breathe, roll your entire body to the side until your mouth and nose come out of the water — imagine that your entire body is on a skewer and must rotate together. Don't lift your head out of the water to breathe — you'll spend a lot of energy doing that, and it'll slow you down in the water.

Swimming tips for rookies

Even if you're the queen of your aerobics class or a champion at cycling uphill, you may still tire quickly in the pool at first. More than almost any other aerobic activity, swimming relies on technique. The following tips can help you get the most out of your swimming workouts.

- **Take a few lessons if you haven't swum in a while.** Beginners waste a lot of energy flailing and splashing around rather than moving forward.

- **Break your workout into intervals.** For example, don't just get into the pool, swim 20 laps, and get out. Instead, do 4 easy laps for a warm-up. Then do 8 sets of 2 laps at a faster pace, resting 20 seconds between sets. Then cool down with two easy laps, and maybe a few extra laps with a kickboard. Mix up your strokes, too. The four basic strokes — freestyle, backstroke, breaststroke, and butterfly — use your muscles in different ways.

- **If swimming is your bag, join a Masters swim club.** These clubs, located at university and community pools nationwide, are geared toward adult swimmers of all levels. A coach gives you a different workout every time you swim and monitors your progress. Best of all, you have buddies to work out with. Don't worry about being slow; the coach will group you in a lane with other people your speed. If you have a competitive spirit, you can compete in Masters meets, where you swim against others who are roughly your speed.

- **If you find swimming a big yawn but enjoy being in the water, try water running or water aerobics.** Water running is a pretty tough workout because the water provides resistance from all directions as you move your legs. It's an excellent workout for injur0ed runners because, even though it's nonimpact and easy on your joints, it helps maintain aerobic conditioning. Don't assume that water aerobics is for little old ladies in flowered caps. With the right instructor and exercise program, you can get a challenging water-aerobics workout. Water running can be even tougher.

Snowshoeing

Suzanne loves the snow but hates downhill skiing. She doesn't understand the point of standing in line for 45 minutes while icy wind whips through your $400 parka — all so you can whoosh down the mountain in three minutes, stand in line, and risk frostbite all over again. Plus, she's a klutz, so she navigates moguls with her skis pointed in that dorky V-shaped position.

For these reasons, Suzanne was thrilled to discover snowshoeing — now her favorite winter sport and one that's booming in popularity nationwide. Snowshoeing takes you into the woods and away from the crowds, burns lots of calories, and generates enough body heat to keep you toasty. Plus, it involves minimal spending, no risk of injury, and, best of all, no skill. Snowshoeing has become so popular that 5K and 10K competitions have sprung up nationwide.

Essential snowshoeing gear

The term *snowshoeing* may conjure up images of bearded Scandinavian trappers slogging across the tundra, their boots strapped to giant wooden tennis racquets. Indeed, that's what snowshoeing was all about — a thousand years ago. Unlike the old 7-foot-long wood-and-cowhide shoes, today's snowshoes are just 2 feet long, and the oblong frames are made of lightweight aluminum. High-tech fabric stretches across the frame, providing a surface area that keeps you from sinking into the snow. (By the way, snowshoes don't directly fit on your bare feet; you strap the snowshoes onto any footwear that's comfortable for you — walking shoes, running shoes, or even lightweight hiking boots.)

Snowshoes run between $120 and $300, and they come in different sizes (heavier people need larger frames) and designs (for casual walking, backcountry hiking, and running on packed snow). Before you make an investment, rent them at a ski shop for $10 to $20. Rent poles, too. They help propel you uphill and help you maintain balance going downhill, and you can decide whether you like them enough to invest in a pair for yourself. (Poles cost from $60 to $140 per pair.)

Be sure to dress in layers. Even in freezing temperatures, you can work up a good sweat and then get chilly fast. Wear a lightweight, breathable top that wicks away sweat. On top of that, wear a fleece pullover or vest. On supercold days, bring a lightweight, water-resistant jacket. (You'll suffocate in a ski parka.)

Snowshoeing the right way

If you can walk, you can snowshoe. Suzanne did manage to fall on her face her first day on snowshoes, but that's because she forgot she was wearing them; her stride was too short, and she stepped onto her own snowshoe and tripped. But after you grasp the fact that snowshoes are longer than hiking boots, you're set.

Still a few handy techniques can help you navigate hilly terrain. When you climb a steep slope, kick the front of your snowshoe into the snow and stomp down to compact the fluffy stuff. To avoid slipping, make sure that each new step is distinct from the previous one. When snowshoeing downhill, keep your knees slightly bent and lean back a bit so your weight is on your heel cleats.

Snowshoeing tips for rookies

Consider these tips before you head out the door:

- **Start on packed snow.** Tromping through fluffy powder can leave you breathless — it's like heading away from the firm, wet shoreline and slogging through deep, dry sand. The deeper the snow and the steeper the terrain, the more exhausted you'll feel.

- **When you're in powder, go single-file, alternating positions to share the burden of *breaking trail* (snowshoeing-speak for being the first person to make a trail through fresh snow).** You may find that you have to take frequent breaks while snowshoeing in powder, because your heart rate is likely to elevate rapidly.

- **Because snowshoeing is taxing and the air at high altitudes is dry, you need to drink plenty of water.** Wear a fanny pack with a water-bottle holster or strap on a hydration pack designed for winter sports.

Part IV
Lift and Curl: Building a Stronger Bod with Weights

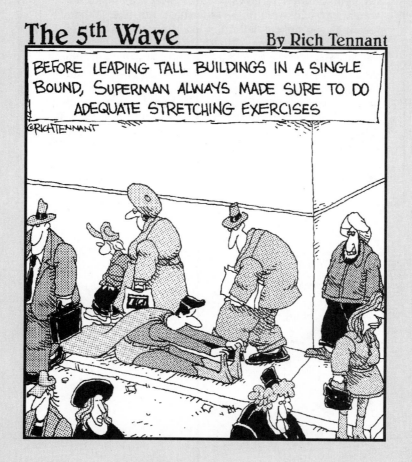

The 5th Wave   By Rich Tennant

BEFORE LEAPING TALL BUILDINGS IN A SINGLE BOUND, SUPERMAN ALWAYS MADE SURE TO DO ADEQUATE STRETCHING EXERCISES

In this part . . .

We give you the know-how to tone and strengthen your muscles, whether you work out at home or at the gym. Chapter 11 gives you five great reasons to lift weights and answers important questions, like: "What if I want to get muscle definition like Buffy the Vampire Slayer or LaBron James?" In Chapter 12, we cover your major muscle groups so that you know your lats from your pecs from your delts. In Chapter 13, we explain the differences between barbells, dumbbells, and weight machines and help you choose the best equipment for you. Chapter 14 helps you get started on a weight-training program. We discuss how much weight to lift, how many exercises to do, and how to use good form so you don't get injured. We also demonstrate a complete weight-training workout that you can perform either at a health club or at home.

Chapter 11

Why You've Gotta Lift Weights

In This Chapter

▶ Understanding five major reasons to lift weights

▶ Busting some weight-lifting myths

▶ Assessing your chances of looking like Jackie Chan or Demi Moore

Maybe you've never considered yourself the weight-lifting type. Maybe you suspect that the size of one's muscles is inversely proportional to the size of one's brain. Maybe when you see a hulking guy on the street, you think, "He may be able to bench-press my minivan, but I can read a menu in French."

The truth is, weight lifting is an incredibly smart thing to do. It's not just a form of narcissism, and it's not just for body builders. Heck, these days, even 80-year-olds are pumping iron. In this chapter, we explain why you should, too. We also dispel popular weight-training myths and tell you what kind of results you can reasonably expect. If you think lifting weight seems too boring, too dangerous, too troublesome, or too likely to transform you into Hulk Hogan, we hope this chapter changes your mind.

First, a quick note: Throughout this book, we use the terms *weight lifting, weight training,* and *strength training* interchangeably, even though you don't necessarily need weight to build strength. *Resistance training* means the same thing, but we spare you that bit of verbiage.

Five Important Reasons to Pick Up a Dumbbell

People who start lifting weights regularly will tell you how much more fit, powerful, and energetic they feel . . . but enough about feelings. There's plenty of good, solid evidence that strength training does all that and more. We bet that at least one of the following reasons will get you to hoist some iron.

Stay strong for everyday life

People who don't exercise lose 30 to 40 percent of their strength by age 65. By age 74, more than one-fourth of American men and two-thirds of American women can't lift an object heavier than 10 pounds, like a small dog or a loaded garbage bag. These changes aren't the normal consequences of aging. They're a result of neglect — of experiencing life from a La-Z-Boy recliner and the front seat of a Winnebago. If you don't use your muscles, they simply waste away. This gradual slide toward wimpiness can begin as early as your mid-20s.

Fortunately, strength is one of the easiest physical abilities to retain as you get older; certainly, you can do a lot more to halt strength loss than you can to prevent wrinkling skin, fading eyesight, or increasing affection for elevator Muzak. One study, which included men up to age 96, found that by lifting weight, most seniors can at least double — if not triple — their muscle power.

So if you rarely lift anything heavier than a cell phone, it's time to build enough brawn to get along in the real world. Increased strength is what you need to unscrew the top off a stubborn jar of pickles, hoist your kid onto the mechanical horsy, and close a suitcase that's too full. Even if you have the stamina to sprint the full length of an airport to catch your plane, it's not going to do you much good if you can't lug along that overstuffed luggage.

Keep your bones healthy

Twenty-five million Americans have *osteoporosis,* a disease of severe bone loss that causes 1.5 million fractures a year, mostly of the back, hip, and wrist. About half of those who break their hips never regain full walking ability, and many of these fractures lead to fatal complications. When bones become extremely weak — picture them like chalk, porous and fragile — it doesn't even take a fall to break them. Someone with osteoporosis doesn't fall and break a hip; she breaks a hip and falls.

Osteoporosis isn't something that happens to you overnight, like becoming eligible for a senior discount at the movies. Most people start out with strong, dense bones — imagine them as poles of steel. But around age 35, most people — men included — begin to lose about ½ to 1 percent of their bone each year. (For women, bone loss accelerates after menopause — 1 to 2 percent a year for the first five years and then about 1 percent annually until age 70. Then the loss slows back to ½ percent a year.) If you do everything right, however, you can decelerate this bone loss significantly — by about 50 percent. If you've already lost a lot of bone, you may even be able to build some of it back. Strength training alone can't stop bone loss, but it can play a big role. Also important are calcium, vitamin D, and aerobic exercise such as walking and jogging. (Swimming and cycling don't work because your body weight is supported, either by the water or the bike; when you have to support your own self, your bones respond by building themselves up.)

Strong muscles and strong bones go hand in hand. The more weight you can lift, the more stress you can put on your bones; this stress is what stimulates them. The first astronauts to spend time in space experienced significant bone-density loss. In space, not only does no one hear you scream, but you're weightless — there's no load placed on your muscles and bones. Today's astronauts prevent bone loss by exercising several hours a day.

Prevent injuries

When your muscles are strong, you're less injury-prone. You're less likely to step off a curb and twist your ankle. Plus, you have a better sense of balance and surefootedness, so you're less apt to take a tumble during a weekend game of touch football. Research shows that one out of every three people over age 65 falls at least once a year. Almost 10 percent of older people who fall are hospitalized for an injury, and about half of those cases involve broken bones.

Look better

Now let's talk about pure, unadulterated vanity. Aerobic exercise burns lots of calories, but weight lifting firms, lifts, builds, and shapes your muscles. A marathon runner may be able to go the distance, but he won't turn any heads on the beach if he has a concave chest and string-bean arms. (He might also be a faster runner if he pumped up a bit.)

We want to be clear here: There's no such thing as spot reducing — that is, selectively zapping fat off a particular part of your body. But you can pick certain areas, such as your butt or your arms, and reshape them through weight training. And if you have wide hips or a thick middle, you can bring your body more into proportion by doing exercises that broaden your shoulders and back.

Weight training also makes you look better by improving your posture. With strong abdominal and lower-back muscles, you stand up straighter and look more svelte even if you haven't lost an ounce.

Speed up your metabolism

Metabolism is all over the news these days. At gyms, health-food stores, and juice bars, you can buy pills, powders, and "thermogenic herbs" touted to rev up your metabolism (and thereby help you burn extra calories without trying). Suzanne's own parents, despite their daughter's eye-rolling and sarcastic snorts, even tried a meat-and-grapefruit diet purported to boost metabolism. All these claims are bogus. The only way to increase your metabolism is to build muscle, which you can best accomplish by lifting weights.

How does this work? First, a couple of definitions: Your *metabolism* refers to the number of calories you're burning at any given moment, whether you're watching The Weather Channel or riding a bike. But when most people use the term, they're referring to your resting metabolism, the number of calories your body needs to maintain its vital functions. Your brain, heart, kidneys, and other organs are cranking away 24 hours a day, and your muscle cells are constantly undergoing repair. All these processes require energy in the form of calories simply to keep you alive.

But here's the key: Your resting metabolic rate depends primarily on your amount of *fat-free mass* — everything in your body that's not fat, including muscle, bones, blood, organs, and tissue. The more fat-free mass you have, the more energy your body expends in order to keep going. So, you want to be muscular. You can't do anything to increase the size of your liver or brain, but you certainly can make yourself more muscular, and lifting weights is the primary way to do just that.

Keep in mind, however, that packing on a few more pounds of muscle isn't going to turn your body into a calorie-burning inferno. For every 1 pound of muscle you gain, your body may burn an extra 30 to 50 calories per day. That's not a lot, especially if you compensate by eating one extra Hershey's Kiss (24 calories) per day. However, in the long run, even that small metabolic boost can be significant. If you burn an extra 25 calories per day, you can burn 9,125 calories in a year — enough to lose nearly 3 pounds, or at least prevent a 3-pound weight gain. And if you add 10 pounds of lean muscle, you can burn an additional 300 to 500 calories per day!

If that's not impressive, consider the flip side: If you don't lift weights, your metabolism will slow down every year, as your muscles slowly waste away. And with a more sluggish metabolic rate, you'll gain weight even if you eat the same amount of food. How's that for incentive to hit the weight room?

One final point: The metabolism-boosting benefits of weight lifting are particularly important if you're cutting calories to lose weight. Dieting alone tends to cause a loss in muscle as well as fat; if you lift weights while cutting back on your calorie intake, you can preserve muscle — and maintain your metabolism — while losing fat.

Building Muscle: Myths and Reality

There sure are a lot of misconceptions about weight training. Many people have no idea what changes to expect when they begin lifting weights, so they ask some not-so-dumb questions, like the ones that follow.

How long does it take to get stronger?

You may be able to lift more weight after just one weight-lifting workout. This isn't because you've built up more muscle; it's mainly because your weight-training skills have improved. The first time you try the bench press, you waste a lot of energy trying to balance the bar, keep it steady, and move it in a straight line. But after you get the hang of the process — typically after one weight-lifting session — you're able to put all your energy into lifting the weight.

Another reason you develop strength after just a few weeks of working out is that, in a sense, your muscles have memory. Your nerves, the pathways that link your brain and muscles, learn how to carry information more quickly — much like the speed-dial feature on your telephone. So after learning an exercise, your brain tells your muscles, "You know what this is. Go for it."

During the first six to eight weeks you lift weight, most of the strength you gain is due to skill and muscle memory. After that time, your muscles begin to grow. In other words, the sizes of your muscle fibers increase — you don't actually grow more muscle cells. Realize that some muscles gain strength faster than others do. In general, large muscles, like your chest and back muscles, grow faster than smaller ones, like your arm and shoulder muscles. Most people can increase their strength between 7 and 40 percent after about ten weeks of training each muscle group twice a week.

Do some people have greater strength potential than others?

How much muscle power you develop depends on many things, including your age, sex, and body type (and, of course, your diligence). Seniors generally can't develop as much strength as young people, but it's not clear whether this is due to the normal aging process or years of inactivity. However, look at Jack La Lanne, who worked out all his life. For his 80th birthday, he towed a rowboat across a river with his teeth. Men typically have the capacity for greater overall strength than women do because their bodies have a higher proportion of muscle and more of the strength hormone testosterone.

Every body type has a different capacity for building strength and muscle. All the training in the world won't change your body type. If you start out short and narrow, weight training won't miraculously make you tall and broad. Weight training may, however, make you a more fit, muscular version of short and narrow.

Strength is one thing, but how long will it take before my body looks better?

Most people start to see changes after six weeks of weight lifting, but we can't give you an exact answer. Results depend on your body type, your starting point, and the amount of time and effort you devote to lifting weight. In general, those who have the furthest to go make the most dramatic changes.

Everyone notices the biggest improvements in the muscles that they use the least. The *triceps* (the muscles at the rear of your upper arm; see Chapter 12) are a classic example: You don't use them much in everyday life, so when you start targeting them with weight they become firmer fairly fast. The same goes for shoulders. Most people don't tend to carry much fat on their shoulders, so shoulders shape and tone relatively quickly.

What if I want to get muscle definition like Demi Moore or Jackie Chan?

Lifting weight diligently will help shape your body, but you'll never see muscle definition if you have a thick layer of fat covering your muscles. *Muscle definition* means that you have so little body fat that you can see the outline of your muscles. You begin to see a hint of definition when your body fat dips into the 20 percent to 22 percent range. At around 18 percent, muscle definition is really apparent. Below 15 percent, you develop an appearance that body builders reverentially refer to as *ripped.* (We tell you all about body fat in Chapter 2.) We're not recommending that you try to get down this low, because it can be dangerously unhealthy; we do, however, want you to be aware that the buff, ripped look doesn't happen for most people. Also, keep in mind that you can still look firm, fit, and sexy even if you aren't ripped to shreds.

Will weight lifting turn me into a WWE contender?

No. About 99 percent of women — and a significant percentage of men — can't develop huge muscles without spending hours a day in the gym lifting some serious poundage. Even then, most women don't have testosterone to add major bulk to their frames unless they take steroids — in which case, they may also end up with acne, a beard, liver cancer, uterus shrinkage, and a voice like Darth Vader's. Just the look you're going for, right?

Lifting may actually make you smaller. Because muscle is a very compact, dense tissue, it takes up less room than fat. At first, you may not lose any weight. You may even gain a few pounds, because muscle weighs more per square inch than fat, but your clothes may fit better. As we explain in Chapter 2, that number on your bathroom scale is an incomplete number.

But what if I want to increase bulk?

Developing huge muscles is difficult for people with certain body types, and usually comes only with a high-calories diet mixed with intensive, consistent training. If you're lean and wiry to begin with, you'll probably add definition but not much size. The people most likely to build up their frames are those who have a muscular body type even before they start lifting.

To bulk up without risking the dangers of steroids, many athletes and recreational exercisers are turning to *creatine,* the apparently more benign substance that was touted by baseball's homerun king Mark McGwire. Some research shows that creatine may indeed make you bigger and stronger; however, the research isn't conclusive, and no one has studied the substance long enough to know if there are long-term side-effects. We also advise against taking *androstenedione* — also known as *andro* — another muscle-building aid that McGwire used. Evidence suggests that andro lowers levels of HDL cholesterol, the good kind, increasing the risk for heart disease, and it's now banned by the U.S. Food and Drug Administration.

Apparently, an increasing number of men are harboring unrealistic expectations about their potential to get huge. A few years ago, a Harvard psychiatrist came up with an interesting theory to explain why: outlandishly muscular toys. Over the last 30 years, G.I. Joe action figures have inflated into hulks with physiques that even top bodybuilders can't attain. The professor measured the waist, chest, and biceps of the action figures and then adjusted the numbers for a 6-foot man. In 1964, G.I. Joe had 12.2-inch biceps; ten years later his "guns" had grown to 15.2 inches. By 1998, G.I. Joe's biceps measured a whopping 26.8 inches — nearly 7 inches larger than Mark McGwire's. For decades, Barbie — with her impossibly small waist and huge chest — has created unrealistic expectations for women and girls; now, it seems that G.I. Joe is doing the same sort of damage in boys and men.

If I stop lifting weight, won't my muscle turn to fat?

Only if silver can be transformed into gold. Fat and muscle are two distinctly different substances. When you look at them under the microscope, fat looks like chicken wire, and muscle looks like frayed electrical wiring. If you stop lifting weight, your muscles simply *atrophy,* a fancy word for shrink. The main reason people may gain fat when they stop lifting weights is that they keep their calorie intake the same but are no longer burning as many calories throughout the day. Those extra calories are stored as fat.

Should I lose weight before I start lifting weights?

Actually, no. Start weight training right away. Weight training can speed up your metabolism and give you more muscle tone, better posture, and better body proportions. In addition, lifting weight enhances your aerobic efforts. With stronger muscles, you have more staying power on the stair-climber, and you're less apt to have a setback due to injury from your aerobic work-outs. For example, you may be working out like gangbusters when, suddenly, you feel a little twinge in your knee. You lay off for a couple days, which turns into a couple years. You may be able to prevent this whole incident by strengthening your knees. Plus, adding weight training to your new exercise program gives you more variety and helps keep you motivated.

Chapter 12

Your Muscles: Love 'Em or Lose 'Em

In This Chapter

▶ Discovering the formal names — and the slang — of your muscles

▶ Looking at nifty muscle illustrations

▶ Finding out our favorite exercises for each muscle

There are 650 muscles in your body. We are happy to report that you don't need to memorize all of them. Consider, for example, the inferior retinaculum of the long extensor of your big toe. We don't want you to remember that one. In fact, we don't even know that one — we had to look it up in our anatomy book. If you have any desire to find out more about that muscle, shut this book and apply to medical school.

Meanwhile, in this chapter, we tell you about the 20 or so muscles that any conscientious exerciser should know. What's the point? For one thing, you won't need an interpreter when a trainer, video instructor, or fellow gym member says, "Let's do lats and pecs today." Before you know it, you may be saying stuff like that, too. And you'll sound really impressive — like wine aficionados who say, "This chardonnay has a superior bouquet."

But more importantly, if you can name your major muscles and understand how each one operates, you can get better results from your workout program. You'll understand, for example, how certain exercises can help you prevent lower-back pain. You'll understand why you should do several different shoulder exercises, rather than just one. And you'll be sure to perform your exercises properly. For example, if you know where your biceps are, you'll realize exactly where you should feel the tension — and you can adjust your form if you don't feel tension in the right spot. With many weight-training exercises, it's easy to emphasize the wrong muscle if you don't understand the purpose of the move. If you simply hop on a machine and pull some lever without knowing which muscle to focus on, you may be cheating yourself out of a good workout. Finally, knowing about all your major muscle groups helps you get a more complete and balanced workout. You'll know not to leave any muscle group out. (See Figures 12-1 and 12-2 for a full view of your muscles.)

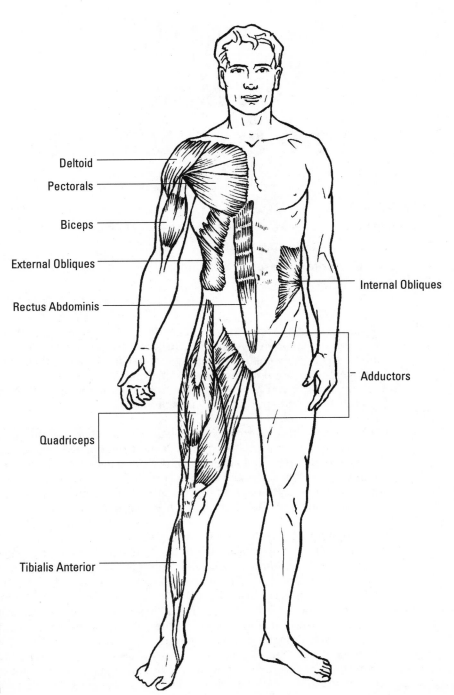

Deltoid

Pectorals

Biceps

External Obliques

Rectus Abdominis

Internal Obliques

Adductors

Quadriceps

Tibialis Anterior

Figure 12-1:
Your
muscles —
front view.

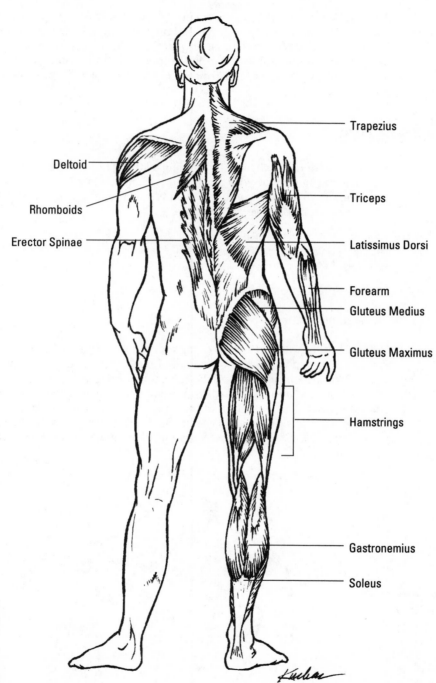

Trapezius

Deltoid

Rhomboids

Triceps

Erector Spinae

Latissimus Dorsi

Forearm

Gluteus Medius

Gluteus Maximus

Hamstrings

Gastronemius

Soleus

Figure 12-2:
Your
muscles —
back view.

This section simply discusses the major muscles of the body; it doesn't show you a weight-lifting technique for that muscle group. However, we do list our favorite exercises for each muscle group, and each exercise is described in Chapter 14. To find out about other exercises that we don't list here, consult a trainer or our book, *Weight Training For Dummies* (published by Wiley).

Shoulders

Strong shoulders are the key to building a strong upper body. Just about every exercise you can do for your chest and back involves your shoulders, too. If your shoulders are weak, you really limit the amount of weight you can use in the rest of your upper-body repertoire.

Deltoids

Given name: Deltoids

Street name: Delts

Whereabouts: Your *delts* wrap completely around the tops of your arms (see Figure 12-3). Cup your hand over your shoulder and you get the idea. Now swing your arm around in a circle, raise it up above your head, and then swing it forward and backward. You can see what a versatile muscle your shoulder is. The front portion of the shoulder muscle is referred to as the *anterior delt,* the side is called the *medial delt,* and the back is called the rear or *posterior delt.* Go ahead, toss those terms around and amaze your friends.

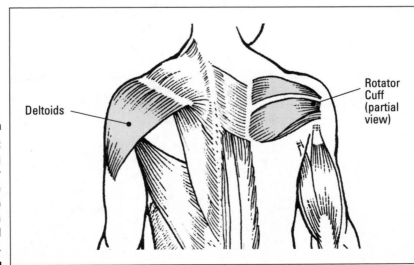

Figure 12-3: Strong shoulder muscles are the key to building a powerful upper body.

Deltoids

Rotator Cuff (partial view)

Job description: Your delts help your arms move in a wide range of directions.

The training payoff: You'll never have to wear shoulder pads if, heaven forbid, they ever come back in style. Also, strengthening your shoulders can help you avoid injuries such as shoulder dislocations or muscle tears. And with strong shoulders, you have no trouble putting that useless "waist trimmer" gadget that you bought for $19.95 on the top shelf in the closet.

Special tips: We tend to like free weights better than machines for strengthening the shoulders. Although most shoulder-press machines have improved in recent years, many other shoulder contraptions, especially lateral-raise machines, tend to be difficult to adjust and uncomfortable to use. Also, machines aren't made for every shoulder movement. For example, no specific machine mimics the front shoulder raise. It's important to target the front, middle, and back of your shoulders, as well as the delts as a whole, so make it a point to master several dumbbell exercises.

Our favorite exercises: Dumbbell shoulder press, dumbbell lateral raise, dumbbell front raise, and dumbbell back delt fly

Rotator cuff

Given name: Rotator cuff

Street name: Rotators

Whereabouts: Four small muscles beneath your shoulder (refer to Figure 12-3); together, they're called your rotator cuff.

Job description: Your rotator-cuff muscles hold your arm in its socket. You use these muscles to rotate the shoulder joint, such as when throwing and catching. Baseball pitchers are constantly sidelined with rotator-cuff injuries.

The training payoff: If you have weak rotators, you can damage them simply by carrying a briefcase or reaching across the table for Rice Krispies Treats — throwing a 90 mph fastball is not a prerequisite for injury (see Chapter 5). By making a special effort to strengthen these commonly injured muscles, you're far less likely to tear or strain them.

Special tips: In addition to doing rotator-cuff exercises, work your shoulders in a variety of directions. Your rotators are put into action whenever your deltoids are working; if your delts are weak and you do a heavy upper-body lift, you may do some serious rotator damage. If you have chronic shoulder pain, check with your orthopedist to see if you've injured your rotator cuff. Sometimes rotator tears can be corrected with exercise; other times, they require surgery.

Our favorite exercises: Internal and external rotation, performed with an exercise band, a dumbbell, or a weight plate, or on a cable crossover machine

Back

Neglecting your back muscles is tempting because you don't face them in the mirror every day. But these muscles are just as important as the muscles in the front of your body, particularly when it comes to injury prevention.

We know a man who injured his back while putting on his underwear in the health-club locker room. He was lying on the floor stark naked for a few hours before he let the staff members call a nurse. Trainers had repeatedly reminded him to strengthen his lower-back muscles and abdominals. After that incident, he finally listened.

Trapezius

Given name: Trapezius

Street name: Traps

Whereabouts: Your *trapezius* is a fairly large, kite-shaped muscle that spans up into your neck, across your shoulders, and down to the center of your back (see Figure 12-4).

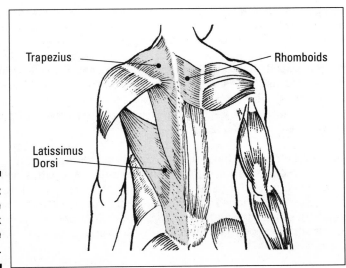

Figure 12-4:
The upper-back muscle team.

Job description: Your trapezius enables you to shrug your shoulders. This muscle is also involved when you lift your arm, such as when hailing a cab.

The training payoff: A toned trapezius adds shape to your shoulders and upper back. Strengthening this muscle may also alleviate the neck and shoulder pain you may get if you sit at a desk all day or if your phone is a permanent appendage to your ear.

Special tips: Give your trapezius extra attention if you often carry a knapsack or heavy bag over your shoulder.

Our favorite exercises: Shrug or shoulder roll with a barbell, two dumbbells, or — if your neck is extremely weak and tight — no weight at all

Latissimus dorsi

Given name: Latissimus dorsi

Street name: Lats (*Note:* Don't make the mistake of saying "laterals," as some less-informed, bookwormish exercisers do.)

Whereabouts: Feel the widest part of your back just behind your armpit — you've just found your *latissimus dorsi,* your largest back muscle. This muscle runs the entire length of your back, from below your shoulders down to your lower back (refer to Figure 12-4).

Job description: Your lats enable you to pull, like when you open a door against the wind or drag your Great Dane into the vet's office.

The training payoff: Well-toned lats make your hips and waist appear smaller by adding shape and width to your upper body. If you play sports — especially a racquet sport, golf, or hockey — strengthening your lats will enable you to power the ball or puck quite a bit further. Runners, walkers, and cyclists also should focus on their lats to help counteract that tendency toward rounded shoulders, which are the result of weak rhomboids (see the following section) and other muscles of the upper and middle back, as well as the result of tight delts (discussed in the "Deltoids" section) and pecs (see the "Chest (the Pectorals)" section).

Special tips: When you do lat exercises, think of your arms simply as a link between your back and the bar or dumbbell. Focus on working your lats, not your arms.

Our favorite exercises: Lat pull-down machine, dumbbell row, dumbbell pullover, T-bar row, seated cable row, chin-up, and pull-up

Rhomboids

Given name: Rhomboids

Street name: None. Almost no one talks about them. (However, we did once hear them referred to as the "rheumatoids," a term we thought was better suited for an octogenarian garage band.)

Whereabouts: Your *rhomboids* are a small, rectangular group of muscles at the center of your back, hidden beneath your lower trapezius (refer to Figure 12-4).

Job description: Your rhomboids pull your shoulder blades together so you maintain good posture.

The training payoff: With strong rhomboids, you're less likely to hunch your shoulders forward.

Special tips: Focus on your rhomboids to avoid poor posture and potential injury.

Our favorite exercises: Chin-up and dumbbell back delt fly

Erector spinae

Given name: Erector spinae

Street name: Lower back

Whereabouts: Your *erector spinae* run the entire length of your spine, but it's the lower third of this muscle group that you strengthen when you perform the exercises we mention later in this section. The rest of this muscle group gets worked when you do upper-back exercises. Figure 12-5 shows where your erector spinae are located.

Job description: Your lower-back muscles are responsible for straightening your spine — for example, when you stand up after tying your shoes. They also work in tandem with your abdominals to keep your spine stable when you move the rest of your body, like when you're sitting in your car and you reach around for something in the back seat.

The training payoff: About 80 percent of adult Americans experience back pain at some point in their lives. You can prevent much of this pain by devoting equal time to strengthening your lower back and abdominal muscles. Strong lower-back muscles are also very important for posture. (Flexibility of the back is also key; see Chapter 6.)

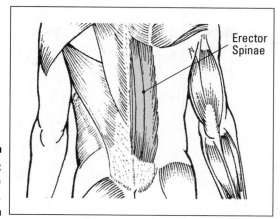

Erector
Spinae

Figure 12-5:
A look at the
lower back.

Special tips: The lower back is an injury-prone area. If you have constant lower-back pain, ask your doctor to recommend exercises for your specific problem.

Our favorite exercises: Pelvic tilt and back extension on the floor or on a hyperextension bench

Chest (the Pectorals)

The fibers of your chest muscles spread out like a fan, connecting to your arms, ribs, collar bone (clavical), and breast bone (sternum). For this reason, your chest muscles respond well when you work them from a variety of angles. For example, you can do chest exercises while lying flat on your back on a bench, reclining at various angles, sitting upright, standing, or lying facedown (like when you do push-ups). Ask a trainer to show you several chest exercises so you can vary your workouts.

Given name: Pectorals

Street name: Pecs

Whereabouts: Place your hand on your chest as if you're pledging allegiance to the flag. You've found your *pecs*. (See Figure 12-6.)

Job description: Thanks to your pecs you can push — a shopping cart, a lawn mover, or some jerk standing in your way. You also use your pecs to wrap your arms around something, like when you give your mom a bear hug.

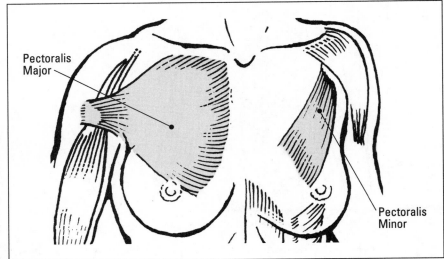

Figure 12-6:
You work
your
pectorals
when you
do chest
exercises.

The training payoff: With strong pecs, you look great in tight t-shirts. You also need strong chest muscles for sports like tennis, golf, and football.

Special tips: For women — it's important to understand that your pecs are not your breasts; in fact they reside directly underneath your breast tissue. However, toning your pecs can lift your breasts and make them appear firmer.

For men — don't become obsessed with bench pressing to the point of excluding all other exercises. Men with overdeveloped chest muscles and wimpy legs resemble hard-boiled eggs on toothpicks. Besides, doing too much chest work sets you up for shoulder injuries.

Our favorite exercises: Bench press, dumbbell fly, push-up, and incline dumbbell press

Arms

Take a survey of today's TV stars, fashion models, and music artists, and you can see that firm arm muscles are in style. Even department-store mannequins now have toned arms. Be sure to give your front and rear arm muscles equal time; if one of these muscle groups is disproportionately stronger than the other, you're at greater risk for elbow injuries.

Biceps

Given name: Biceps

Street name: Bi(s) or guns

Whereabouts: Your *biceps* are the two muscles at the front of your upper arm (see Figure 12-7) — the ones that pop up when you flex like a bodybuilder.

Job description: Your biceps are responsible for bending your elbow. When you pick up this book or when you turn the pages, you use your biceps.

The training payoff: With strong biceps, lifting a stack of newspapers or carrying an armload of wood is easier. Your biceps also help out your back muscles when you pull a really stubborn weed out of your garden. Plus, strong biceps make you look buff.

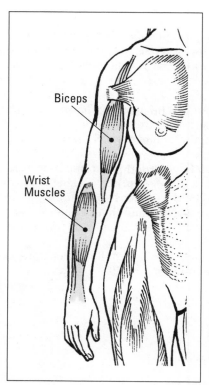
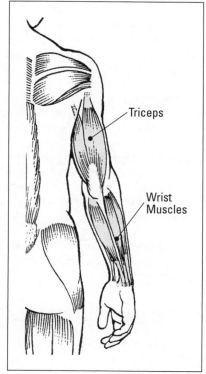

Figure 12-7:
Your arm
muscles
(front and
rear view).

Special tips: Many people have sloppy posture when they do biceps exercises — they rock their bodies back and forth to hoist the weight up. Not only is this posture dangerous for your lower back, but it also makes life too easy for your biceps. Pay special attention to form on bicep exercises, and don't use more weight than you can handle.

Our favorite exercises: Dumbbell biceps curl, concentration curl, barbell biceps curl, and machine arm curl

Triceps

Given name: Triceps

Street name: Tri(s)

Whereabouts: Your triceps are located at the back of your upper arm (refer to Figure 12-7).

Job description: Your triceps do the opposite of what your biceps do; that is, your triceps straighten your elbow. Your triceps help out your chest muscles when you push something, like your 1966 Volkswagen Bug that has stalled at an intersection.

The training payoff: Triceps exercises help firm up *bingo arms*. That's when the backs of your arms flap loosely away from the bones — a condition common among people whose main form of physical activity is playing bingo.

Special tips: The triceps make up two-thirds of your upper-arm size, so if you want a nice pair of arms, work these muscles. Working your triceps is especially important if you often hold a briefcase or handbag while your arm is straight. If your triceps are weak — and that's common because these muscles don't get much work in daily life — you may be prone to elbow pain.

Our favorite exercises: Triceps kickback, bench dip, triceps press-down, and triceps-extension machine or dumbbells/barbells.

Forearm muscles

Given name: Wrist extensors and flexors

Street name: Wrist or forearm muscles

Whereabouts: These muscles run from the bottom of your elbow to your wrist (refer to Figure 12-7).

Job description: Your forearm muscles bend and move your wrists. They're also a link between your upper body and any barbell, lever, or dumbbell you move. If you don't have the wrist strength to grip a barbell, you're certainly not going to be able to bench-press, even if your chest muscles are strong.

The training payoff: Powerful wrist muscles give you a stronger grip for weight lifting. Wrist strength also can help prevent or alleviate tennis elbow (see Chapter 5) and _carpal tunnel syndrome_ — a painful irritation of wrist nerves resulting from repetitive motions such as typing or certain assembly-line tasks, such as tightening a bolt with a wrench.

Special tips: To ensure that you develop adequate wrist strength, wrap your hand firmly around the barbells or dumbbells you use.

Our favorite exercises: Dumbbell wrist curl and reverse wrist curl

Abdominals

Developing a toned, flat abdomen has become somewhat of a national obsession. Most fitness magazines don't let a month go by without an article titled "Midriff Madness!" or "Flatten Your Tummy in 3 Minutes a Day!" But don't delude yourself: All the abdominal exercises in the world won't make your tummy pancake flat; in order to whittle your middle, you need to lose the extra body fat stored on top of your abdominal muscles. Still, ab training is a must, both for good posture and for the prevention of lower-back pain.

Rectus abdominis

Given name: Rectus abdominis

Street name: Abs (**_Note:_** Don't refer to your abdominals as your stomach, which is the organ responsible for digesting food.)

Whereabouts: Your rectus abdominis is a flat sheet of muscle that runs from just under your chest down to a few inches south of your belly button (the top of your pelvis) (see Figure 12-8). This is one long, continuous muscle; you don't have "upper abs" and "lower abs," as many people mistakenly think. Although you can do exercises that emphasize the upper or lower portions of your rectus, all abdominal exercises do involve the entire muscle.

The muscle just below the rectus abdominis is the _transverses abdominis,_ the deep stabilizer of the trunk. It's responsible for protecting the trunk and spine; think of it as the body's internal weightlifting belt.

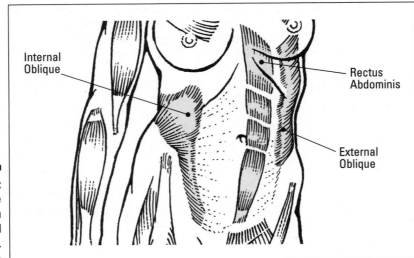

Internal Oblique

Rectus Abdominis

External Oblique

Figure 12-8: These are your main abdominal muscles.

Job description: Your rectus allows you to flex your spine and pull your torso or chest toward your hips, and it works with your lower-back muscles to keep your torso stable while you move the rest of your body. For example, when you're shoveling dirt in your garden, your arms are moving, but you have to brace your body to get enough leverage and to protect your lower back.

The training payoff: The obvious reason to train your abdominals is to firm up your midsection. If your abs are really toned and you don't have much excess fat around your middle, you can see six distinct sections of the muscle. This is known as *washboard abs* or the *six pack.* But having such a firm midriff is not worth fixating on — for most people, washboard abs are not a realistic proposition. Even people with relatively low body fat tend to store at least some fat around the middle. Appearances aside, strong abs improve your posture by making it easier to stand up straight. Plus, they're important for guarding against lower-back pain.

Special tips: Those full sit-ups you did back in high school gym class won't do the job — plus they're hard on your back, especially if you lock your feet under a couch. Although many gyms have abdominal machines, we feel that floor exercises, including the ones we name later in this section, are more effective. We also like doing abdominal exercises while leaning against an oversized plastic ball known as a *physioball.* To prevent yourself from sliding off the ball, you have to keep adjusting your body position; this forces you to work your abs more completely, hitting some deeper muscle fibers that don't get much of a workout while doing conventional crunches. As for those ab-strengthening gadgets advertised on TV infomercials, you're better off spending your money on a Miracle Mop.

Our favorite exercises: Abdominal crunch, reverse crunch, and physioball crunch

Internal and external obliques

Given name: Internal and external obliques

Street names: Obliques or the waist

Whereabouts: Your internal and external obliques run diagonally down the sides of your rectus abdominis (refer to Figure 12-8).

Job description: Your obliques enable you to twist from the waist or do a side bend.

The training payoff: Strong obliques are essential for preventing lower-back pain. They work with your rectus abdominis and lower-back muscles to support your spine.

Special tips: Doing side bends while holding a weight in each hand is not a good idea unless you want to build a thicker waist. In addition, placing a pole across your shoulders and twisting from side to side can wreak havoc on your lower back, especially if you do this movement a zillion times.

Our favorite exercise: Crunch with a twist, plus side bends with an exercise ball

Butt and Hips

If your rear end and hips are larger than you'd like them to be, don't be afraid to strengthen these muscles with weights. With the right workout program, these muscles can look firmer and more shapely, not bigger and bulkier. Also, strengthening your butt and hip muscles can help prevent hip and lower-back injuries. If your job requires you to sit on your rear end all day, doing exercises that target these muscles is a good idea.

Gluteus maximus

Given name: Gluteus maximus

Street name: Glutes, buns, or butt

Whereabouts: The largest muscle in your body — as if you need anyone to tell you that. Your two glutes (left and right cheeks) span the entire width of your derriere (see Figure 12-9).

Job description: Your glutes extend your hips and help you jump, climb stairs and hills, and straighten your leg behind you. You also use your gluteus maximus when you stand up from a sitting position.

The training payoff: Training your glutes can lift your butt, make it rounder, and give it more shape. You also need your glutes to get off the couch so you can go work out.

Special tips: Some glute exercises, such as the squat and the lunge (elongated variations of deep knee bends), can be hard on your knees, so pay extra attention to your form. When you bend your knees, your kneecaps should move in the direction that your toes are facing, and they should not shoot out past your toes.

Our favorite exercises: Squat, lunge, and leg-press machine

Hip abductors

Given name: Hip abductors

Street name: Outer thighs or outer hip

Whereabouts: The meatiest part of the side of your hips (refer to Figure 12-9)

Job description: Your abductors help you slide your leg out to the side, like when you go skating or step aside so someone can get past you. These muscles also help your gluteus maximus (or butt) rotate your hips outward.

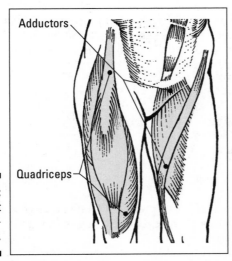
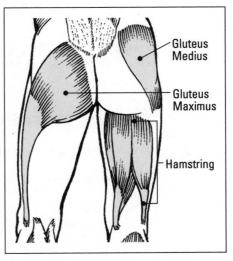

Figure 12-9:
Your butt and upper-leg muscles.

Adductors

Quadriceps

Gluteus Medius

Gluteus Maximus

Hamstring

The training payoff: Working your abductors can firm up your outer thighs and prevent hip injuries. Athletes and seniors should pay special attention to strengthening their hip muscles. You need strong abductors for running, jumping, pedaling, kicking, and skating — just about any movement that involves your lower body. Strong abductors also are important for maintaining a natural walking stride. If your hip abductors are weak, you tend to shuffle along.

Special tips: Some exercise programs advise you to do hundreds of leg lifts to tone this area. But as we explain in Chapter 14, following this advice won't get you anywhere. Work your outer thighs as you would any other muscle group — by doing 8 to 15 moderately challenging repetitions.

Our favorite exercises: Outer-thigh machine and internal hip rotation

Leg adductors

Given name: Leg adductors

Street name: Inner thighs

Whereabouts: Your *adductors* are several muscles that run from inside your hip to various points along your inner thigh (refer to Figure 12-9). You don't need to know each by name.

Job description: Your adductors help you move one leg in front of the other, especially moving your leg to the midline of your body.

The training payoff: When you sit astride a horse or motorcycle, your inner hips squeeze inward to keep you from sliding off. You also use your inner-thigh muscles for skating, soccer, and swimming the breaststroke.

Special tips: Forget the ThighMaster and the other "thigh toner" gadgets you see advertised on TV. You can work your inner-thigh muscles more effectively by adding exercise bands to floor exercises or by using machines in the gym specially designed to focus on these muscles. Don't become fixated on toning your inner thighs; the *New England Journal of Medicine* reported about a woman who had overused a thigh-toning gadget to the point that all the tendons of her inner thighs became inflamed. Ouch.

Our favorite exercises: Inner-thigh machine and side-lying inner-thigh lift

Legs

Keep in mind that, if all goes well, your legs will be carrying you from here to there for the rest of your life. So treat them with respect. By strengthening your leg muscles, you can head off many common knee and ankle injuries. And by staying healthy, of course, you can stay active. You can work out more and develop lean, toned legs that power you up a hill and look good in shorts.

Quadriceps

Given name: Quadriceps

Street name: Quads

Whereabouts: Your quadriceps are the four muscles at the front of each thigh (refer to Figure 12-9).

Job description: Your quadriceps straighten your knee.

The training payoff: You need strong quads for walking, running, climbing, skiing, skating, hopping, skipping, and jumping. Keeping your quads strong can help prevent knee problems. (If you already have knee pain, check with your doctor to find out which exercises are best for you.)

Special tips: Don't worry if you feel an intense burning sensation when you do the leg extension, shown in Chapter 14. This is one of the few exercises that completely isolates the quads, which causes them to tire quickly. Waste products like lactic acid flood into the muscles, causing you to really feel the burn.

Our favorite exercises: Squat, lunge, leg press, and leg-extension machine

Hamstrings

Given name: Hamstrings

Street name: Hams

Whereabouts: Your hamstrings are the three muscles at the back of your thigh (refer to Figure 12-9).

Job description: Your *hamstrings* work in opposition to your quadriceps; in other words, your hamstrings bend the knee. They also help out your glutes when you move from a sitting to a standing position (see the "Gluteus maximus" section earlier in this chapter).

The training payoff: Hamstring injuries are pretty common (if not properly strengthened and flexible) because hamstrings tend to be weak compared to quads. Weekend warriors are especially prone to hamstring pulls, usually when they sprint or jump suddenly, like when they leap for a fly ball during a game of pick-up softball. Suzanne even had a friend who pulled a hamstring muscle while bowling, just as he released the ball.

Special tips: Because your hamstrings are susceptible to pulls, make sure they're adequately warmed up before you perform strengthening exercises, and always stretch them after a workout. For tips on warming up, see Chapter 8.

Our favorite exercises: Seated-leg-curl machine, lying-leg-curl machine, lunge, and dead-lift. For a good hamstring stretch, see Chapter 5.

Gastrocnemius and soleus

Given names: Gastrocnemius and soleus

Street name: Calves

Whereabouts: Your *gastrocnemius,* also called your gastroc, is the large diamond-shaped muscle that gives shape to the back of your lower legs. (To see precisely what the gastroc looks like, pedal behind any top-notch cyclist.) The *soleus* resides underneath the gastroc (see Figure 12-10).

Job description: Your calf muscles allow you to stand on your tiptoes and spring off the ground whenever you jump for joy.

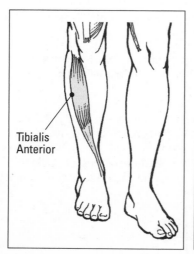
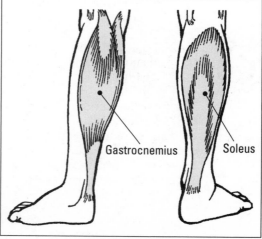

Tibialis Anterior

Gastrocnemius

Soleus

Figure 12-10:
Your lower-leg muscles.

The training payoff: Strong and shapely calves don't just look good; they also give you staying power when you take those long, romantic walks or wait in a three-hour line for Garth Brooks tickets. Plus, you need strong calves for dancing, jumping, running, and hopping.

Special tips: With calf exercises, some people find it more effective to use slightly lighter weights and do a few more repetitions — say, up to 25 — than with most other muscle groups. The muscle tissue in your calves is made specifically for endurance (walking and standing), so it takes more repetitions to reach the deepest fibers.

Our favorite exercises: Standing calf raise, seated calf raise, and standing-calf-raise machine

Tibialis anterior

Given name: Tibialis anterior

Street name: Shins

Whereabouts: The *tibialis anterior* is the largest of several muscles that run from the top of your foot up the lower leg to the outside of the shin bone, near the knee (refer to Figure 12-10).

Job description: Your shin muscles enable you to pull your toes toward your shin, as when you pick up your foot when walking or running.

The training payoff: *Shin splints* — throbbing pain at the front of your ankles caused by any sort of irritation or inflammation in the shins — are fairly common among walkers, runners, dancers, and aerobicizers who overdo it (see Chapter 5). You're especially prone to this injury if your shin muscles are weak compared to your calf muscles.

Special tips: If you do get shin splints, stay off your feet for a few days until the pain subsides. Icing and stretching can help speed recovery. For tips on icing, see Chapter 5.

Our favorite exercises: You're not likely to find a special machine at the gym to work your shins, so try the following exercise, called the toe lift: Stand flat on your feet and lift your toes off the floor 8 to 15 times. If you don't have access to this machine, you can stand on a step or a stair, balancing on your heels and arches, with your toes hanging off the edge of the step. Hang on for support, and lift your toes 8 to 15 times.

Chapter 13

Demystifying Strength Equipment

Some weight-lifting contraptions look like the convergence of a gynecological examination table, a minimalist sculpture, and an all-terrain vehicle. It's only natural to stare at them and think: Where do I sit? What do I push? Has anyone ever been killed on one of these things?

As far as we know, no one has ever exploded on the Butt Blaster or been mashed into lunchmeat by the leg-press machine. Weight equipment is not as complicated as it appears. Still, you need to know what the heck you're looking at and how to use each machine safely. In this chapter, we cover the vast array of strength-training equipment that you can use at home or at health clubs, including the latest developments in gym machines and free weights. We explain the pros and cons of each type of device and help you choose the right equipment for your goals. For advice on buying strength equipment for your home, see Chapter 20.

Weight Machines

If you can unfold a lawn chair, you're more than qualified to operate a weight machine. It all comes down to two relatively simple acts: You adjust your seat and then you either push or pull a bar or a set of handles. These handles are connected to a cable, chain, or lever, which, in turn, is attached to a stack of rectangular weight plates. Each plate in the stack weighs between 5 and 20 pounds, depending on the make and model, and has a hole drilled in the center. If you want to lift 30 pounds, you stick a metal peg, called a *pin,* into the hole on the plate marked "30." When you pull the machine's handles, the cable picks up 30 pounds.

You may also come across machines that don't have a weight stack. Instead, you adjust the poundage by sliding donut-shaped weight plates onto a thick peg. Jargon-heads call these *plate-loaded machines.* The weight plates are the same ones used for loading up barbells. (See the "Free Weights" section later in this chapter for details about weight plates.) The two most popular brands of plate-loaded machines are Hammer Strength and CYBEX. Many plate-loaded machines are designed so that each arm or leg works independently of the other, a feature we like because it forces your weaker side to work hard.

Weight machines have been around for more than a hundred years. Back in the '60s, Arthur Jones, inventor of the Nautilus machines, created the most significant innovation in weight machines to date. Jones realized that when you lift a barbell or dumbbell, there are certain points during the exercise that feel very heavy and certain points that feel light. (Try a biceps curl with a dumbbell, and you see that the dumbbell is hardest to move when your forearm is parallel to the floor.) Because your muscle is only fully working at the instances where the weight is difficult to lift, Jones concluded, traditional exercises don't give your muscles a complete workout. Then Jones realized that if you use a machine with a kidney-shaped pulley rather than a round one, your muscles feel resistance during the entire exercise and can be strengthened more completely.

Most of today's weight machines still work under the same principles that Jones discovered, but they have become smoother, safer, and more comfortable to use. Most of the top brands, including Body Masters, CYBEX, Hammer Strength, Nautilus, LifeFitness, and ICARIAN do an excellent job. The brands generally differ in the size and shape of the pulleys; the angles of the bars, seats, and weight stacks; and the type of seat and handle adjustments. You may like the Nautilus chest press but prefer the CYBEX back machine. Try every machine in your gym at least once. Even if the machines are all the same brand, you may feel more comfortable using, say, the vertical chest press rather than the horizontal one.

The weight machines designed for home use — called *multi-gyms* — generally aren't as sophisticated as health-club machines, but in many cases, your muscles won't know the difference.

The advantages of machines

Machines are ideal for beginners, because they're quite safe. If you can't muster the strength to finish an exercise, you don't have to worry about dropping a bar on your chest. But one caveat: Don't stick any body part near a weight stack that is being lifted or lowered. Liz saw a woman place her hand on a weight stack as she pulled out the pin. Sixty pounds of weight came crashing down on the woman's palm. She was rushed to the hospital, where her hand was repaired with eight stitches. Liz also saw a woman with long hair lean over to pull out a pin before lowering the weight stack; the last

4 inches of her hair got pressed between the weights. Fortunately, Liz and other staff members were able to rectify the situation without giving the woman a new hairstyle.

Most machines require little coordination; they basically hold your body in position and guide you through the motion. Consider the shoulder-press machine. You simply sit in a chair and push the handles up — all your effort goes into lifting those handles. But if you're shoulder pressing with a barbell (defined in the "Free Weights" section later in this chapter), you not only have to push the bar up but also have to keep it balanced and steady. Initially, your arms may wobble back and forth. Even after you get the hang of it, the exercise always requires a certain amount of balance and coordination.

You may come across one type of machine that does require coordination. These "free-floating" machines look like regular weight machines, but the levers don't move in a fixed pathway. You have to control the motion so the bar doesn't wobble. These machines are designed to give machine users a free-weight feel while retaining the safety aspect of machines. But we're not high on the concept. We think these machines are too complicated for beginners and not very satisfying for advanced lifters. If an experienced lifter wants the feel of free weights, he'll likely prefer the real McCoy.

Another plus for traditional machines: They're helpful for isolating a particular muscle group. *Isolating* is just gymspeak for zeroing in on one muscle (actually, using a single joint in a motion) rather than getting several muscles or joints into the act. This is helpful if you're trying to correct a specific weakness. For example, if your hamstrings (rear-thigh muscles) are underdeveloped, you can use a machine that holds your whole body still while you bend your legs to target your hamstrings. With free weights, you'll have a harder time strengthening your hamstrings without working your front-thigh and butt muscles, too.

Finally, machines — at least those with weight stacks — let you get in a faster workout with less stopping and starting to adjust the weights. Instead of sliding weight plates on and off or removing free weights from the rack, you simply place a pin in a hole and adjust the seat. If your gym has 10 or 12 machines grouped in a circle, square, or similar shape, you can move from one right to the other, exercising your whole body in less than 20 minutes. Typically, machines that work your larger muscle groups (chest, back, butt, and thighs) come before machines that work your shoulders and arms.

The drawbacks of weight machines

You may want to stick to machines initially, but plan to mix in some free weights after a month or two of working out two or three days a week. Machine circuits can get pretty boring — for you and your muscles. You need to stimulate your muscles with at least occasional changes in your workout. Typically, a gym has only two or three machines for each muscle group; with free weights, you can strengthen each muscle with dozens of exercises.

Weight machines for women

Many women don't fit into conventional weight-training machines. Either their legs dangle off the floor when they hop up into the seats, or their arms are too short to reach the bar they're supposed to grab.

About ten years ago, Nautilus recognized these problems and designed weight-training machines especially for women. Today you can find these machines in women-only gyms and in many large gyms that have several lines of equipment. Some gyms carry only one or two pieces, usually chest machines because they're the ones smaller women have the most trouble using.

In addition to downsizing the frames, Nautilus researchers studied the way women lift weights. They found that, like men, women are stronger at certain points in an exercise and weaker at other points; however, they also discovered that for men and women these points are not the same. So, they set up the machines' pulleys differently from conventional machines to give women a better workout. They also made the weight increments smaller — you can go up by 5 pounds instead of 10.

Liz likes the Nautilus women's line a lot because she is, shall we say, not anyone's first choice to play center on a basketball team. The line includes the only *pec deck* (a type of chest machine with a butterfly motion) she has ever used that didn't make her feel as if her shoulder was going to be ripped out of its socket.

Realize, too, that every weight machine won't fit every body. Most machines are designed for people of average height, so if you're shorter than 5'4" or taller than 6'2", you may not be able to adjust the seat to fit your body. (Figuring out which machines don't fit may take you a while, however. Unlike amusement parks, gyms don't post height-requirement signs.) Manufacturers have tried to get around the height problems by offering a variety of pads to sit on or stick behind you, but they don't work for everyone. If a machine feels uncomfortable to you — even if you're of average height — try another machine that targets the same muscle group or head for the free-weight area. As we describe in the "Weight machines for women" sidebar, Nautilus makes a line of machines scaled for women's bodies.

Another drawback of machines is that many of them isolate each muscle group. We know we said this was an advantage, but it can be a flaw. Because you rarely isolate your muscles in everyday life, some experts believe it doesn't make sense to train them that way in the gym. If muscles become used to working as separate entities, the theory goes, they don't cooperate with one another to the extent they should — a situation that may set you up for injuries.

Consider the lying leg curl, a popular hamstring machine. You lie flat on your stomach and then bend your knees until your heels approach your rear end. This exercise does a nice job of focusing on your hamstrings, but when in real life do you lie on your stomach and kick yourself in the butt? (Actually, we have relatives who do this when they throw tantrums, but apparently they don't need to train for them.) Some experts believe you're better off strengthening your hamstrings with exercises such as squatting, a motion you use often in daily life, like when you pick up a heavy box. Because each has its advantages, we recommend doing both free-weight and machine exercises.

One final reason to venture beyond machines: You can't take 'em with you. If you're on vacation and your hotel gym has nothing more than a pile of dumbbells, you need to know what to do with them. Don't give yourself another excuse to blow off a workout.

Special tips for machines

Don't let weight machines scare you. Use the following tips to look like an old pro next time you go to the gym:

- ✔ **Make the adjustments.** Don't just hop on a machine and start pumping away. If the last guy who used it was a foot taller than you are, you may find yourself suspended in midair in the middle of the exercise.

  To adjust a machine, you usually have to pull out a pin, shift the seat up or down, and then reinsert the pin. Adjusting the seat is a hassle at first, but if you don't do it, you set yourself up for an injury. Also, you cheat yourself out of a good workout. For instance, if you don't adjust the biceps-curl machine correctly, you may compensate by using your back muscles, thereby defeating the purpose of the exercise.

  Let a trainer show you how to adjust each machine to fit your body. In general, line up the joint that you're trying to move (your knees, for example) with the joint of the machine that's moving. You shouldn't have to strain in any way to do the movement. If you begin to feel any discomfort, particularly in your joints, stop the exercise and readjust the set or position, as needed.

- ✔ **Check the weight stack before you lift.** Never begin the exercise without checking where the pin has been inserted. If someone has *racked* the machine (put the pin all the way on the bottom so the entire weight stack is captured), either your eyes are going to pop out of your head or you're going to be mighty embarrassed when you can't budge it. When you first learn to use a machine, write down the weight and seat adjustment ("leg extension: 30 lbs., second setting") on a card or in a workout log. Carry these notes with you and update them regularly.

✓ **Remember the name of each machine.** You should not refer to the lat pull-down as "that one where you pull down that bar thingy." Knowing what to call each contraption reminds you what the heck you're doing — you'll remember that you're working your lats, assuming you remember what those are. (If you don't, see Chapter 12.) Most machines have some sort of name plaque or label. Check that the name of the machine you're using corresponds to the name of the machine on your workout card.

✓ **Stay in control.** If the weight stack bangs and clangs like a junior-high marching band, you're probably lifting too fast, and you're definitely annoying the guy on the machine next to you. Many machine manufacturers recommend taking two slow counts to lift the weight stack up and four slow counts to lower the weight stack down. You may feel more comfortable speeding it up to a 2-2 count. When you become a more advanced lifter, you may want to try SuperSlow training, a method that involves a full 20 seconds per repetition. We describe this controversial technique in Chapter 14.

✓ **If the machine has a seat belt, use it.** We're not aware of any gyms that enforce seat-belt laws, but that belt is there for a reason: to keep you stable while you move through an exercise. Not every machine has one, so check carefully.

✓ **Change the weight in the smallest increment possible.** Most machines have half plates hanging on the frame. Instead of increasing your weight by an entire plate, you can place this thin rectangle on top of the stack. CYBEX and other equipment manufacturers have come up with an ingenious way to increase weight by one-third of a plate, a system used on some of its machines. Each machine has an abacus-like apparatus linked to the stack of 20-pound weight plates. To increase the weight, you slide a weighted disk toward the stack, increasing the weight by 5 pounds. There are three disks per abacus, allowing you to go from 10 pounds to 15 pounds to 20 before moving on to a new plate.

Free Weights

Free weights are nothing to be afraid of. They're simply bars with weight plates on each end, and they're perfectly suitable for people who don't envision a Mr. Olympia title in their future. The long bars are called *barbells,* and the short bars are called *dumbbells* (see Figure 13-1). It takes two hands to hoist a barbell. You can lift a dumbbell with one hand, although you may do some exercises using two hands on a single dumbbell.

Barbells and dumbbells are called *free weights* because they're not attached to any chains, cables, or weight stacks. You're free to do with them whatever you want, although we recommend using them for strength training rather than, say, banging nails into a wall.

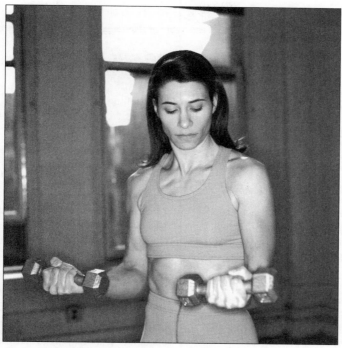

Figure 13-1:
You can use dumbbells for hundreds of exercises.

Photograph by Sunstreak Productions, Inc.

At most gyms, you find a wide array of dumbbells, lined up from lightest, usually 3 pounds, to heaviest, as much as 200 pounds. At larger gyms, you also find a selection of bars with plates welded to each end, starting with 20 pounds and increasing in 10-pound increments.

Virtually every gym has bars without weight plates on each end. The *long bar* (also called an *Olympic bar*) alone usually weighs 45 pounds. To increase the poundage, you slide *weight plates* — round plates with a hole through the center — to each end. You then secure the plates with clips called *collars*. An assortment of these weight plates, typically from 2½ pounds to 45 pounds, sits on a rack near the bars. If you want to lift 75 pounds, you add a 10-pound plate and a 5-pound plate to each side of the 45-pound bar. After you finish, be sure to remove these plates and put them back in their proper place. Otherwise, you risk unfriendly stares from the staff and the guy or gal who uses the bar after you.

If you're lucky, your gym will have weight plates made by Iron Grip. These plates are easier to carry than the traditional ones because they have handles built in. Imagine the difference between carrying a suitcase with a handle and without. We suspect they prevent back problems caused by improperly lifting standard weight plates. The handles also keep the plates from slipping and dropping to the floor. A few other brands have copied this concept, but we like Iron Grip the best.

How to spot and be spotted

If you spend enough time in the gym, sooner or later someone is going to ask you, "Hey, mind giving me a spot?" He's not asking you to buy him a puppy; he would like assistance with his next set. You should be flattered at the request, but be aware that spotting is an awesome responsibility. It falls on your shoulders to prevent the weight from, well, falling on the guy's shoulders.

By the way, don't hesitate to ask for a spot yourself if you think you may have trouble completing a set. A spotter is particularly helpful when you graduate to a heavier weight. You can enlist help from a health-club staff member; or better yet, ask anyone nearby who doesn't look too busy. (This is a good way to make friends at the gym, too.) Fill your spotter in on your game plan. Mention how many reps you think you can do and on which rep you think you'd like to call in the cavalry.

Here's how to handle the job of spotting a fellow weight lifter:

✔ **Pay attention at all times.** Don't get into a heated discussion about the war in Iraq. You need to be ready, on a split-second's notice, to lift the bar off your spottee's chest if his arms give out. Politely tune out the rest of the world until your spottee completes his set.

✔ **Ask your spottee where he'd like you to place your hands.** There are several schools of thought on this subject. You can rest a fingertip or two on the bar at all times so you can give instantaneous help when your spottee calls for it — usually during the last repetition or two. Some people, including us, find that position annoying, because it diminishes the feelings of glory you experience when you complete a set by yourself. We prefer the ready-willing-and-able spotting technique. That is, have your hands poised a couple inches from the bar; touch the bar only when your spottee begins to struggle. Some spotters also place their hands on the joint or limb doing the movement, as close to the bar as possible (for example, on the wrists).

✔ **If you don't think you can handle spotting someone, say so.** This is no time for heroics. In order to spot someone bench-pressing 100 pounds, you need not be able to bench 100 pounds yourself — you're just there to help out. However, if you have trouble lifting the 5-pounders off the rack, you're not a candidate for this job.

✔ **Use proper posture.** This means not rounding your spine, keeping a good center of gravity, and making sure you're in a stable position.

✔ **Don't over-spot.** You're there to help the guy, not do the work for him. When you're spotting someone on the bench press, don't lean directly over the bar, grip it with both hands, and pull it up and down. With a little experience, you'll be able to provide just the right amount of additional effort that the person needs to complete the exercise. (If you're the one being spotted, you may want to say something like, "Don't help me until I really need it." You can also scream, "I got it! I got it!" if it looks like your spotter is going to prematurely swoop in to help.)

✔ **Always offer encouraging words.** Say things like "It's all yours! You got it! You got it! All you!" This gives your spottee inspiration to squeeze out that last repetition. Plus, it makes everyone else in the gym glance over in admiration.

✔ **No matter which end of the spot you're on, pleasant breath is a must.** Remember, you'll be breathing forcefully right into someone's face. You don't want to find a bottle of Scope waiting for you in your locker.

The advantages of free weights

Free weights are much more versatile than machines. Whereas a weight machine is designed for one particular motion, a single pair of dumbbells can be used to perform literally hundreds of exercises. For instance, you can push dumbbells overhead to work your shoulders, press them backward to tone your triceps, or hold one in each hand while you squat to strengthen your thighs and butt muscles. You can change the feel and emphasis of an exercise by simply altering the way you grip the bar.

Another important benefit of free weights is that they work your muscles in a way that closely mimics real-life movements. Machines tend to isolate a particular muscle so the rest of your muscles don't get any action. But free-weight training requires several muscles to move, balance, and steady a weight as you lift and lower it. Free-weight exercises allow you to strengthen muscles that wouldn't get much work if you were doing isolation exercises with machines. Some people find they gain strength and increase in size faster when they do the majority of their exercises with free weights.

The drawbacks of free weights

For some novices, free-weight exercises are hard to get the hang of. You need more instruction than you do with machines — there are a lot more mistakes to make and injuries to avoid. Also, free-weight exercises require more balance than machine moves. If you're short on time, a free-weight workout probably will take you longer than a machine workout. Instead of simply putting a pin in a weight stack, you may have to slide weight plates on and off a bar. But if a gym has various free weights available without having to change plates, this may not be the case.

Special tips for free weights

Anyone using free weights needs to be very careful, even with light weights. Debbie Bacon of Phoenix, Arizona, learned this lesson the hard way. While waiting for her husband to come home late one night, Debbie decided exercising might help her stay awake. She was doing shoulder exercises with 7-pound dumbbells when she got so tired that she lost control of the weights and they crashed together. Unfortunately, her right index and ring fingers got in the way. The incident involved a fractured fingertip and a piece of acrylic nail that got lodged where it shouldn't have been. But we'll spare you the gory details. Suffice it to say that free weights require your full attention. Here are a few other tips to make free-weight training safe and fun:

WARNING!

✔ **If you're using very heavy weights, enlist a spotter.** (See Figure 13-2 and the sidebar "How to spot and be spotted" in this chapter.)

✔ **Be careful when you lift a weight from a rack and when you put it back.** Never pick up a weight off the floor without bending your legs.

✔ **Never drop the weights carelessly when you've completed a set.** The loud clang is sure to annoy your fellow lifters, and the weights may roll away and land on someone's toes.

✔ **Use two hands when lifting weight plates.** Remember that plates are weight, too, and you can just as easily hurt yourself placing a weight on a bar as you can performing an exercise. Don't attempt to lift a weight plate onto a bar if it's too heavy for you.

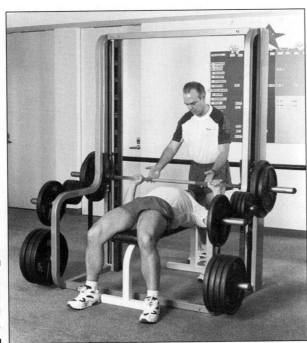

Figure 13-2:
Spotting
the bench
press.

Photograph by Sunstreak Productions, Inc.

A word about benches

A bench can help you get a better workout. Some benches are flat, and some are upright, like narrow chairs with high, padded backs. Others are adjustable so you can slide them to an incline or decline position. Here are some tips for using benches:

✔ **Experiment with the angle of the bench, especially for chest exercises.** Inclining the bench a few degrees allows you to work the muscle fibers of your upper chest. (But attempting chest exercises at too high an angle can put your shoulder joint in jeopardy.) Declining the bench emphasizes your lower chest. You can use a slightly different angle each workout if you want.

✔ **Use a bench for support.** When you're doing overhead lifts or bicep curls, adjust the seat so it's upright, and sit snugly against it. This position protects your back and prevents you from cheating. You won't be able to rock your body back and forth to build momentum to hoist the dumbbell. You have to rely solely on the muscle power of your biceps. However, you'll still have to stop yourself from arching the small of your back off the bench when the weight gets heavy.

✔ **Use weight-lifting benches for one activity only: lifting weights.** Don't use a bench to change a light bulb at home and don't use it at the gym to take a nap. Never use a weight bench for step aerobics. You can, however, use your step bench as a weight bench as long as you're not lifting dumbbells heavier than, say, 30 pounds.

✔ **Keep your feet flat on the floor or flat on the bench — whichever is more comfortable.**

✔ **Don't put your feet up in the air, especially if you're a beginner.** This creates an unstable position and looks like you want your stomach scratched. Instead, keep your feet firmly planted on the floor.

Cable Pulleys

At most gyms, you see a box full of ropes, straps, handles, short bars, long bars, V-shaped bars, and bars shaped like a handlebar mustache. This paraphernalia looks like a pile of junk excavated from someone's garage. But in fact, these are the attachments you can clip onto a cable machine to do a wide variety of exercises. The cable machine consists of a cable and a round pulley attached to a metal frame.

To strengthen your back, you can pull down a bar clipped to a high pulley — one that's attached all the way at the top. To strengthen your biceps, you can pull up on a low pulley — attached near the bottom of the frame, typically a few inches from the floor. To strengthen your chest, you can grab a high pulley on each side of the frame and pull both handles toward your chest, as if you're going to wrap your arms around someone.

Cable pulleys are a cross between machines and free weights. On the one hand, the cable is hooked up to a stack of weights, so nothing can come crashing down. On the other hand, the motion isn't guided — you're free to pull the bar down the way you want to, and you're free to make lots of mistakes. Like free weights, cable machines require a certain amount of control.

Don't be afraid to play around with the different types of adjustments. Attaching a new bar is easier than it looks, and you may find that, when working your triceps, a V-shaped bar feels more comfortable than a straight bar. When you do make the switcheroo, you may need to adjust the amount of weight you're using. Even if you're doing the very same exercise, you may use more weight pulling down the V-shaped bar than you would pulling down the straight bar.

Tubes and Bands

Exercise tubes are like the thick rubber tubes you can find in a medical-supply store — they just come in brighter colors. Some exercise tubes have handles or buckles attached to each end (see Figure 13-3), or they come in a kit with attachable plastic bars and door attachments. You also can buy *exercise bands,* which are long, flat sheets of strong rubber.

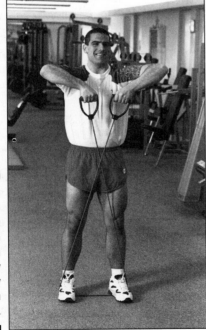

Figure 13-3:
You can use
exercise
tubes to
strengthen
virtually
every
muscle in
your body.

Photograph by Sunstreak Productions, Inc.

You can exercise virtually every muscle group in your body with bands and tubes, although tubes work better for some exercises, while bands work better for others. You just have to experiment. Here's how you can use bands to work both of your biceps at once: You stand on the center of the band and hold an end in each hand, with your elbows by your sides. Bend your arms and curl your hands up toward your shoulders. Lower your arms slowly so the band doesn't just snap back into place. (You can find a whole chapter full of band exercises in our book *Weight Training For Dummies,* published by Wiley.)

The advantages: Bands and tubes take up zero space, and they're portable. They give you an instant strength workout, whether you're in a small studio apartment, in a hotel room, or on a camping trip in the Mojave Desert. Bands and tubes are easy to adjust, too; to make an exercise tougher, just use a shorter or thicker band or step farther away to stretch the band further and increase the level of resistance. They're also cheap: You can purchase a couple of bands for around $10. Even if you go hog wild, you'd have trouble spending more than $60 on a set of bands, a travel bag, and a video explaining how to use the bands.

The drawbacks: If a band or tube slips, you can get snapped in the face or groin. Ouch. Also, reproducing the same amount of work from one workout to the next is difficult. You know when you're lifting a 20-pound dumbbell or a 50-pound weight stack, but bands and tubes have no comparable measuring system. They simply come in different resistances: usually light, medium, heavy, and extra-heavy. (There's no universal code for color. One company's yellow band may be the easiest resistance, whereas another company's yellow band may be the most difficult. Look for band thickness.) Also, know that there's a limit to how much strength you can gain with bands.

When you're using bands and tubes, keep the following tips in mind:

- ✔ **Lift and lower the band or tube slowly.** If you move carefully, you'll feel your muscles working in both directions.

- ✔ **Don't wrap the band or tube so tightly around your palms or feet that you cut off the circulation to your hands or feet.** Instead, wrap it loosely several times so that it forms loops, the way you wind a dog's leash around your hand.

- ✔ **When you wrap a band or tube under your feet, make sure that it's secure.** You don't want a band to slip out from under you.

- ✔ **Use bands or tubes that are specifically designed for exercising.** Inspect them frequently for holes and tears and replace them when they're worn.

Your Body

Yes, your very own body can function as strength equipment. You can lift it, lower it, curl it, twist it, and bend it in all sorts of ways that are designed to increase your strength. We're talking leg lifts, push-ups, pull-ups, and the like. When you move your body weight, you're fighting gravity — and that can be a considerable fight.

The advantages: You don't require any storage space and you certainly can take yourself anywhere. Plus, push-ups and pull-ups are impressive, and they call upon just about every muscle in your upper body. If you're really serious about building upper-body strength, add push-ups and pull-up-type exercises to your strength-training routine.

The drawbacks: Ever try a pull-up? They're darned hard. Most people can't do pull-ups until they've spent at least a few months lifting weights. And then, eventually, they have the opposite problem: The pull-ups become too easy. To continue making progress, you may need to invest in equipment or join a gym.

Chapter 14

Designing a Strength-Training Program

Scan the fitness aisle in any bookstore or video store and you find fitness experts who claim to have discovered the Secret, the Answer, the world's best solution to building a new you. "I can't stand to know a secret that can help others without telling them about it," says one popular instructor.

Well, we have a secret, too: There are no secrets to weight training. To find a program that works for you, you need to experiment with a variety of training methods. Lifting weight is an art, not an exact science.

In this chapter, we present an array of tools you can use to custom-design a strength-training program. We address questions such as, "How much weight should I lift?", "How many exercises do I need to do?", and "How many days a week should I work out?" There's no single answer to any of these questions. You need to decide what your goals are, which techniques you like best, and which ones your body responds to. Also, we recommend consulting with a qualified trainer at least once before you embark on a strength-training program. (See Chapter 4 for tips on finding a competent trainer.)

The Building Blocks of a Weight Workout

You can't begin to design a strength-training program without knowing two terms: rep and set.

> ✔ *Rep* is short for repetition — one complete motion of an exercise. Suppose you're doing a leg lift. When you lift your leg and then lower it back down, you've completed one rep.
>
> ✔ A *set* is a group of consecutive repetitions. For example, you can say, "I did two sets of ten reps on the chest press." This means that you did ten consecutive chest presses, rested, and then did another ten chest presses.

How many reps should I do?

The number of reps you should do depends on where you are in your training (new, experienced, coming back from a long layoff) and your goals. To become as strong and as big as your body type will allow, do fewer than eight or ten reps per set. To tone your muscles and develop the type of strength you need for everyday life — moving furniture or shoveling snow — aim for 10 to 12 repetitions. Doing dozens of reps with ultralight weights (weights you can barely even feel) doesn't bring good results of any kind, because you're not stressing your muscles enough.

No matter how many repetitions you do, always use a heavy enough weight so that the last rep is a struggle, but not such a struggle that you compromise good form. After about a month of strength training, you may want to go to *muscular failure* (that is, your last repetition is so difficult that you can't squeeze out one more).

If you have a few different goals in mind, you can mix and match the number of reps you do per workout. If you want to get bigger and stronger and also improve the endurance of those muscles, you can do a heavy workout one day and a lighter workout the next time out. Keep track of how you feel; your body may respond better to one type of training than another.

Be sure to adjust the amount of weight you use for each exercise. In general, use more weight to work larger muscles like your thighs, chest, and upper back, and use less weight to exercise your shoulders, arms, and abdominals. But even when doing different exercises for the same muscle group, you're likely to need a variety of weights. For example, you typically can handle more weight on the flat chest-press machine than you can on the incline chest-press machine.

Write down how much weight you lift for each exercise so that next time around, you don't have to waste time experimenting all over again. But don't lock yourself into lifting a certain amount of weight every time. Everyone feels stronger on some days than on others. Just because you can bench-press 80 pounds on Monday doesn't mean you'll be able to do it on Wednesday. Listen to your body. It'll tell you what it can and can't handle.

How much should I lift?

To increase strength, you need to lift an amount that stresses your muscles. So, although we can't tell you a specific amount to lift, we can tell you that it has to be enough so that you feel challenged as you're lifting, and so that the last rep is difficult to complete (difficult, but still possible and still using good form).

After about age 30, you lose bone mass for the rest of your life. But don't let that frighten you, because there is a solution. To maintain bone density (that is, to build enough bone density to offset the loss of bone density that occurs as you age), you need to perform weight-bearing exercise. *Weight-bearing exercise* means that your skeleton is supporting any sort of weight, as it does when you walk, run, or — yes — lift weights. Theories abound as to why weight-bearing exercise builds bone density, but the most probable is that your body creates *osteoblasts,* or cells that form more bone when muscles are stressed. This phenomenon occurs when muscles flex and the tendons to which they're attached pull on the bone to which they are connected. This means that when your muscles (and, thus, your bones) are placed under pressure, as they are during weight-bearing exercise, your bones adapt to the pressure and become more dense (and that means they're stronger). Weight lifting is one of the best ways to build bone density, because you're loading your muscles (and, therefore, your bones) with weights. But keep in mind that as your muscles gain strength, you need to gradually increase the load on them by increasing the amount of weight you lift.

How do I know when I'm ready to lift more weight?

It won't take long to outgrow the weights you use during your first workout. When you can easily do the maximum number of reps you're aiming for, increase the weight by the smallest increment possible and drop down to fewer reps. You know you're lifting too much weight if you can't complete your repetitions with good form and if you feel the need to grunt.

Not all muscles improve at the same rate. After a month of weight training, you may jump up 20 pounds on a chest exercise but only 5 pounds on a shoulder exercise.

How fast should I do my reps?

Take a full 2 seconds to lift a weight and 2 to 4 seconds to lower it. If you lift more quickly than that, you may hear a lot of clanging and banging (of the weights). Plus you'll end up relying on momentum rather than muscle power. Going slow and steady yields better results because more of your muscle gets into the act.

Some trainers take this notion even further, advocating repetitions that last an excruciating 20 seconds or more, a technique called *SuperSlow* training. We think that SuperSlow workouts may have a place in advanced exercise routines but are too challenging and result in too much muscle soreness for novice exercisers.

SuperSlow works like this: You take 20 more seconds (which means moving in super-slow motion) to do each repetition and perform 3 to 5 reps. Although the number of reps may seem low, keep in mind that SuperSlow lifters spend about twice as much time on each exercise as do traditional weight lifters, and some swear they see more rapid improvements in strength, although those improvements haven't been borne out in studies.

This technique can be done with machines, free weights, or body weight (such as push-ups), and it's very, very hard, because you can't use any momentum the way you can with traditional weight lifting. In fact, SuperSlow is so exhausting that at one New York gym that advocates this approach, a sign on the wall warns exercisers not to drive for at least 30 minutes after a workout. SuperSlow training requires more patience than most people have, and even people who try it and like it rarely continue with the training. If you decide to try SuperSlow, it's best if you're coached through your reps by a trainer with experience using this technique.

We also disagree with many of the beliefs promoted by a group of trainers called the SuperSlow Exercise Guild. These trainers maintain that one or two weekly SuperSlow workouts are the best way to achieve fitness and that cardiovascular exercise is not a necessary part of fitness training, even to prevent conditions like heart disease and high blood pressure. We couldn't disagree more! As we explain throughout this book, the ideal fitness program includes a combination of cardiovascular, flexibility, and strength workouts.

How many sets should 1 do for each muscle group?

There's no simple answer. Several studies show that doing one set per muscle builds just as much strength as doing three sets per muscle, at least for the first three or four months of training. So here's our advice: If you're a novice or if you're starting again after a layoff, begin with one set of 10 to 12 repetitions, and make sure your last rep feels challenging. You should feel like you have control of the weight but if you did one more rep, you may not be able to make it all the way. Most people can increase their initial weights after two to four weeks of training; at that point, consider adding a second or even third set for each muscle group. However, if your goal is simply to build enough strength for good health, one challenging set may be sufficient.

If you're aiming for maximum strength or a physique like the ones you see on ESPN body-building competitions, you need to do at least 10 to 20 sets per muscle group!

How long should I rest between sets?

The amount of rest you take in between sets is another variable that you can toy around with. If you're a beginner, rest about 90 seconds between sets to give your muscles adequate time to recover. As you get in better shape, you need less rest — only about 30 seconds — before your muscles feel ready for another set. If you follow a chest exercise with, say, a thigh exercise, you typically need less rest than if you do consecutive exercises for the same muscle group, such as two chest exercises in a row.

After the first few weeks of training, you can fine-tune the amount of rest you take between sets according to your goals. If you're using really heavy weights and doing fewer reps in order to bulk up, you can take up to 5 minutes between sets so that your muscles can pump out their greatest effort each time.

If you're short on time or you like a fast-paced workout, try *circuit training:* You move quickly from exercise to exercise with little or no rest at all. Circuit training does a decent job of building strength, and can be a good substitute for an aerobic workout, especially if you start and end with a fairly long aerobic warm-up and cooldown. See Chapter 15 for details.

In what order should I do my exercises?

In general, exercise larger muscles before smaller ones. Work your back and chest before your shoulders and arms, and your butt before your thighs and calves. Smaller muscles assist the larger muscles. If the smaller muscles are too tired to pitch in and do their job, they give out long before your big muscles get an adequate workout. For example, your biceps help out your upper back when you do a *lat pull-down,* an exercise where you pull a bar down to your chest. If you work your biceps first, they'll be too tired to do their job during the pull-down, and your back muscles won't get as good a workout.

As for which muscles to start with — chest, back, or legs — that's up to you. You may want to begin with all your chest exercises and then move on to your back. Or you can alternate chest and back moves. You can fit your abdominal exercises in whenever you like, as long as you remember to do them. (See the "All about Abs" section for more on exercising your abdominals.)

How many times a week do I need to lift weights?

Start by lifting two or three days per week for several weeks, completing one set of 10 to 12 reps. Increase to two or three sets. If your aim is maximum strength, targeting each muscle three times a week may not give your muscles enough chance to rest. In that case, cut back to two workouts per muscle group per week.

If you really get into weight training, consider doing a *split routine,* in which you exercise some of your muscles during one workout, and then come back a day or two later to exercise the others. You still work each muscle at least twice a week, but because you don't train every muscle during every workout, you can devote more energy to the muscles you're focusing on that day — and each of your muscles still gets enough rest.

Splitting your routine is a good idea, especially if you're serious about building muscle and if you have free time in small chunks. You may be fresher and more motivated if you walk into the gym knowing that, today, you have to work only your chest, triceps, and shoulders. You probably work these muscles harder than if you try to fit all your muscle groups into one workout.

Here are the two most popular ways of splitting a routine:

✔ **Push/pull:** Work your *pulling muscles* (your back muscles and biceps) on one day, and during the next session, work your *pushing muscles* (your chest and triceps). You can fit in your leg, shoulder, and abdominal exercises whenever you want. Following is an example of a push/pull routine. In Chapter 12, we list several exercises for each muscle group; you can learn them from a trainer or a book.

Day	*Muscles Worked*
Monday	Push (chest, triceps, shoulders, lower-body exercises)
Tuesday	Pull (back, biceps, abdominals)
Wednesday	REST
Thursday	Push (chest, triceps, shoulders, lower-body exercises)
Friday	REST
Saturday	Pull (back, biceps, abdominals)
Sunday	REST

✔ **Upper body/lower body:** You work your upper body one day and your lower body the next. You fit in your abs two to four times a week whenever it's convenient. (See Chapter 12 for definitions of gluteals, quadriceps, and the like.)

Day	Muscles Worked
Monday	Upper body (back, chest, shoulders, triceps, biceps)
Tuesday	Lower body (gluteals, quadriceps, hamstrings, calves, abdominals)
Wednesday	REST
Thursday	Upper body (back, chest, shoulders, triceps, biceps)
Friday	REST
Saturday	Lower body (gluteals, quadriceps, hamstrings, calves, abdominals)
Sunday	REST

Whatever workout schedule you design, make sure each muscle group gets at least one full day of rest between sessions. You can lift two days back to back, but you don't want lift with your upper body, for example, two days in a row. Lifting weight literally creates tiny little tears in your muscles. They need those 48 hours to recover and rebuild. (You can do aerobic training on consecutive days because it's much easier on your muscles than weight training.) If you don't rest in this way, you may wind up sore and more prone to overuse injuries. (Keep in mind that perpetual soreness can be a sign of overtraining.) Besides, overworking a muscle may weaken it, defeating your purpose for training.

How often should I change my routine?

Some people change some or all of their exercises every time they work out. There's no hard-and-fast rule on this subject, but we recommend that you try at least one new exercise every month. After you learn a basic routine, such as the one we demonstrate in the last section of this chapter, expand your repertoire so that you have more options to choose from. Varying your exercises keeps you more interested and can help you get better results. If you stick with the same routine month after month, year after year, your muscles adapt to those exercises; but by working your muscles from a variety of angles, you involve more muscle fibers and keep your muscles challenged.

Changing your exercises isn't the only way to keep you — and your muscles — stimulated. You also can play with other variables, such as how many sets and reps you perform and how much rest you take between sets.

Advanced weight-training techniques

We call the following techniques advanced, but novices can use them, too (most of them, anyway — we let you know which ones are off limits for beginners).

✔ **Super set:** You do two consecutive sets of different exercises, preferably ones that exercise opposite muscle groups (like quadriceps and hamstrings) without resting in between. For example, you can do one chest exercise immediately followed by a different chest exercise and then take a rest. The idea is to completely tire out the muscle — to work it so hard that you reach the deepest muscle fibers. You also can do a super set with exercises that target different muscle groups, like a chest exercise followed by a leg exercise. With this type of super set, you don't rest between exercises — the purpose is simply to save time.

✔ **Pyramids:** You do multiple sets of an exercise, increasing the weight for each set while decreasing the number of reps. You may do a light warm-up set for ten reps, then a heavier set for eight reps, then an even heavier set for six reps, and so on, until you reach a weight at which you can do only one rep. You don't have to go all the way down to one rep for your workout to be considered a pyramid. The idea is to work up slowly and fatigue the muscle.

✔ **Negatives:** Someone helps you lift a weight, and then you're on your own for the lowering, or *negative,* phase of the lift. Your muscles generally can handle more weight when you lower a weight than when you lift it, so this technique gives you a chance to really tire out your muscles. *Note:* If you're a beginner, don't try negatives. They can cause significant muscle soreness.

✔ **Breakdowns (also called *drop sets* or *descending sets*):** You lift a heavy weight, and as soon as you exhaust the muscle — however many reps it takes — you pick up a lighter weight and squeeze out a few more reps. You might do ten reps of an exercise and then drop 5 pounds and try to eke out three or four more reps. The theory is that you use more of your muscles this way. You have to dig deeper because the muscle fibers you normally use are already pooped out.

✔ **SuperSlow training:** See the "How fast should I do my reps?" section earlier in this chapter for details. *Note:* It's generally not for beginners.

Consider trying *periodization,* a method of organizing your workout program into several periods, each lasting about four weeks. Each phase has a different emphasis:

✔ The first month you may do a basic routine, using moderate weights and performing one set of eight to ten reps of each exercise.

✔ In the next period, you may go for more strength, lifting heavier weights, doing six to eight repetitions and taking more rest between sets.

✔ In the third phase, you may focus on building stamina, doing 10 to 12 repetitions and taking less rest between sets.

Periodization is great if you're a beginner, because it helps you focus on one goal at a time.

All about Abs

Abs are everywhere these days, from infomercials featuring "ab-flattening" products to the covers of fitness magazines, promising ten steps toward washboard abs. To have great-looking abs — and who doesn't want that? — you need to develop the abdominal muscles through strength training. But keep in mind that even rock-hard, six-pack abdominal muscles won't look like a washboard if they have a layer of fat over them. If you're overweight, abdominal strength training will hone your abs, but you won't see those ab muscles until you lose body fat.

There are more theories about abdominal strength training than there are about the Kennedy assassination. Here's our take on getting your midsection into shape. (Read Chapter 12 to discover the names and functions of your four abdominal muscles; see "The strength workout" section in this chapter for step-by-step instructions for the exercises mentioned here.)

- ✔ **Don't do abdominal exercises every day.** Your abs, like all your other muscle groups, need a day of rest between workouts. And be sure that, just like strengthening any other muscle group, your last few reps are difficult to complete.

- ✔ **Do up to 3 sets of 10 to 25 reps.** If you're able to whip off 100 ab exercises without breaking a sweat, chances are you're doing the exercises too quickly or are engaging muscles other than the abs to complete the exercise. See the following section for two exercises (Basic Crunch and Ball Crunch) that isolate the abdominal muscles.

- ✔ **Stay away from abdominal machinery.** Instead, stick with exercises performed on the floor, such as the crunch and moves performed with a physioball (both demonstrated in the following section). We're not fond of most abdominal weight machines because they tend to bring the lower-back or hip muscles into the act. Nor do we like those abdominal infomercial gadgets that you can strap over your knees or stick under your butt; they force you to pay money for something you don't need.

The only type of ab device we're not entirely opposed to are ab-roller contraptions. You've probably seen them on TV: You lie in the center of a semi-circular metal frame, rest your head on a foam pad, place your arms atop the curve of the frame, and curl upward in a crunching motion. An ab roller can function like training wheels on a bike, guiding you through the correct path of motion until you're strong enough and skilled enough to perform it on your own. Also, it supports your head to reduce neck pain. However, when you're past the remedial stage of ab training, foregoing the ab roller and performing crunches under your own power is more effective. (Still, some trainers like to use the ab roller on occasion for the sake of variety.)

✓ **If you can do more than 12 reps of an abdominal exercise, you're either doing the reps too quickly or with poor form, or the exercise is too easy for you.** As with any other exercise, you should be struggling on the last repetition. Doing 100 continuous reps of any ab exercise is inefficient.

✓ **To make abdominal exercises more challenging, you can do them at a slight incline, so that your head is lower than your legs.** This is more effective than holding a weight plate on your abdomen. However, don't fix your feet in place; this shifts the work from your abdominals to the muscles in your lower back and at the front of your hips.

A Simple Functional Workout

In this section, we provide you with a *total-body workout* — a snazzy term referring to a routine that covers all the major muscle groups in your body. You can perform this routine either at home or at the gym. All you need for this workout are dumbbells (four to eight pairs should suffice) and a weight bench. In case you have access to health-club machines, we include a second exercise, which we call a gym alternative, for each muscle group.

This section also offers general rules for lifting weights safely as well as tips on how to progress after you master this workout.

Reading the exercise instructions

Don't worry: Our directions are in plain English, not like those assemble-it-yourself furniture manuals. For each exercise, we tell you which muscles the move targets. Then, where appropriate, we include a Warning icon that identifies potential joint injuries and reminds you to pay special attention if you've ever injured the joint in question. Never work through an injury; if you feel pain, review your technique and slow down the pace to make sure you're performing the move correctly. If you're using good form and you still hurt, skip the exercise for now. You may want to try it again after you've been exercising for a few weeks. Or, you may need to try a different exercise that targets the same muscle.

You notice that in the exercise descriptions, we use a few phrases over and over again. Here's a brief explanation of these phrases, which you're likely to hear from trainers and group-exercise instructors:

✓ **"Pull your abdominals in."** This doesn't mean to suck in your gut so hard that you can't breathe. Simply pull your abs slightly inward, a movement also known as tightening or contracting your abs. You're pulling your belly button up and in toward your spine. Imagine that you're wearing a pair of underwear that's one size too small; when you pull your abs in, it's like tightening the underwear another two sizes down. This position helps hold your torso still while you exercise, protecting your lower back from injury and ensuring that you're actually using the muscle you're intending to work.

✔ **"Stand up tall."** You don't need to stand like a guard at Buckingham Palace, but do lift your chest and keep your head centered between your shoulders. No slumping allowed!

✔ **"Tilt your chin toward your chest."** Tilt your chin just enough to fit your closed fist between your chest and chin. This position lines up the vertebrae of your neck with the rest of your spine. If you tilt your chin back or drop it toward your chest like you're sulking, you put excess pressure on your neck.

Lifting weights the right way

The way some people lift weights, you'd think they were in labor or impersonating a mountain gorilla. Grunting, screaming, and rocking back and forth are not indications of proper weight-lifting technique. We've seen people invent some pretty outrageous exercises. One guy bent over, picked up a very heavy dumbbell, lifted it straight over his head so that he almost fell backward, and then threw it to the ground so hard that it bounced and broke a mirror. He seemed quite pleased with himself.

Whether you're performing the exercises that we feature in this chapter — or any other exercise you try — the following rules always apply:

✔ **Always warm up.** Before you lift a weight, do at least five minutes of aerobic exercise to get your muscles warm and pliable. If you're going to do arm exercises and there aren't any upper-body aerobic machines around (such as a VersaClimber, rower, or cross-country skier), you can even do a few minutes of arm circles.

✔ **Good form is always more important than lifting a lot of weight.** Don't arch your back, strain your neck, or rock your body to generate momentum. Not only can these maneuvers cause injury, but they also make the exercises less effective.

✔ **Increase your weight by the smallest possible increment.** Jumping from a 5-pound weight to a 10-pounder doesn't sound like a big leap, but think about it: You're doubling the load on that muscle. If you're using a 5-pound weight, move up to a 6-, 7-, or 8-pounder. If your health club or home gym doesn't have interim weights, buy a pair of PlateMates — nifty magnets that you stick on each end of a dumbbell or barbell. (See Chapter 25 for details.)

✔ **Remember to breathe.** In general, exhale forcefully through your mouth as you lift the weight and inhale deeply through your nose as you lower it. Just don't overdo it because overly forceful breathing can leave you feeling lightheaded. Although proper breathing is important for speeding oxygen to your muscles, don't get hung up on the mechanics. Some people spend so much time trying to get the correct breathing pattern down that they lose track of what they're doing. Just don't hold your breath. You can bring about sharp increases in your blood pressure, and you can even faint from lack of air.

Do, however, hold your breath during extremely heavy lifts. This protects your spine by bracing it with the pressure from the held breath. We mention this information on the outside chance that some world-class power lifter reads this section and becomes incensed by the omission of it. Don't hold your breath unless you're aiming to lift world-record amounts of weight.

✔ **Use a full range of motion.** In other words, pull or push as far as you're supposed to. (If you're not sure, a trainer can show you the correct range of motion for each exercise. See Chapter 4 for tips on finding a personal trainer.) Using the full range of motion enhances your flexibility. However, you don't want to go past a natural range of motion because this can cause injury to the joint. For example, lifting dumbbells out to the side above shoulder level puts too much stress on the shoulder. Sitting down too far when you squat can cause knee injuries.

✔ **Pay attention.** Remind yourself which muscle you're working, and focus on that muscle. It's easy to do lat pull-downs without challenging your lats. And it's easy to do abdominal crunches without really working your abs. Suzanne recently watched a guy perform abdominal crunches with the sports section of the newspaper lying on his lap. He tried to steal a glance at the paper every time he curled his torso up. We suspect his abs aren't getting much in the way of results.

A word about the exercises

The 18 exercises described in this section aren't your only options. We could write an entire book about strength training exercises. In fact, we did write that book: *Weight Training For Dummies* (published by Wiley), which features more than 130 exercises using a vast array of equipment. So how did we choose the moves that we demonstrate in this book?

We emphasize dumbbell exercises because you can easily perform them at home or at the gym. The particular dumbbell exercises that we show here are all suitable for beginners; they don't require the brawn of an NFL defensive end or the coordination of an Olympic gymnast. Also, many of these moves perform double or triple duty; for example, the squat works three lower-body muscles — your front thighs, rear thighs, and derriere — in a single exercise.

The machines we show here generally mimic the dumbbell moves, working your muscles with a similar movement and from similar angles. Virtually every health club has these machines, in addition to other contraptions that work your muscles in different ways, and we highly recommend exercising each muscle group from a variety of angles. After you become familiar with the basic exercises shown here — in about six to eight weeks — we suggest you consult a trainer, a video, or other books to expand your repertoire.

The strength workout

In the following sections, we introduce you to some of our favorite strength exercises.

Squat

In addition to strengthening your butt muscles, the squat also does a good job of working your quadriceps and hamstrings. If you have hip, knee, or lower-back problems, restrict the distance your knees travel during this exercise by bending only part of the way down.

Getting set

With either your hands on your hips or holding dumbbells with your arms down at your sides, stand with your feet as wide apart as your hips and place your weight slightly back on your heels. Let your arms hang down at your sides. Pull your abdominals in and stand tall with square shoulders. (See Figure 14-1a.)

The exercise

Sit back and down, as if you're sitting into a chair (refer to Figure 14-1b). Lower as far as you can without leaning your upper body more than a few inches forward. Don't lower any farther than the point at which you're parallel to the floor, and don't allow your knees to shoot out in front of your toes. Once you feel your upper body fold forward over your thighs, straighten your legs and stand back up. Don't lock your knees at the top of the movement.

Technique tips

Keep these tips in mind as you perform the squat:

- **Keep your head up and eyes focused on an object directly in front of you.** Your body tends to follow your eyes, so if you're staring at the ground, you're more likely to fall forward. Imagine balancing a book on top of your head.

- **When you stand back up, push through your heels rather than shifting your body weight forward.** Don't let your heels (or toes) lift off the floor.

- **Try not to arch your back as you stand up.**

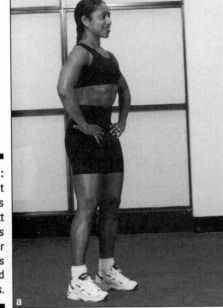
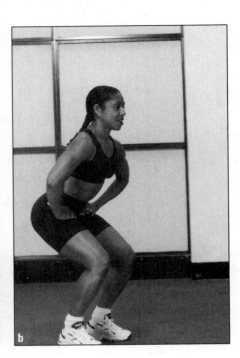

Figure 14-1:
The squat strengthens your butt and works your quadriceps and hamstrings.

Photograph by Sunstreak Productions, Inc.

Gym alternative: Leg-press machine

This is an excellent squat alternative for those who have chronic knee problems or who don't have good balance. Set the leg-press machine so that when you're lying on your back, your shoulders fit snugly under the shoulder pads, and your knees are bent to an inch or so below parallel to the foot plate. Place your feet as wide as your hips with your feet pointing forward. Grasp the handles. (See Figure 14-2.)

Pull your abdominals in and keep your head and shoulders on the back pad. Push upward until your legs are nearly straight, just short of locking. Then bend your knees, controlling the weight as you go down, until your thighs are parallel to the foot plate.

Standing calf raise

The standing calf raise targets your calf muscles, particularly the larger, outermost muscle that is responsible for the shape and size of your calves.

Getting set

Stand on the edge of a step. (Or, if you have a step-aerobics platform, place two sets of risers underneath the platform.) Stand tall with your abdominals pulled in, the balls of your feet firmly planted on the step, and your heels hanging over the edge. Rest your hands against a wall or a sturdy object for balance.

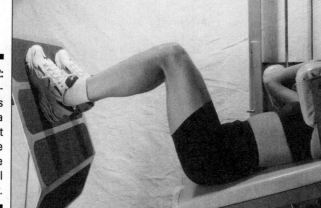

Figure 14-2:
The leg-press machine is a great alternative to the traditional squat.

Photograph by Sunstreak Productions, Inc.

The exercise

Raise your heels a few inches above the edge of the step so that you're on your tiptoes (see Figure 14-3a). Hold the position for a moment, and then lower your heels below the platform, feeling a stretch in your calf muscles (see Figure 14-3b).

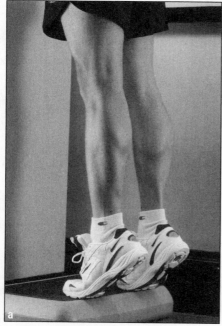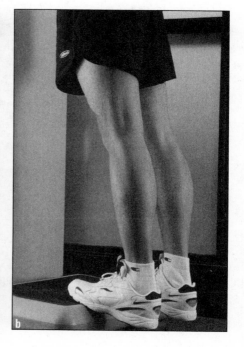

Figure 14-3:
The standing calf raise works your calf muscles.

Photograph by Sunstreak Productions, Inc.

Technique tips

Keep these tips in mind as you perform the standing calf raise:

- ✔ **Lift as high as you can onto your toes and lower your heels down as much as your ankle flexibility allows.**

- ✔ **Push evenly through the entire width of your foot.** Don't push off from your big toe or the outside edge of your feet.

Gym alternative: Toe press on the leg-press machine

Lie on the leg-press machine with your shoulders snugly underneath the pad. To lift the weight stack, straighten your legs completely, and carefully walk your feet down the foot platform until your heels hang off the end. Keeping your legs straight, rise up on your tiptoes as high as you can (see Figure 14-4) and then lower down until your heels are below the level of the foot plate. After you complete all the reps, carefully walk your feet back to the center of the foot plate before bending your knees and lowering the weights.

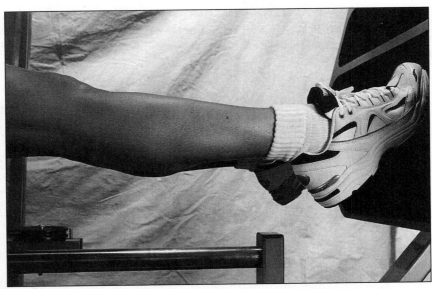

Figure 14-4:
As an alternative to the standing calf raise, try the toe press on the leg-press machine.

Photograph by Sunstreak Productions, Inc.

One-arm dumbbell row

Exercising your upper back without machinery isn't easy, but this move is one that does a good job. The one-arm dumbbell row also strengthens your biceps and shoulders. Be especially careful if you have lower-back problems.

Getting set

Stand to the right of your weight bench, holding a dumbbell in your right hand with your palm facing in. Place your left knee and your left hand on top of the bench for support. Let your right arm hang down and a bit forward. Pull your abdominals in and bend forward from the hips so that your back is naturally arched and roughly parallel to the floor, and your right knee is slightly bent. Tilt your chin toward your chest so that your neck is in line with the rest of your spine. (See Figure 14-5a.)

The exercise

Pull your right arm up until your elbow is pointing to the ceiling, your upper arm is parallel to the floor, and your hand comes to the outside of the ribcage (refer to Figure 14-5b). Lower the weight slowly back down.

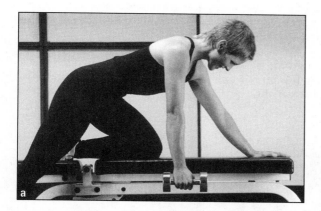

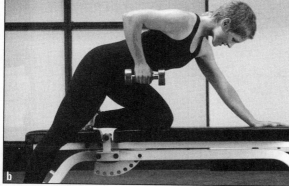

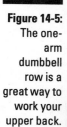

Figure 14-5: The one-arm dumbbell row is a great way to work your upper back.

Photograph by Sunstreak Productions, Inc.

Technique tips

Keep these tips in mind as you perform the one-arm dumbbell row:

- **Concentrate on pulling from your back muscles (right behind and below your shoulder).** Don't just move your arm up and down. Although your arm is moving, this is a back exercise. Think of your arm as a hook that connects to the weight and is pulled by the back.
- **Keep your abs pulled in tight throughout the motion.**
- **Don't let your back sag toward the floor or hunch up.**
- **Pull your shoulders back and down to set the shoulder blades.**

Gym alternative: Seated row machine

Set your seat height so that when you grasp the handles, your arms are level with your shoulders (see Figure 14-6). Sit tall in the seat facing the weight stack with your chest against the pad.

Remaining tall, pull the handles toward you to lift the weight stack. When your hands are a few inches in front of your chest, slowly straighten your arms to lower the weight.

Figure 14-6:
Try the seated row machine as an alternative to the one-arm dumbbell row.

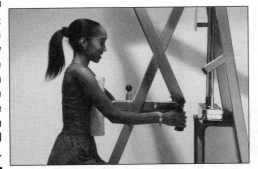

Photograph by Sunstreak Productions, Inc.

Dumbbell chest press

The dumbbell chest press closely mimics the bench press — the all-time favorite exercise among serious weightlifters everywhere. This exercise works your chest muscles, along with your shoulders and triceps. If you have shoulder, elbow, or lower-back problems, limit the range of motion. You should lower and lift the dumbbells only a few inches to avoid over-straining these joints.

Getting set

Lie on the bench with a dumbbell in each hand and your feet flat on the floor (or up on the bench if it's more comfortable). Push the dumbbells up so that your arms are directly over your shoulders and your palms up. Pull your abdominals in, and tilt your chin toward your chest. (See Figure 14-7a.)

The exercise

Lower the dumbbells down and a little to the side until your elbows are slightly below your shoulders (refer to Figure 14-7b). Roll your shoulder blades back and down, like you're pinching them together and accentuating your chest. Push the weights back up, taking care not to lock your elbows or allow your shoulder blades to rise off the bench.

Technique tips

Keep in mind the following tips as you perform the dumbbell chest press:

- ✔ **Let your back keep a natural arch so that you have a slight gap between your lower back and the bench.**

- ✔ **Don't contort your body in an effort to lift the weight.** Lift only as much weight as you can handle while maintaining good form.

- ✔ **When pressing the dumbbells up, have them form a triangular motion; they don't need to touch each other.**

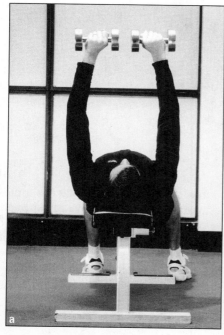 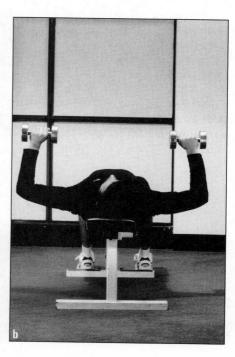

Figure 14-7: The dumbbell chest press works your chest muscles, shoulders, and triceps.

Photograph by Sunstreak Productions, Inc.

Gym alternative: Vertical chest-press machine

Sit so that the center of your chest lines up with the center of the horizontal set of handlebars. Press down on the foot bar so that the handles move forward. Grip the horizontal handles and push them forward, straightening your arms. Lift your feet from the foot bar so that the weight of the stack transfers into your hands. Slowly bend your arms until your elbows are slightly behind your chest (see Figure 14-8), and then push the handles forward until your arms are straight. After you complete the set, put your feet back on the foot bar and let go of the handles before you lower the weight stack all the way down.

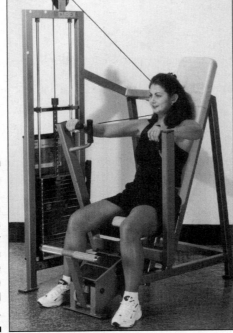

Figure 14-8:
The vertical chest-press machine is our pick for a gym alternative to the dumbbell chest press.

Photograph by Sunstreak Productions, Inc.

Dumbbell shoulder press

The dumbbell shoulder press targets your shoulders, placing some emphasis on your triceps and upper back. Use caution if you have lower-back, neck, or elbow problems.

Getting set

Hold a dumbbell in each hand and sit on a bench with back support. Plant your feet firmly on the floor about hip-width apart. Bend your elbows and raise your upper arms to shoulder height so the dumbbells are at ear level. Pull your abdominals in so there is a slight gap between the small of your back and the bench. Place the back of your head against the pad. (See Figure 14-9a.)

The exercise

Push the dumbbells up and in until the ends of the dumbbells touch lightly, directly over your head, and then lower the dumbbells back to ear level. (Refer to Figure 14-9b.)

Technique tips

Keep these tips in mind as you perform the dumbbell shoulder press:

- ✔ **Keep your elbows rigid without locking them at the top of the movement.**

- ✔ **Press your back against the back support without flattening out the curve in your back.**

- ✔ **Bring your arms and elbows down, keeping your elbow joints in line with your shoulders.**

- ✔ **If the bench is tall enough, keep your head against the back rest.**

- ✔ **Don't wiggle or squirm in an effort to press the weights up.**

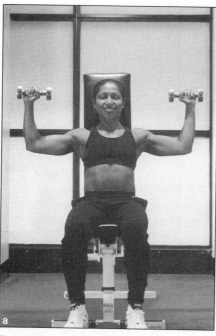
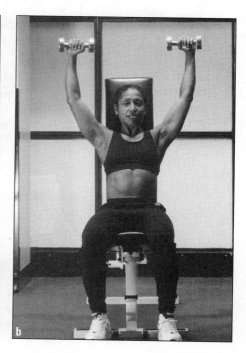

Figure 14-9: The dumbbell shoulder press works out your shoulders, triceps, and upper back.

Photograph by Sunstreak Productions, Inc.

Gym alternative: Shoulder-press machine

Set your seat height so that the shoulder-press machine's pulley is even with the middle of your shoulder. Hold onto each of the front handles (see Figure 14-10). Pull your abdominals in tight, but allow a slight natural gap to remain between the small of your back and the back pad.

Press the handles up without locking your elbows. Lower your arms until your elbows are slightly lower than your shoulders.

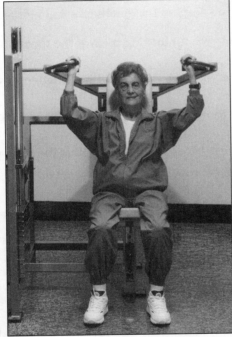

Figure 14-10:
Try the shoulder-press machine as an alternative to the dumbbell shoulder press.

Photograph by Sunstreak Productions, Inc.

External and internal rotation exercises

External and internal rotation exercises target your rotator-cuff muscles but strengthen your shoulder muscles as well. If these movements bother your neck, try resting your head on your outstretched arm.

Getting set

Hold a dumbbell in your right hand and lie on the floor on your left side. Bend your right elbow to a 90-degree angle and tuck it firmly against your side so that your palm is facing downward. Pull your abdominals in. Bend your left elbow and rest the side of your head in your left hand (see Figure 14-11a).

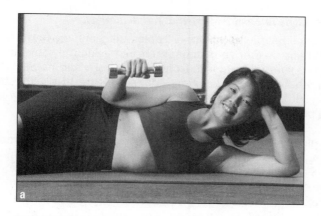

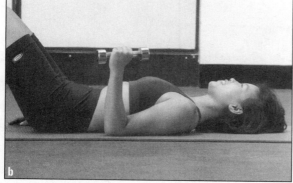

Figure 14-11:
Rotation
works your
rotator-cuff
muscles.

Photograph by Sunstreak Productions, Inc.

The exercises

Keeping your right elbow glued to your side, raise your right hand as far as you comfortably can. Slowly lower the weight back toward the floor. This exercise is *external rotation*. After you complete all the repetitions, switch the weight to your left hand and lie on your back (refer to Figure 14-11b). (You can also do this exercise lying on one side on the bench, with your forearm hanging off the bench.) Bend your elbow so your forearm is perpendicular to the floor and your palm is facing in. Lower your hand down and out to the side as far as you can, and then lift the weight back up. This exercise is *internal rotation*.

Technique tips

Keep these tips in mind as you perform external and internal rotation:

✓ **Use a very light weight.**

✓ **Imagine that your shoulder is the hinge of a door that is opening and closing.**

✓ **Keep your wrist straight.**

Gym alternative: Cable internal and external rotation exercises

Attach a horseshoe handle to the upper cable pulley and grasp the handle with your right hand so that your right arm is alongside the cable tower. Bend your arm so your forearm is in front of your body and parallel to the floor, and your elbow rests against your side (see Figure 14-12). Pull the handle across your body to lift the weight, and then slowly return your arm to the starting position. This exercise is *internal rotation*.

After you complete your reps, do *external rotation* with your left rotator cuff: Without changing position, hold the horseshoe handle in your left hand, so your forearm is across your waist. Keeping your left elbow against your side, pull the handle outward to lift the weight. To lower the weight, return to the starting position. To complete internal and external rotation on both arms, switch to the other side of the cable tower or turn your body around.

Figure 14-12:
Cable internal and external rotation exercises target your rotator-cuff muscles.

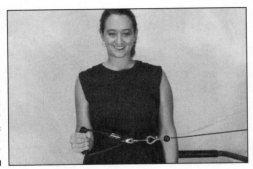

Photograph by Sunstreak Productions, Inc.

Dumbbell biceps curl

The dumbbell biceps curl targets your biceps, the muscles you rely on to hold heavy objects and look buff in sleeveless shirts. Use caution if you have lower-back or elbow problems.

Getting set

Hold a dumbbell in each hand and stand with your feet as wide apart as your hips. Let your arms hang down at your sides with your palms forward. Pull your abdominals in, stand tall, and keep your knees slightly bent. (See Figure 14-13a.)

The exercise

Curl both arms upward until they're in front of your shoulders (refer to Figure 14-13b). Slowly lower the dumbbells back down.

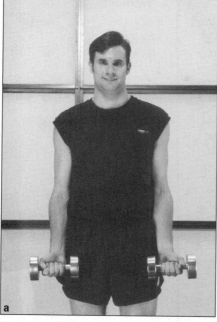
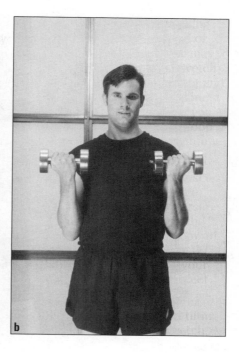

Photograph by Sunstreak Productions, Inc.

Figure 14-13: Keep your elbows close to your body while performing the dumbbell biceps curl.

Technique tips

Keep these tips in mind as you perform the dumbbell biceps curl:

- ✔ **Keep your knees slightly bent and your posture tall.** Don't lean back or rock your body forward to help lift the weight.

- ✔ **Keep your elbows as close to your body as you can without supporting your elbows on the sides of your stomach for leverage.**

- ✔ **Don't rest when you reach the top or bottom of the exercise; instead, keep a constant tension on the biceps.**

- ✔ **Lower the weight back to the starting position slowly and with control.**

Gym alternative: Arm-curl machine

Adjust the seat so when you sit down and extend your arms straight out, they're level with your shoulders, and your elbows are lined up with the moving hinge or pulley of the machine. Sit down and grasp a handle in each hand with your palms facing up.

Bend your elbows and pull the handles until they're just above your shoulders (see Figure 14-14). Then slowly lower the handles back down.

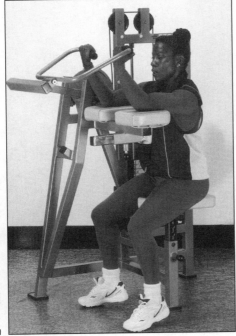

Figure 14-14:
We suggest
the arm-curl
machine as
a gym
alternative
to the
dumbbell
biceps curl.

Photograph by Sunstreak Productions, Inc.

Triceps kickback

The triceps kickback works your triceps, which assist the chest in just about every pushing movement. Use caution when doing this move if you have elbow or lower-back problems.

It's all in the wrists

Chapter 5 discusses two ways to avoid a painful injury known as tennis elbow, and one involves strengthening your wrists. One of the simplest weight-lifting exercises for your wrists is the dumbbell wrist curl:

1. Form a 90-degree angle between your forearm and bicep and lay your forearm on a table or weight bench, palms facing up.

2. Placing a dumbbell in your open hand, close your fingers and hand around the dumbbell and roll the dumbbell up until your wrist is flexed.

3. Return to your starting position and repeat for a set of eight to ten reps.

Getting set

Stand to the right of your weight bench, holding a dumbbell in your right hand with your palm facing in. Place your left lower leg and your left hand on top of the bench. Lean forward at the hips until your upper body is at a 45-degree angle to the floor. Bend your right elbow so your upper arm is parallel to the floor, your forearm is perpendicular to it, and your palm faces in. Keep your elbow close to your waist. Pull your abdominals in and bend your knees slightly. (See Figure 14-15a.)

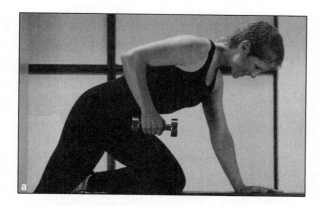

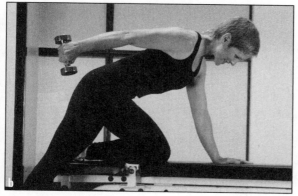

Figure 14-15:
Make sure your shoulder doesn't drop below waist-level during the triceps kickback.

Photograph by Sunstreak Productions, Inc.

The exercise

Keeping your upper arm still, straighten your arm behind you until your entire arm is parallel to the floor and one end of the dumbbell points toward the floor (refer to Figure 14-15b). Slowly bend your arm to lower the weight. After you complete the set, repeat the exercise with your left arm.

Technique tips

Keep these tips in mind as you perform the triceps kickback:

- ✔ **Keep your abdominals pulled in and your knees relaxed, and don't allow your back to round.**
- ✔ **Don't lock your elbow at the top of the movement.** Straighten your arm, but keep your elbow slightly bent.
- ✔ **Don't allow your upper arm to move or your shoulder to drop below waist-level.**
- ✔ **Keep your wrist straight.**

Gym alternative: Triceps-extension machine

Adjust the seat so when you sit down with your arms straight out, they're level with your shoulders and your elbows are lined up with the moving hinge or pulley of the machine. Sit down and tip the handles back so the hand grips are alongside your shoulders.

Grasp a handle in each hand with your palms facing inward. Straighten your arms out in front of you to lift the weight stack, and then slowly bend your arms to lower the weight. (See Figure 14-16.)

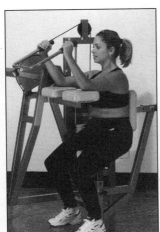

Figure 14-16:
Use the triceps-extension machine at the gym as an alternative to the triceps kickback.

Photograph by Sunstreak Productions, Inc.

Basic crunch

The basic crunch is the consummate abdominal exercise. Pay special attention to your form if you have lower-back or neck problems. We don't offer a machine alternative for the basic crunch because we think abdominal crunch machines are difficult to use correctly, and we don't think machines are as safe or effective as abdominal floor exercises. Instead, our alternative abdominal move uses a large plastic ball known as a physioball.

Getting set

Lie on your back with your knees bent and feet flat on the floor, hip-width apart. Place your hands behind your head so your thumbs are behind your ears. Don't lace your fingers together. Hold your elbows out to the sides but rounded slightly in. Tilt your chin slightly, leaving a few inches of space between your chin and your chest. Gently pull your abdominals inward. (See Figure 14-17a.)

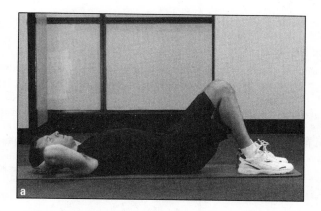

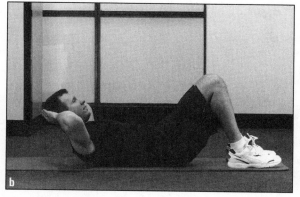

Figure 14-17: Curl up to work on your abs.

Photograph by Sunstreak Productions, Inc.

The exercise

Curl up and forward so that your head, neck, and shoulder blades lift off the floor (refer to Figure 14-17b). Hold for a moment at the top of the movement and then lower slowly back down.

Technique tips

Keep the following tips in mind as you perform the basic crunch:

- ✓ **Keep your abdominals pulled in so you feel more tension in your abs and so you don't overarch your lower back.**
- ✓ **Don't pull on your neck with your hands or draw your elbows in.**
- ✓ **Do curl as well as lift.** In other words, don't yank your head, neck, and shoulder blades off the floor; you also need to curl forward, as if you're doubling over. Think of bringing your ribs to your pelvis and exhale as you crunch up; inhale as you lower back down, keeping your belly button drawn in.
- ✓ **Perform crunches very slowly and with control, doing 12 reps.**

Gym alternative: Ball crunch

Sit on a physioball and roll your torso down so that your back — from your shoulder blades down to your tailbone — is resting on the curve of the ball and your head, neck, and shoulders are above the ball. Your knees are bent, and your feet are planted on the floor, hip-width apart. (See Figure 14-18.)

Perform the same abdominal curling movement as you do for the basic crunch. You have to move slowly and keep your abdominal muscles fully engaged to keep yourself from wiggling around on the ball or rolling off of it.

Figure 14-18:
You can
perform the
basic-
crunch
movement
on a
physioball
as an
alternative
to the
traditional
exercise.

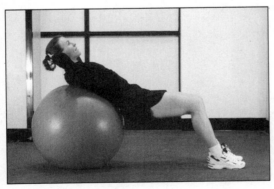

Photograph by Sunstreak Productions, Inc.

Back extension

The back extension both stretches and strengthens your lower back. It's the perfect complement to the basic crunch to develop a strong, balanced mid-section. Use caution if you have a lower-back problem or experience lower-back pain while performing this exercise. If you do feel pain, try lifting only your legs and leaving your arms flat on the floor.

Getting set

Lie on your stomach, facedown, arms straight out in front of you, palms down, and legs straight out behind you. Pull your abs in, as if you're trying to create a small space between your stomach and the floor. (See Figure 14-19a.)

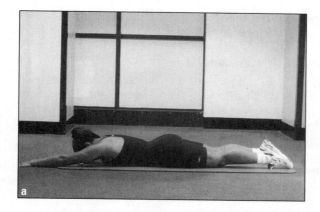

Figure 14-19: The back extension stretches and strengthens your lower back.

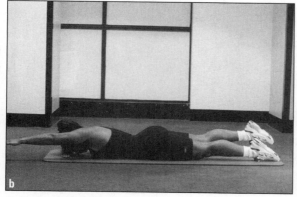

Photograph by Sunstreak Productions, Inc.

The exercise

Lift your left arm and right leg about 1 inch off the floor, and stretch out as much as you can (refer to Figure 14-19b). Hold this position for five slow counts and then lower your arm and leg back down. Repeat the same move with your right arm and left leg. Continue alternating sides until you complete the set.

Technique tips

Keep the following tips in mind as you perform the back extension:

- ✔ **Exhale as you lift your arm and leg, and inhale as you lower them.**
- ✔ **Pretend that you're trying to touch something with your toes and fingertips that's just out of reach.**
- ✔ **Work for precision rather than height.** Lift your arm and leg at the same time and to the same height.

Gym alternative: Ball back extension

Kneel on a physioball and place your hands behind your head. Lean forward and lengthen your body so your torso is resting against the ball and you're firmly balanced on your toes (see Figure 14-20). Make sure your spine forms a straight line from your tailbone to your neck. Lift your chest upward a few inches, hold a moment, and then slowly lower back down.

Cross your arms over your chest, pull your abs in, and lower your upper body a few inches by bending forward at the hips. Raise back up, using your lower back, so your body is parallel to the floor.

Figure 14-20: Perform the back extension on a physioball to add variety to your workout.

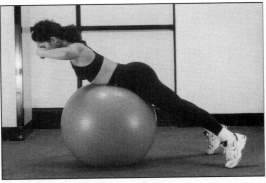

Photograph by Sunstreak Productions, Inc.

Part V
Cardio-Strength Workouts: Getting the Best of Both Worlds

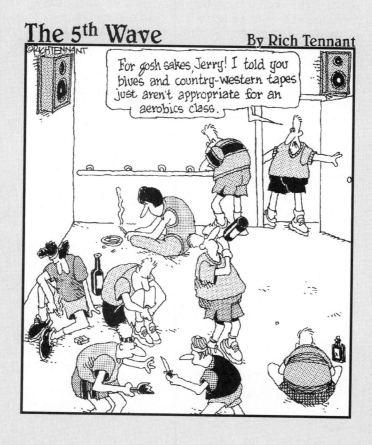

In this part . . .

You find out about workouts that combine aerobic activity and strength-building exercises. These days, everyone's short on time, so workouts that combine cardio and strength training are increasingly popular. In Chapter 15, you get a short course on circuit training, one of the most interesting and popular ways to get and stay fit. Chapter 16 introduces you to the many different varieties of yoga, an approach that not only calms your mind but also invigorates your body. Finally, Chapter 17 familiarizes you with Pilates, a strength and cardio workout that sculpts your body in exciting ways.

Chapter 15

Circuit Training for Fitness and Fun

In This Chapter

▶ Setting up strength-building stations

▶ Getting a step-by-step look at circuit training

▶ Taking a peek at a sample circuit

C ircuit training is a unique method of working out that combines cardiovascular exercise with strength training. Circuit training includes a
warm-up, followed by a succession of strength-building exercises at *stations*
(in between which you walk fast or run), followed by a cooldown. (Note that
a station can be just a spot where you do pushups; it doesn't have to be
anything fancy.) You get to decide how long your total workout will be, how
many stations you'll include, and what exercises you'll do at those stations.
Workouts are fun, the time flies by, and within just a few weeks of doing
circuits two days per week, most people notice a big difference in the
strength of their arms, legs, abdomen, and buttocks. This chapter helps
you decide how to set up your workouts.

Setting Up Stations and Knowing Which Exercises to Do

Have you even seen a circuit-training area at your local park: Along a trail,
stations appear periodically, and at those stations are instructions for doing
push-ups or pull-ups or a variety of other strengthening exercises.

You don't need to use the stations set up at your local park, though. Your
local gym may have a circuit-training class or may have a self-paced circuit
routine that you can do on your own time. You can also easily set up stations
in your own home. If you have a weight machine, you're way ahead of the
game and can do most of the weight-lifting exercises there. But if you don't,

gather up the following inexpensive equipment and set up stations in your exercise room, spare bedroom, (dry) basement, garage, backyard (in good weather), or any other place you can think of:

- ✔ A sit-up mat or thick towel (for sit-ups, push-ups, crunches, Pilates exercises)

- ✔ One pair each of 5-, 8-, 10-, 12-, and/or 15-pound weights (for curls, shrugs, upright rows, punches, and so on)

- ✔ A weight bar with however much weight you can handle for squats

- ✔ A sturdy chair or ledge (for chair dips)

- ✔ A pull-up bar secured in a doorway (for pull-ups, hanging abs)

- ✔ A stairway or step (for step-ups, single-leg squats, toe raises)

Arrange each of these so that they're 10 to 20 feet apart; a circle or square can work, but so can a zigzag pattern, as long as you have some room to walk quickly or run between stations. If you need to place the stations closer than this — say, right next to each other — that's fine. Just do jumping jacks, jump rope, or run in place with high knees for ten seconds between exercises.

To choose which exercises to do at each station, see the following sections, check out Chapter 14 for illustrations of many of these exercises, or — for detailed coverage of all these exercises — get a copy of our book, *Weight Training For Dummies,* 2nd Edition (published by Wiley).

At each station, you can do several different exercises, as described in the following sections. However, you can easily forget what exercise you're supposed to do when you get to a station, so I suggest putting a sheet of paper at each station that lists, in order, the one, two, or three exercises that you're planning to doing there.

Arm-strengthening stations

Because the warm-up, cooldown, and movement between stations work your leg muscles, many people emphasize arm-strength stations in their circuit routines, focusing as many as half of the total number of stations on their arms.

This list is not meant to be exhaustive. If you get results from other arm-strengthening exercises, put those on your circuit. This list is also not meant to imply that you'll include all these exercises in your circuit. You can pick and choose from the list, as best suits your needs.

If you don't have the space to store weights, you can also use exercise bands or tubes (see Chapter 20) to do many of the weight-intensive exercises.

Dumbbell biceps curl

This exercise, as you may expect, works the biceps. Hold a dumbbell in each hand and stand with your feet as wide apart as your hips. Let your arms hang down at your sides with your palms forward. Pull your abdominals in, stand tall, and keep your knees relaxed. Curl both arms upward until they're in front of your shoulders. Slowly lower the dumbbells back down and repeat.

Punches

Punches work your shoulders and upper arms. Take a dumbbell in each hand, put each hand in front of its respective shoulder, and stand with your legs wider than shoulder-width apart, abdominals pulled in. Take your right hand, cross it over your body, and punch out to the left. To keep your knees healthy, roll up to your toes on your right leg as you punch out your right arm. Repeat with your left side and vice versa.

Upright rows

Upright rows work the shoulders. While standing, hold a dumbbell in each hand and put the ends of the two weights together, holding your hands right in front of your thighs. Pull your abdominals in. Keeping the weights together, pull your hands up to your collarbone. Lower and repeat.

If you've had any shoulder (specifically, deltoid) injuries, steer clear of upright rows. Instead, do shoulder presses (see Chapter 14).

One-arm dumbbell row

This exercise works the lats (the widest part of your back just behind your armpit) and biceps. Stand to the right of your weight bench, holding a dumbbell in your right hand with your palm facing in. Place your left knee and your left hand on top of the bench for support. Let your right arm hang down and a bit forward. Pull your abdominals in and bend forward from the hips so your back is naturally arched and roughly parallel to the floor, and your right knee is slightly bent. Tilt your chin toward your chest so that your neck is in line with the rest of your spine. Pull your right arm up until your elbow is pointing to the ceiling, your upper arm is parallel to the floor, and your arm brushes against your waist. Lower the weight slowly back down and repeat.

Push-ups

Push-ups work all the upper-body muscles. Facing the ground, rest your body on your hands and tiptoes, and keep your back and legs perfectly straight. Pull in your abdominals, lower your chest to the ground, and raise your chest back up again by pushing against the ground until your elbows are nearly locked. Repeat. As push-ups become easier for you, try elevating your feet, which makes this exercise much harder.

Pull-ups

Pull-ups work all the upper-body muscles. For this exercise, you need a bar that can hold your body weight. Place your hands (palms facing away) wider than your shoulders on the bar and hang. To do one pull-up, pull yourself up until your chin reaches over the top of the bar. Lower yourself to the hanging position and repeat. Don't be surprised if, on your first attempt, you can do only one pull-up (or, maybe, not even one!). With repeated attempts, you'll quickly improve.

Shrugs

Shrugs work your trapezius and upper-back muscles. Plant your feet shoulder-width apart. Take a dumbbell in each hand, relax your arms by letting them hang down at your sides, and relax your shoulders. Pull in your abdominals. Without bending your elbows, raise and lower your shoulders. Repeat.

Dumbbell chest press

Working the chest, triceps, and shoulders, this exercise is an all-time favorite. Lie on a bench with a dumbbell in each hand and your feet flat on the floor. Push the dumbbells up so that your arms are directly over your shoulders and your palms up. Pull your abdominals in, and tilt your chin toward your chest. Lower the dumbbells down and a little to the side until your elbows are in line with or just slightly below your shoulders. The weights should be directly above the elbow joints, which should create a 90-degree angle. Push the weights back up in a triangular motion to where the weights are directly above your chest, taking care not to lock your elbows or allow your shoulder blades to rise off the bench. Repeat. You can also substitute the bench press if you have a weight machine handy.

Dumbbell shoulder press

Shoulder presses work your shoulders, as well as your triceps and upper back. Hold a dumbbell in each hand and sit on a bench with back support. Plant your feet firmly on the floor about hip-width apart. Bend your elbows and raise your upper arms to shoulder height so that the dumbbells are at ear level. Pull your abdominals in so that there is a slight gap between the small of your back and the bench. Place the back of your head against the pad. Push the dumbbells up and in until the ends of the dumbbells touch lightly directly over your head, and then lower the dumbbells back to ear level. Repeat.

Triceps dips

Triceps dips really work your triceps; in fact, you may find that you can do only one or two dips the first time you attempt this exercise. Use a sturdy chair, ledge, or seat of a weight bench. Extend your legs with your heels on the ground and rest your hands on the outside edge of the chair with your elbows locked. Pull in your abdominals; keep your shoulders back, down, and not rounded; and pull your chest up. Bending your elbows, lower your butt to the ground and then push yourself back up until your elbows lock again. Repeat.

If you find that you can't lower yourself all the way to the ground and still come back up, lower just half the distance to the ground and do as many that way as you can.

Triceps kickback

Not to be exceedingly obvious, but this exercise works your triceps! Stand to the right of your weight bench, holding a dumbbell in your right hand with your palm facing in. Place your left lower leg and your left hand on top of the bench. Lean forward at the hips until your upper body is at a 45-degree angle to the floor. Bend your right elbow so that your upper arm is parallel to the floor, your forearm is perpendicular to it, and your palm faces in. Keep your elbow close to your upper arm. Pull your abdominals in and relax your knees. Keeping your upper arm still, straighten your elbow behind you until your entire arm is parallel to the floor and one end of the dumbbell points down. Slowly bend your arm to lower the weight. Repeat. On the second circuit, do the exercise with your left arm.

Leg-strengthening stations

Because your warm-up, cooldown, and travel between stations is leg-intensive, you don't need to include a lot of leg-strengthening exercises in your circuit routine. The exercises in this section, however, are some of our favorites.

If you have a weight bench with attachments at your disposal, you can add leg extensions, leg curls, leg presses, and any other exercises the machine supports.

Step-ups

Step-ups work nearly every muscle in your leg, as well as your butt muscles. To do this exercise, you need a step — one of the steps on the bottom of a stairway can work well. However, buying a step-aerobics platform and placing two sets of risers underneath the platform (to a height of 10 to 12 inches) may be more convenient (because it's portable). You simply keep walking or running up and down the one step. Step up on one step and then bring the other leg up on that step, too. Then step back down, following with the other leg. Then up the step again, then back down, and so on.

Single-leg squats

Single-leg squats work your butt and upper legs and help develop balance. Stand on your right leg at the edge of the step, so that the instep of your right foot comes right to the edge of the step and your left leg is dangling off the step. Pull in your abdominals and bend your right leg on the step at the knee as you push your hips back, sinking into your right heel, until the heel of your left leg just touches the ground. Lead with your right heel, not your toes; straighten the leg on the step. Repeat. On the second circuit, use the other leg.

The heels of both feet should be along the same horizontal line. Also, you may need to hang on to something (perhaps a railing) to keep yourself from falling.

Standing calf raise

Standing calf raises work your calves and shins and help develop balance. Stand on the edge of a step or, if you have a step-aerobics platform, place two sets of risers underneath the platform. Stand tall with your abdominals pulled in, the balls of your feet firmly planted on the step, and your heels hanging over the edge. Rest your hands against a wall or a sturdy object for balance. Raise your heels a few inches above the edge of the step so you're on your tiptoes. Hold the position for a moment, and then lower your heels below the platform, feeling a stretch in your calf muscles. Repeat. On the second circuit, use the other leg.

If you find one-legged calf raises too challenging at first, try doing this exercise with both legs.

Abdomen, butt, and lower-back strength stations

These exercises help you develop great abs, a nice tush, and a healthy lower back. This list is not anywhere near all-inclusive, however. In fact, setting up Pilates stations to work your core is an excellent circuit-training option. For a brief introduction to Pilates, check out Chapter 17. To get the full lowdown, pick up a copy of *Pilates For Dummies* by Ellie Herman (published by Wiley).

Basic crunch

Crunches primarily work the upper region of the abs. Lie on your back with your knees bent and feet flat on the floor, hip-width apart. Place your hands extended out toward your knees, across your chest, above your head, or behind your head so your thumbs are behind your ears — depending on what's comfortable for you. Don't lace your fingers together. Hold your elbows out to the sides but rounded slightly in. Tilt your chin slightly, leaving a few inches of space between your chin and your chest. Gently pull your abdominals inward. Curl up and forward so that your head, neck, and shoulder blades lift off the floor. Hold for a moment at the top of the movement and then lower slowly back down. Repeat.

Leg raises

Leg raises work primarily the lower portion of the abs. Lie on your back and place your hands, palms down, under the area where your pelvis and lower back meet. (Find a spot where your hands are comfortable.) Pull in your abdominals. Raise your legs (your knees can be slightly bent) about 12 inches off the floor and hold. Lower your legs to just barely above the floor, and then raise them again to 12 inches. Repeat.

Hanging abs

Hanging abs work the lower region of the abs. Using a pull-up bar or hanging-ab apparatus (ask about it at your gym), hang from the bar, pull in your abdominals, and then lift your knees toward your chest, tucking the pelvis under and causing your spine to round. Lower your legs slowly back to the hanging position. Repeat.

Obliques curls

These curls work the *obliques,* the sides of your core area midsection. Lie on your right side with your arms crossed in front of you. Bending sideways at your waist, lift your upper body off the ground a few inches. You may need to brace your feet under a bar or sturdy piece of furniture. Repeat. On your second circuit, lie on your left side.

Back extension

Back extensions are a great exercise for your lower back. Lie on your stomach, looking down at the floor, arms straight out in front of you, palms down, and legs straight out behind you. Pull your abs in, as if you're trying to create a small space between your stomach and the floor. Lift your left arm and right leg about 1 inch off the floor, and stretch out as much as you can. Hold this position for five slow counts and then lower your arm and leg back down. Repeat the same move with your right arm and left leg. Continue alternating sides until you complete the set.

Squat

Squats work your butt and upper legs. Either with your hands on your hips or holding dumbbells with your arms down at your sides (you can also hold your arms out in from of your torso or your fists in at your chest to create a counterbalance, or put them in the overhead position to challenge your posture), stand with your feet as wide apart as your hips and place your weight slightly back on your heels. Let your arms hang down at your sides. Pull your abdominals in and stand tall with square shoulders. Sit back and down, as if you're sitting into a chair. Lower as far as you can without leaning your upper body more than a few inches forward. Don't lower any farther than the point at which you're parallel to the floor, and don't allow your knees to shoot out in front of your toes. When your thighs are parallel to the floor, straighten your legs and stand back up. Don't lock your knees at the top of the movement.

Lunge

Lunges are amazing for your butt, hips, and upper legs. Stand upright with your feet shoulder-width apart. Take a large step forward, and plant your foot on the ground. Keeping your front knee completely stable and your upper body perfectly vertical, lower your body straight down until your back knee nearly touches the ground. Raise your body straight up and repeat with another step. Keep repeating.

Don't allow your torso to lean forward and be sure to evenly distribute your body weight on both legs. Think of your torso as having a pole placed directly down the center, like a horse on a merry-go-round and go up and down, not back and forth. Also keep in mind that the farther you step out, the more emphasis is placed on the butt and hamstrings; the more shallow your step, the more emphasis is placed on the quads. Finally, when you're in the down position, both knees should form a 90-degree angle, and you should be able to see the tip of your shoe or toes.

Moving through Sample Stations

The beauty of circuit training is that you can set up the stations any way you want, using only a few of the exercises in this chapter, all of them, and/or other exercises from other sources. You can do each exercise once in the circuit, or you can repeat an exercise two or more times in one circuit. Your circuit can include 5 exercises or 25. You get to decide, see what works for you, tweak the circuit, do it some more, and so on.

Be sure to arrange your circuit so you alternate stations that use similar muscles. In other words, do an exercise for your abdomen, then arms, then legs, then your back, and then go back to abdomen, arms, and so on. Or, if you want to do an arm-intensive circuit, set up a station for your arms, then legs, then arms, then back, then arms, then abdomen, then arms, and so on. Either way, give your muscles a little time to rest before working them again.

Here's a sample way of ordering the exercises listed in this chapter. This gives you 21 exercises for your circuit. See the following section for step-by-step instructions on how you work these 21 exercises into a circuit-training workout.

- Triceps kickbacks
- Basic crunches
- Dumbbell biceps curls
- Step-ups

- ✔ Dumbbell shoulder presses
- ✔ Back extensions
- ✔ Pull-ups
- ✔ Single-leg squats
- ✔ Push-ups
- ✔ Hanging abs
- ✔ Tricep dips
- ✔ Leg raises
- ✔ One-arm dumbbell rows
- ✔ Lunges
- ✔ Dumbbell chest presses
- ✔ Obliques curls
- ✔ Upright rows
- ✔ Standing calf raises
- ✔ Shrugs
- ✔ Squats
- ✔ Punches

Putting the Stations Together into a Circuit

After your stations are set up and you've determined an order to follow, follow these circuit-training steps:

1. **For your warm-up, either outside or on indoor equipment, run, walk, cycle, swim, or do any other cardiovascular activity for 5 to 20 minutes, depending on how much you're currently working out each day, and how long you want your overall workout to be.**

2. **When you get back, *immediately* begin your circuit-training workout.**

   You can stop for a quick drink of water, if you absolutely need it. But don't walk around or chit-chat with neighbors or anything like that. Do your warm-up, and then go right to the first station, where you want to ease into your first few strength exercises by using slow, methodical movements.

3. **Set the timer on your watch for 20 to 45 seconds (start on the low end, and gradually build up) and before you begin doing an exercise at the first station, start the timer.**

4. **When your watch beeps, briskly walk or run to the next station, set the timer again, and immediately begin doing the next exercise.**

5. **When the watch beeps again, proceed to the next station, and so on.**

6. **Repeat the entire circuit (all the exercises) at least once.**

   You can do as many circuits as you choose. If you've set up five stations with three different exercises you're going to do at each, and you've set your timer for 30 seconds, the circuit routine is going to take you 7½ minutes, plus walking/running time between stations, so the entire circuit may take you 10 minutes. Given this scenario, you could do three circuits, which gives you a 30-minute workout, plus your warm-up and cooldown, which gives you a grand total of 50 to 75 minutes of exercise! Not bad.

7. **When you finish the last circuit, immediately begin your 10- to 15-minute cooldown.**

8. **Stretch immediately after finishing your cooldown.**

Chapter 16

All about Yoga: Mind and Body

In This Chapter

▶ Understanding asanas

▶ Exploring the different forms of yoga

▶ Finding yoga classes

▶ Looking at a yoga workout

*H*ere in the West, we tend to view exercise as way to improve your body — to strengthen your heart, tone your muscles, and make your joints more flexible. Only in the last ten years or so has the mainstream fitness community come to accept what many other cultures have known for thousands of years: Exercise can also be good for your mind.

This realization has spawned a new fitness catchphrase — mind-body exercise — and yoga is at the forefront. We think everyone can benefit from adding a mind-body activity to their exercise repertoires. You can substitute these workouts for your regular program once or twice a week. For example, instead of lifting weights or doing your regular stretching routine, do a session of yoga. Some mind-body classes are intensely demanding, so make sure that you don't overload your workout schedule.

Take yoga for a while and you'll become much more aware of your body — how you stand, sit, and walk. Most people begin to see and feel improvements in their flexibility, strength, and stress levels after only a few classes. Over the long term, yoga can keep your body looking and feeling remarkably young. Suzanne took a class from an older man who pranced around the room with incredible grace and agility. After class, Suzanne was shocked to learn that the instructor was 80 years old!

Knowing Your Asana from Your Elbows

Developed in India more than 5,000 years ago, yoga consists of a series of poses (known as *asanas*) that you hold from a few seconds to several minutes. The moves — a blend of strength, flexibility, and body-awareness exercises — are intended to promote the union of the mind, body, and spirit. Most forms of yoga focus on relaxation and deep breathing as you perform and hold the poses.

Yoga classes have a different feel than the usual Western workouts, often including a spiritual element such as chanting or burning candles or incense. (However, many classes these days dispense with the traditional Indian touches and just get right down to the business of kicking your butt.)

The most common misconception about yoga is that you have to be as flexible as Gumby to do it. In fact, there are many, many variations on the poses, and a good teacher can teach you to do them in a way that accommodates your level of flexibility. As you improve, you'll need fewer modifications.

Finding a Yoga Style That's Right for You

There are many forms of yoga. Most include the same fundamental poses but differ in terms of how quickly you move, how long you hold each pose, how much breathing is emphasized, and how much of a spiritual aspect there is. Some styles offer more modifications to the really bendy and twisty moves, so they're more accessible to new exercisers and the flexibility-challenged. Others are for people who can already touch their toes with their tongue. If you find that you dig yoga, experiment with some of the different styles. You may find you like one more than the others.

Here's a brief look at the main yoga options.

- **Ananda:** Ananda yoga requires less strength and flexibility than most other styles, so it's a great place to start. The moves are fairly straightforward, and ananda doesn't involve much chanting.

- **Anusara:** Anusara, a relatively new form of yoga, has a deep spiritual element and a heavy focus on good posture and body alignment.

- **Astanga:** Astanga, sometimes called Power Yoga, is one of the most physically demanding forms of yoga in terms of flexibility, strength, and stamina. You move from one posture to another without a break, so we don't recommend this style for beginners.

- **Bikram:** Bikram, an intensely physical style of yoga, includes a lot of breathing exercises. The same 26 poses are performed in the same order during 90-minute classes that are usually conducted in a room heated to 100 degrees. (The heat is intended to make it easier to stretch.) If you have high blood pressure, are at high risk for developing heart disease, or already have heart disease, get your doctor's permission before taking a class conducted in a room at a high temperature.

- **Integral:** Integral classes involve lots of meditation and chanting. However, integral yoga is one of the easier forms to learn because the postures are relatively simple with plenty of modifications offered for the flexibility-challenged.

- **Iyengar:** Iyengar yoga instructors must complete a rigorous two- to five-year training program for certification, so the quality of teaching tends to be consistently good. Iyengar yoga involves props such as foam blocks and stretching belts. Instructors pay close attention to body alignment.

- **Kripalu:** Kripalu, a less physical and more meditative style of yoga, emphasizes body alignment and breath and movement coordination. There are three stages in kripalu yoga. Stage One focuses on learning the postures and exploring your body's limits of strength and flexibility. Stage Two involves holding the postures for an extended time, developing concentration and inner awareness. Stage Three involves moving from one posture to another without rest.

- **Kundalini:** Kundalini yoga was one of the first "Westernized" forms of yoga. Because it's designed to release energy in the body, it involves a lot of intense breathing exercises. Most of the poses are classic flexibility exercises.

- **Sivananda:** This classic style of yoga is one of the most widely followed in the world and follows well-known poses, with an emphasis on relaxation and breathing.

Taking Yoga Classes

Most health clubs offer yoga classes at no additional charge. You can find a wider variety of styles and techniques at yoga-only studios, which charge $8 to $25 per class. You'll likely also find classes aimed at different experience levels.

If you're a yoga novice, make sure that you take a beginning class, and don't try to keep up with anyone else. Yoga can be extremely demanding, both in terms of flexibility and strength. Even if you can bench-press a heavy load in the gym, you may find yourself lacking the strength to hold a yoga pose for a minute. Yoga requires a different type of strength than weight lifting does. For instance, many yoga poses require you to call upon the strength of your abdominals, lower back, and dozens of small spinal muscles that don't get much action in a weight-machine workout.

There's no national yoga certification, so we can't list certain credentials to look for in a teacher. In the yoga world, it usually means a lot if you've studied with a certain yogi master, but most people have trouble evaluating this type of credential. Rely on your own judgment and word-of-mouth recommendations. A good yoga instructor wanders around the room correcting class members' techniques and offering variations that allow less-flexible people to accomplish all the poses.

Learning the ropes: Yoga equipment and clothing

Yoga doesn't require a large commitment of equipment and clothing. Some people wear leotards; others wear baggy clothes; still others go without clothing altogether (an option if you're working out at home, but you won't find many clothing-optional classes).

The one piece of equipment you absolutely do need is a *yoga mat,* one that's sticky or tacky (that is, nonslip), as opposed to smooth or slippery. Look for a mat that's at least 68 inches long by 24 inches wide — longer is better, if you can

find one. If you'd like to try yoga once or twice without investing in a mat, you can use a thick towel or blanket. Look for a yoga mat at your local sporting goods store, yoga specialty shop, gym, yoga studio, or at online shops (search for "yoga mat" on Google or some other search engine).

Unlike most other fitness activities that require a major investment in footwear, yoga is generally practiced barefoot, although some practitioners do wear socks.

Some yoga instructors don't take into account individual differences in fitness and flexibility, so it's up to you to know your own limits. Suzanne learned this lesson the hard way when her sister, Jennifer, a longtime yoga devotee, dragged her to an advanced yoga class. The 2-hour session involved hanging upside down from a rope for 20 consecutive minutes, an activity that was intended to be relaxing but left Suzanne feeling as if her brain was going to burst through her skull. The class also included demanding hamstring stretches that made Suzanne so sore that she couldn't ride her bike for four days.

Some classes may be too spiritual for you if that's not what you're after. Liz once took a class in which the instructor asked students to reveal their innermost fears. Liz didn't feel like sharing that bit of information with a group of strangers sitting around the room with their legs twisted around their necks.

Yoga offers an active time-out to energize your body and calm your mind. Most yoga classes end with several minutes of lying facedown on the floor. This come-down time, called shivasana, is low-key enough to make some people fall asleep, but after you get up, you feel recharged.

A Yoga Routine

The following sections describe several basic yoga poses; however, these step-by-step instructions are for demonstration purposes only. From here, you want to pick up a book, rent a video, or take a class to obtain guidance on how long to hold these poses, how often to repeat them, and how to combine them with other poses.

Yoga For Dummies by Georg Feuerstein and Larry Payne (published by Wiley) discusses most of the poses and includes very helpful photos. Wiley has also published the two following yoga workout videos:

- *Basic Yoga Workout For Dummies,* led by Sara Ivanhoe, teaches 12 basic poses and additional modifications to those poses.

- *Beyond Basic Yoga For Dummies,* another video led by Sara Ivanhoe, builds on the first video with additional poses and challenges.

Taking a yoga class is another way to master the many yoga poses that make up a yoga workout. See the preceding section for more on finding yoga classes.

Easy pose

This is one of the simplest poses you'll do — it's a simple sitting pose in which many workouts begin. Here's what you do:

1. **Sit on the floor.**

2. **Bend your knees, keeping your feet flat on the floor, and then wrap your arms around your knees.**

3. **Pull your knees to your chest to straighten your spine.**

4. **Release your arms when you no longer feel any stretch in your spine, cross your legs, and let your knees drop to the floor.**

   Be sure to keep your head and body in a straight line.

Forward bend

The forward bend is extremely relaxing, because you stretch your back and legs. Here's how you do it:

1. **Start in a sitting position, with your legs out in front of you in a V (whatever width of V is comfortable for you), toes pointed up toward the ceiling.**

2. **Pull up on your butt, so that you're resting on your pelvic bone.**

3. **Stretch your arms straight up, trying to lengthen your spine as you stretch, and inhale.**

4. **As you exhale, lean your chest forward, keeping your back straight.**

5. **Try to bring your chin to your shins and your chest to your thighs, as shown in Figure 16-1.**

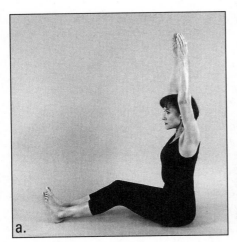
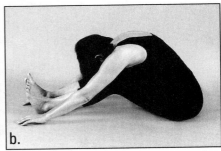
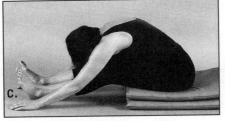

Figure 16-1:
Forward
bend.

Photograph by Blaine Michioka/Rainbow Photography

Child's pose

This move stretches your lower back and arms and relaxes your entire body. If you have knee problems, lower yourself into position with extra care. Here's what to do:

1. **Start in a kneeling position.**

2. **Drop your butt toward your heels as you stretch the rest of your body down and forward.**

3. **In the fully stretched position, rest your arms in a relaxed position along the floor, rest your stomach comfortably on top of your thighs, and rest your forehead on the mat (see Figure 16-2).**

   You should feel a mild stretch in your shoulders and buttocks and down the length of your spine and arms.

Ease into this stretch by keeping your shoulders and neck relaxed. Don't force your derriere to move any closer to your heels than is comfortable.

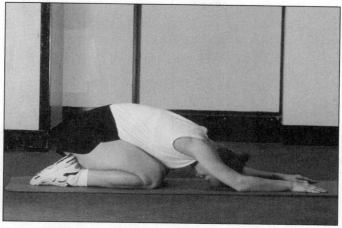

Figure 16-2:
Child's pose.

Photograph by Sunstreak Productions, Inc.

Sage twist

This unique pose rotates the spine from left to right, toning and relaxing as you go. Here's what to do:

1. **Start in the sitting position and extend both legs forward.**

2. **Bend your right knee and place your right foot on the floor, next to your inside left thigh.**

3. **Place your right hand on the floor behind you, palm down.**

4. **Take your left palm and wrap it around the outside of your right knee (see Figure 16-3).**

5. **Inhale, extending and lifting your spine upward; exhale and twist your torso and head to your right side (see Figure 16-3).**

Cat pose

The cat tilt elongates your spine and eases tension in your back. Try it by following these steps:

1. **Rest on your hands and knees, with your belly facing the floor.**

2. **Inhale deeply.**

3. **Exhale and pull in your abdominal muscles, tailbone, and butt.**

4. **Pressing down on your hands, press your back toward the ceiling so your spine rounds, as shown in Figure 16-4.**

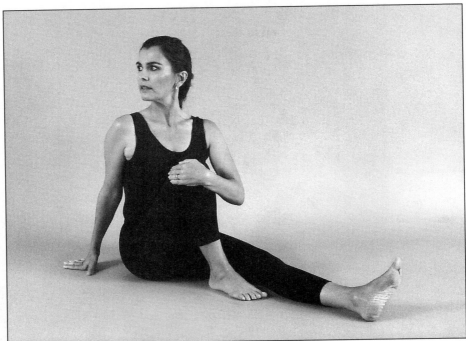

Figure 16-3:
Sage twist.

Photograph by Blaine Michioka/Rainbow Photography

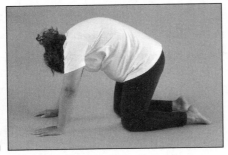

Figure 16-4:
Cat pose.

Photograph by Blaine Michioka/Rainbow Photography

Triangle pose

Moving from a sitting or lying position to standing, the triangle pose stretches your spine and abdomen. Here's how you do it:

1. **Stand with your feet much wider than your shoulders, and place both arms straight out to the side, parallel to the floor, with palms facing up.**

   Both feet can sit flat on the floor, or you can point your left foot, keeping your heel off the floor.

2. **Inhale deeply.**

3. **Exhale and bend to the right, as shown in Figure 16-5.**

   Keep your knees straight and your hips facing forward. Don't twist your lower body; simply bend at your waist.

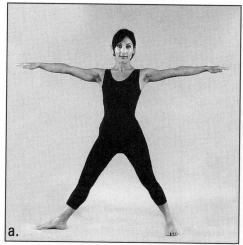 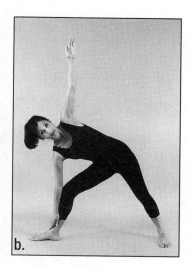

Figure 16-5: Triangle pose.

Photograph by Blaine Michioka/Rainbow Photography

4. **Slide your right arm down your right leg as you bend, and then hold your leg or ankle.**

5. **Hold this position, slowly breathing in and out several times.**

   If you're able to, now lift your left leg off the floor, anywhere from 3 to 18 inches, keeping your knee straight.

Sun salutation

This move stretches your abdominal, lower-back, front-hip, and thigh muscles. If you're prone to lower back pain, make a special point of tightening your abdominals, and don't arch your lower back. Here's how to do it:

1. **Kneel on the floor and then bring your left leg forward so that your foot is flat on the floor, your knee is bent, and your thigh is parallel to the floor.**

2. **Lift your arms straight up with your palms facing in.**

3. **Pull your abdominals gently inward, and keep your shoulders down and back.**

4. Look to the ceiling, and as you stretch upward with your upper body, push your weight slightly forward from your hips into your front thigh (see Figure 16-6).

You should feel this stretch travel through your torso and upper body, including your arms. You should also feel it at the very top of your back thigh. Repeat with your right leg forward.

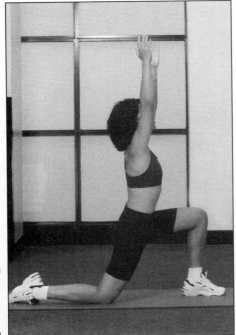

Figure 16-6:
Sun
salutation.

Photograph by Sunstreak Productions, Inc.

Keep in mind the following tips as you perform the sun salutation:

✔ Hold onto something solid, like a sturdy chair, with one hand if you have trouble maintaining balance.

✔ Don't lean so far forward that your front knee moves in front of your toes.

✔ Don't arch your lower back.

Chapter 17

Pilates: Sculpting and Strengthening

*F*irst things first: This form of exercise is *not* pronounced *pie*-lates but rather pih-*lah*-teez. It's named after its inventor, Joseph Pilates, a former carpenter and gymnast who invented the technique for injured dancers. Many of the moves were inspired by yoga or patterned after the movements of zoo animals such as swans, seals, and big cats.

Zoo animals aside, this chapter gives you a quick overview of Pilates, from understanding how it works to finding a gym or video, to taking a stab at a quick workout.

Understanding How Pilates Works

Pilates tends to emphasize your body's *core,* that is, the abdomen, obliques, lower back, inner and outer thigh, butt, and so on. For this reason, Pilates develops much of what exercisers need — strength, flexibility, muscular endurance, coordination, balance, and good posture — with a much lower chance of injury than with other forms of exercise. The discipline emphasizes correct form instead of going for the burn. Plus, with so many exercise variations and progressions, we think you'll have a hard time getting bored with this creative form of exercise. The moves require you to engage virtually your whole body. At times, you may try to strengthen one muscle while stretching another. Pilates moves take lots of concentration; you can't simply go through the motions like you can on gym equipment. And then, for every move you think you've mastered, Pilates has another version that's a little different and a little harder.

Consider a move called "rolling like a ball" (see Figure 17-1): You balance on your rear end, roll backward, and then roll back up into the balanced position again. This move requires a good balance of abdominal and lower-back strength and is deceptively tough. Liz has seen many muscular bodybuilders taken down by this move. Pilates teaches you to think about how you use your muscles during your workout so you use them better in daily life. For instance, because much of the focus is on good posture and body mechanics, you stand and sit taller and walk more gracefully. Liz always leaves her Pilates classes feeling a few inches taller.

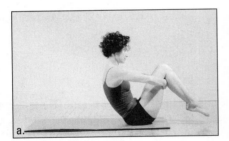
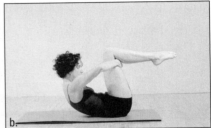
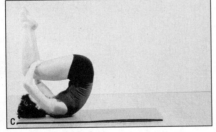
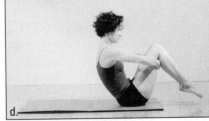

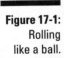

Figure 17-1:
Rolling
like a ball.

Return to the Balance Point.

Photograph by David Herman and Jordan Levy

Anybody can benefit from Pilates. Liz has been taking Pilates classes for years. Although she has always been strong and has plenty of endurance from all the running, hiking, and weight training she does, she continues to find Pilates very challenging.

Finding a Class or Instructor

You can practice Pilates three ways:

- You can take a group class that involves performing specialized calisthenics exercises, with or without a mat (refer to Figure 17-1).

- You can take private lessons on a series of machines with exotic names like the Cadillac and the Reformer. The Cadillac, with its array of springs, straps, poles, and bars, looks like a bed that the Marquis de Sade might have enjoyed. The Reformer looks like a weight bench souped up with assorted springs, straps, and pads.

- You can pick up a copy of *Pilates Workout For Dummies,* a workout video by Michelle Dozois (published by Wiley), that demonstrates Pilates techniques for beginners but also offers challenging workouts as you advance.

  Also pick up a copy of *Pilates For Dummies* by Ellie Herman (published by Wiley), a step-by-step guide for everything from basic Pilates to super-advanced exercises.

There are nearly 500 Pilates studios nationwide, and the explosion continues. Instructors of the official Pilates Method must complete a rigorous training program that includes more than 600 apprenticeship hours. Other Pilates factions have created their own certifications, which may or may not be as rigorous. To find a good Pilates instructor, you're going to have to rely on your own judgment and recommendations from people you trust.

Pilates is expensive. Private lessons will set you back $40 to $200 a session. Yes, you read correctly: Some instructors charge $200 for a single session. That's because there are many more personal trainers who don't have a Pilates specialization than do, and when they get a following, their prices tend to skyrocket. Mat classes are a relative bargain, running from $12 to $25 per session, but that's still more than many monthly gym memberships. Some gyms offer Pilates classes to members at no additional charge and offer private instruction at a discount. If you like to master athletic activities quickly, this may not be the workout for you. Like dance, yoga, and martial arts, learning Pilates is a long-term process.

If you can afford it, we recommend taking a private session or two on the machines. It is both an enlightening and humbling experience — enlightening because you discover that your body can move in ways you never imagined, and humbling because you discover ways your body should be able to move but can't.

Looking at Some Pilates Exercises

Pilates includes hundreds of movements and exercises (and many have numerous steps), and different combinations of these moves make up a Pilates workout. Because of a lack of space, however, we can't show you anything but a small sampling here. But you can get some idea of what a few basic Pilates moves look like, and you can try them in your own living room before shelling out the big bucks for classes and/or equipment.

You may require several weeks to become comfortable with your Pilates workout, and several months to become skilled at it. It's a difficult activity, but one that pays off handsomely if you stick with it.

Upper-abdominal curls

Many people struggle with abdominal curls, usually because of weak abs. Although you may struggle at first to do this exercise, by staying with it, you encourage a strong core.

1. **Lie on your back with your knees bent, feet flat on the floor, and your fingers behind your head, as shown in Figure 17-2.**

2. **Pull your navel toward your spine.**

3. **Lift your shoulders just barely off the mat and pull your chin toward your chest, as shown in Figure 17-2.**

4. **Hold, and then relax and lower yourself to the mat. Repeat eight times. (Okay, repeat only three or four times until you get used to this activity and can handle eight reps!)**

Bridge

The bridge strengthens and stabilizes the core muscles, especially your butt and the back of your legs. Be careful, however, not to arch your back.

1. **Lie on your back, knees bent, feet flat on the floor.**

2. **Breathe in deeply.**

3. **Exhale and push your feet into your yoga mat, squeeze your butt, and thrust your hips toward the ceiling, forming a straight line from your shoulders to your knees (see Figure 17-3).**

4. **Return to the mat and repeat four times.**

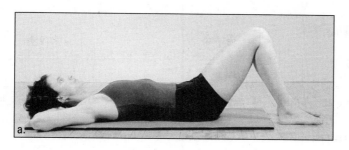

Figure 17-2:
Upper-
abdominal
curls.

Photograph by David Herman and Jordan Levy

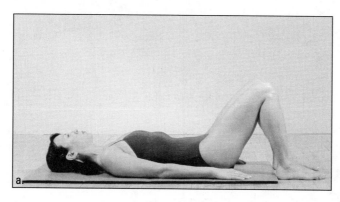

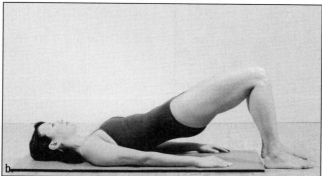

Figure 17-3:
The bridge.

Photograph by David Herman and Jordan Levy

Basic cat

Looking much like a yoga pose (see Chapter 16), basic cat lengthens and stretches the muscles around your spine.

1. **Start on all fours, hands directly below your shoulders, with a natural sway in your spine (see Figure 17-4a).**

2. **As you inhale, arch your back a little (see Figure 17-4b).**

3. **Exhale, pull your navel in, tucking your butt under and pushing the middle of your back up toward the ceiling, and then push your hands into your mat. Round out your back, dropping your head and making your back look like the letter *c* (see Figure 17-4c).**

4. **Return to Step 1 and repeat three more times.**

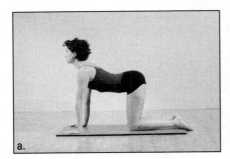 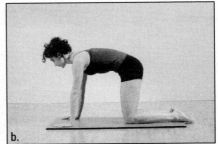

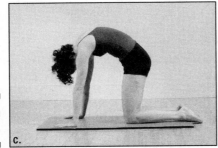

Figure 17-4:
Basic cat.

Photograph by David Herman and Jordan Levy

Part VI
Conquering the Gym (Even at Home)

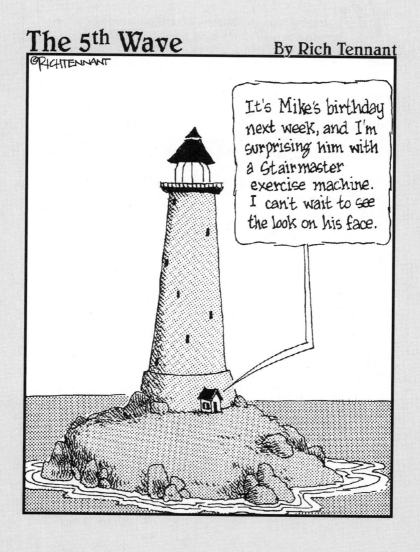

The 5th Wave   By Rich Tennant

@RICHTENNANT

It's Mike's birthday next week, and I'm surprising him with a Stairmaster exercise machine. I can't wait to see the look on his face.

In this part . . .

We prepare you to take the health-club plunge — or create the best home gym for your budget and goals. Chapter 18 explains how to choose the best gym for you and how to recognize slimy sales tactics; we also update you on the latest health-club trends and share the unwritten rules of the gym: what to say, what to wear, and what to do about that pool of sweat you left on the leg-press machine. Chapter 19 helps you sort through the wide range of classes you're likely to find — from spinning to kickboxing to circuit training — and also gives you the lowdown on exercise DVDs and videos, including how to build a first-rate library, where to get the best deals, and which instructors to try.

To create your own home gym, take a look at Chapter 20, which covers the basics: where to shop, how to get a good deal, and where to put your equipment so you'll actually use it, with special sections that focus on cardiovascular machinery and strength and flexibility equipment. We even tell you which brands and features to look for and how to distinguish the quality equipment from the contraptions that will collapse the first time you use them.

Chapter 18

Health-Club Primer: Getting the Most Out of Your Gym

*W*hen it comes to health clubs, we're biased: We like 'em. Liz likes them so much that she's a member of four different clubs. Suzanne likes them so much that she brings weight-lifting gloves on vacation and always hunts down the nearest gym, even if it's in the basement of a crummy hotel in Morocco.

We like health clubs because there's always someone around to give you help and encouragement. You also can get a much wider variety of workout choices than you would in your living room. Of course, to reap the benefits of a health club, you have to actually show up. The reality is, most people don't. If every member of your gym worked out regularly, the place probably would look like the floor of the New York Stock Exchange. About half the people who join a club quit exercising within two months, and only 20 percent work out three times a week.

To boost your odds of becoming a regular, it's important to choose a gym that suits your schedule, your goals, and your personality. This chapter covers the latest trends in health clubs and helps you choose the right club for you. And to make sure you pay a fair price, we explain some of the sneaky sales tactics and hidden costs you may encounter. Finally, we fill you in on health-club etiquette and help you move to the head of the class when taking advantage of the fitness classes offered at most health clubs.

Should You Join a Health Club?

A health club isn't for everybody. Before you shop around, consider whether you're the sort of person who will thrive at a gym. This may save you plenty of money and guilt in the long run. If you decide that a gym isn't for you, that's fine. There are other places to get fit (see Chapter 10 and Part V for more ideas).

Three reasons to sign up

Joining a gym requires a fair amount of guts. It took our friend Chivas Clem two years to venture into his neighborhood health club. "I almost turned around and walked out," recalls Chivas, who's a very svelte 5'8". "The room was full of these tanned, perfect bodies in spandex cat suits, and I'm totally emaciated. Finally, I get the nerve to ask this hulk-like man behind the counter if I can join. He says, 'So, you've never been to a gym before?' I say, 'No, is it that obvious?'" Don't be put off by insensitive comments like that. If you're debating whether to join a gym, remember the following great reasons to sign up.

You need inspiration

At home you can always drum up an excuse not to exercise, even if it means dusting your bread maker or reading your VCR/DVD universal TV remote manual. But at the gym, what else is there to do but exercise? Even if you never talk to a soul, you can feed off the energy of those around you. You may even find a workout partner. Some gyms will scout out a buddy for you.

You want variety

Even if you can afford $10,000 to build an elaborate home gym, you can still find more options at a health club. At home, you may have a stationary bike, a treadmill, or a stair-climber. At a gym, you have all three and more. The same goes for weights. You can strengthen your triceps just fine with a pair of dumbbells in your living room, but at a gym you also have the option of using machines, barbells, and cable pulleys. Gyms frequently update their equipment, so you can try strength and aerobic machines that haven't yet hit the home market or are still too expensive. You can also choose from a long list of classes.

You want expert advice

At a good gym, a trainer is always on hand to help you figure out the chest machine or tell you how to firm up your butt. You also have a room full of other exercisers to watch, although they may or may not be good instructors to learn from.

Three reasons to say, "No thanks"

Some people collect gym memberships like Elizabeth Taylor collects husbands — with about as much success. They figure that if they keep joining, one of these days they may actually go, but inevitably the affair is short-lived. Don't bother buying a membership if you have no serious intention of using it. If you fit the following categories, you're better off finding an alternative way to work out.

You want to exercise alone

If you can't bear the thought of working out in public just yet, start off at home and consider a gym again in a few months when you feel more confident. Or, if you're someone who prefers solitude and uses your workout time to think, don't waste your money on a health-club membership.

Your schedule won't allow time

If you don't have the time to drive to a club or if you can't find one to accommodate your work hours, don't force the issue. Exercising at home makes more sense. (Know, however, that 24-hour gyms are becoming more popular. Even Kingston, New York, Liz's hometown, has had one for years — and the place doesn't even have a Starbucks.)

You hate exercising indoors

If indoor workouts make you feel like a hamster in a Habitrail, head outside and walk, run, skate, or cycle. Keep in mind that you have to be pretty creative to get a great strength-training workout outdoors, but if you use your body weight (push-ups, pull-ups), benches, outdoor circuit-training or fitness courses, and so on, you can put together a pretty decent strength workout.

Knowing How to Judge a Gym

Don't join a club simply because your accountant goes there or because the club is promoting a special discount. Shopping around before you part with any money is important. Here are ten factors to consider (some may matter to you; others won't) when judging a gym.

Location

This is probably the most important consideration. If your gym is on the other side of town, you won't go — even if it's the Taj Majal of health clubs. Ideally, join a club within a ten-minute walk or drive from your home or office.

The only exception may be a gym with special facilities that the nearest club doesn't have, like Pilates or boot-camp classes. But if you're a beginner who hasn't yet made exercise a habit, you may still be better off at a nearby club that doesn't have all the amenities.

Size

The big trend here is the super-club — the health club equivalent of Wal-Mart. You can find low prices, an enormous selection of equipment and classes, plenty of energy, and a large staff of trainers. For an experienced exerciser, a super-club can be as fun as an amusement park; you can never get bored, roving from the golf clinic to the climbing wall to the Middle Eastern belly dancing class. Chelsea Piers in New York City has two floors of ice-hockey rinks, a bowling alley, an equestrian center, a gymnastics studio for kids, and a 10,000-square-foot climbing wall.

If you're a beginner, however, these mega-clubs can be overwhelming. You can get lost trying to find your way from the locker room to the T'ai Chi class. In that case, a smaller, cozier gym may be a better choice. You can get to know the entire staff on a personal basis, and they may even notice if you don't show up for a while.

Super-clubs tend to take a "jack-of-all-trades, master-of-none" approach. These clubs may have a small yoga room, a limited boxing program, and a small climbing wall that would bore you after a week. If you're trying to familiarize yourself with a specific skill or technique, a mega-club isn't the place to get in-depth knowledge. Yoga, for example, is best learned at a studio that teaches only yoga. But if you want a smorgasbord of activities, a super-club is the place to be.

Some larger health clubs tend to take a "no-frills" approach, which means you may not have a spa, day-care center, pool, and 20 different types of workout classes, but you do have cardio and strength equipment, plus a locker room in which to change and shower. If no-frills is appropriate for you, you'll pay far less than at a health club that offers all the amenities.

Cost

Membership fees vary greatly. Large clubs often charge less than small ones because they have more members. (They also tend to pay their staff less.) But the dollar figure doesn't mean everything. Fifty bucks a month may seem outrageous for a small neighborhood club with old equipment; on the other hand, if the club is half a mile from your house, it's a bargain because you may actually go. It's a much better investment than a $30-a-month club that's 20 minutes away.

Consider these other money matters when you choose a gym:

✔ **Hidden costs:** The monthly membership may be reasonable, but will you pay out the wazoo in extras? A few years ago, Suzanne checked out a club that cost $25 a month. What the sales guy didn't happen to mention was the $1.35 daily parking fee. If Suzanne went to the gym five days a week, she would have paid more per month in parking — $27 — than in membership fees. She ultimately found a gym with free parking (a prized commodity in Los Angeles).

Some gyms charge extra for specialty classes, such as boxing. Other clubs don't have membership dues but charge hefty fees for trainers; the catch is, you can't use the club without one. This type of club could run you $10,000 a year. On the other hand, you're bound to get plenty of attention.

✔ **Initiation fees:** In addition to the monthly membership fee, many clubs require an initiation fee. At least they claim to require it. If you insist strongly enough, many clubs waive this fee. Or clubs use this initiation fee as a marketing ploy — something they don't really intend for you to pay. Some salesperson may say, "Just because you seem like a terrific person, and I really want you to get in shape, I'll waive the initiation fee. But shh — don't tell my boss. He'll kill me." Initiation fees can range from $25 to $1,500.

✔ **Bargaining:** Many clubs make special deals if you ask, although they don't advertise this fact. The best time to ask is during slow periods like summer and the end of the month, when clubs are hungrier for sales. You may also get a break if you join with a family member or friend. If you have friends who are already members, ask what they paid; if the sales rep cites you a higher fee, don't be afraid to say, "My friend Jane Smith paid $30 a month, and I'd like the same deal."

✔ **Trial memberships:** If you're unsure about the club, ask for a two-week free trial period before joining, or at least a day pass. Some clubs lead you to believe that you're joining for only a month when you're actually paying by the month and joining for a year. This is why you need to read your contract. If you choose to pay by the month, we recommend using your credit card instead of writing a check. The credit-card company can protect you from incorrect charges.

✔ **Long-term memberships:** Don't even think about it. You don't know where you're going to be in three years (although some club chains do allow you to transfer your membership) — or whether the club will even be in business. One club in New York was selling lifetime memberships until the day before it closed its doors. Never sign up for more than one year. You may even want to sign up on a month-to-month basis if the club allows it; you'll probably pay more, but you give yourself an out if the club doesn't suit you.

Four slimy sales tactics to recognize

Some clubs will try anything to rope you in. Be prepared to combat these sales strategies:

✔ **Limited offers:** "You must join right now," the salesperson may say, "or I can't give you this special deal. I'm really sorry, but the sale ends today." The truth is that if you come back tomorrow, the club may offer you an even better deal so that you don't walk out again. Suzanne's gym seems to have a membership "special" going on every day of every month. If it's not the "Valentine's Day Join-with-Your-Partner Special" or the "March Madness Special," it's the "April After-Taxes Special" or the "May Get-Ready-for-Summer Special." What prospective members may not realize is that these specials aren't so special. Month after the month, the offers are pretty much the same.

✔ **Creating fear or insecurity:** The salesperson may rattle off death statistics for men your age who don't exercise, or tell you that women just a few years older than you disintegrate from osteoporosis because they don't work out. The salesperson may even tell perfectly healthy women that they're fat. This was a common practice at a gym where Liz used to work as a trainer. The salespeople would try to get the trainers to test the body fat of prospective

members — and then inflate the numbers. Liz, of course, refused to participate in this scheme. Watch out: Some clubs try to make you feel as if you can't go on living one more minute without a gym membership.

✔ **An answer for everything:** If you say that you have to ask your wife, the salesperson may attack your manhood: "What's the matter? You need her to tell you what to do about your health? Okay, here's the phone." Then the sales associate sits there while you make the call. If you say you can't afford the membership, the salesman may say, "How can you not afford to invest in your health?" Then he'll whip out the contract and keep inching it across the desk toward you. Be prepared to walk out, even as he tells you how insane you are for doing so.

✔ **The bait-and-switch:** The newspaper ad tells you one price, but when you go in, the salesperson says, "Oh, that sale ended yesterday, but I can give you this offer." Or, "You misunderstood the woman on the phone — we can't give you the first three months free." Always ask whom you're talking to so you can name names. Bring the newspaper ad along so you can use it for proof.

✔ **Cancellation policies:** Salespeople won't always tell you this, but in most states the law requires a three-day cooling-off period. In other words, if you change your mind within three days, the club must refund your money in full. If the club won't, get your lawyer to shoot off a letter; that should do the trick. Also, ask what happens if you quit three months after joining. Some clubs will refund your money for any reason. But most will offer a refund only if you move more than 25 miles from the club, if you can prove that you have a medical condition that will prevent you from exercising for several months, or if the club stops offering the services promised in the contract (although many even have a way around this).

Equipment

You may not consider yourself qualified to judge the equipment at a gym, but even a novice can make some important assessments. If you wouldn't know a hamstring machine even if you were sitting on one, ask your tour guide specifically about the following factors:

- ✔ **Variety:** Do you want three varieties of bikes, or will you settle for one? Some clubs have 10-, 15-, and 20-pound dumbbells; at other clubs, you'll also find 12-pounders, 17½-pounders, and 22½-pounders. Some gyms have a single hamstring machine; others have four, so you can work these muscles standing, sitting, leaning forward, or lying facedown.

- ✔ **Quantity:** Is there enough equipment to support the membership? You don't want your wait for the treadmill to be like the line at the Department of Motor Vehicles. Take a tour at the same time of day you plan to work out, and notice whether the machines are overbooked. Many gyms enforce a rush-hour policy that limits you to 20 minutes on the cardio equipment if others are waiting. This restriction can be frustrating if you've planned a longer workout that day.

- ✔ **Quality and upkeep:** Is the place in a state of disrepair? Is the stuffing coming out of the weight benches? Lots of duct tape is not a good sign. Get on a couple of weight machines and see how smoothly the weight stacks work. Pick up a few free weights and see whether the ends are loose. Listen to the cardiovascular equipment: Are the treadmills loud and whiny? That noise means that the motors need a tune-up. Don't be afraid to test-drive a good portion of the equipment — or to ask other members whether they feel the machinery is well-maintained.

- ✔ **Equipment turnover:** Is the equipment older than the anchors of *60 Minutes?* Or does the club have a new fleet of stationary bikes with built-in heart-rate monitors? Most gyms can't afford to replace all their equipment every year, but at least 10 to 30 percent of the machines should be new.

However, you can still break a decent sweat on equipment that's not state-of-the-art. Sooner Fitness in Norman, Oklahoma, bought the world's oldest Lifecycle at an auction in 1978, and the machine has been in daily use ever since.

Classes

Make sure that the club offers what you want, whether it's the latest and greatest, like Pilates, circuit training, Woga (yoga in the water), or triathlon training, or more-basic strength-training and aerobics classes. (Some no-frills clubs don't offer any classes.) See whether the classes meet at convenient times. To assess whether classes are any good, ask if you can sample a few before joining. Also, ask other members for their opinions. For more on qualities to look for in specific classes, and to read about trends in fitness classes, see Chapter 19.

Members

If you're new to a club, you may initially be intimidated by some of the other members. Our friend John recalls his second day at his new club: "I was in the locker room when this guy with the most perfect body — the biceps, the abs, the whole thing — walked up to the scale and weighed himself. He must have weighed an ounce over what he wanted because he went into a complete rage, punched the wall, and then walked away. I looked down at my body and thought, 'Oh, man. I'm going to be the wimpiest guy at this gym.'"

Fortunately, John didn't give up his membership. He soon found out that there are all types at his gym and that the narcissists are easy to avoid. So don't be too judgmental about the members of your gym. Sure, you may feel more comfortable at some clubs than others; some gyms cater to people over 40, and others attract bodybuilders who could open a door from the hinged side. But people are people, and most of them are nice, even if they look like underwear models for Calvin Klein or Victoria's Secret. Don't give the membership factor too much weight, unless you're joining a gym primarily to socialize.

Besides, you may be surprised by who becomes your friend. "The members I was most intimidated by ended up being just regular guys," says one friend of ours. "One guy had his head shaved except for a rat tail in the back. He looked really mean and scary, but he was a doll when you talked to him. It turned out he was a nurse."

If you're a woman and prefer to work out with other women, consider joining a Curves club. Many of the clubs are efficient (read that: small), so that they can be located in small towns and still turn a profit, but they offer a 30-minute total-fitness program in an environment that's often quite comfortable for women. The focus here is on working out; in fact, you may not be able to do your own individual workout but instead join classes or structured circuit workouts.

Staff

If you're inexperienced, the staff is going to play an important role in your success. Ask the same questions you'd ask when hiring a personal trainer (see Chapter 4). Are the trainers certified by a reputable organization? Are they experienced? Look around: Are the staff members sitting around telling jokes to each other while some poor guy is pinned under a barbell? Is the only visible trainer doing his algebra homework at the front desk? Does anyone acknowledge your existence when you walk through the door?

When you're taken on a tour of the club, notice whether your tour guide actually answers your questions, instead of spewing fitness jargon in hopes of impressing you. Suzanne was pedaling on the recumbent bicycle at her gym when one of the sales staff came by with a prospective member. "These are the recumbent bikes," the sales guy said, to which the woman replied, "What's the difference between these bikes and the other ones?" The sales guy's response: "These are different because they're recumbent." Ideally, staff members should be able to provide a wee bit more information. (To find out what a recumbent bike actually is, see Chapter 8.)

Cleanliness

Is the place clean and well-ventilated? Pay special attention to the locker rooms: Are the bathrooms spotless, or is it foot fungus city? Open the shower curtains and check the floor, the soap dish, and the walls for gunk and mold. If a club isn't clean, don't join — it's not worth the health risk. Ask how often the cleaning crew makes its rounds. And take a gander at the air vents to see whether they're dirty or full of mildew.

One club in Florida has banned soap, shampoo, and shaving cream in the showers to stem the tide of lawsuits filed by members who claimed to have slipped and fallen. Although we sympathize with the management, we do wonder what sort of odors emanate from the club.

Hours

There are 24-hour gyms and gyms that close at 8 p.m. Check your club's hours, particularly on weekends, when most gyms close earlier. Generally, the larger the club, the longer the hours.

Extra amenities

Competition is forcing many clubs to offer more than a Jacuzzi, towel service, and juice bar. A club may organize hikes, ski trips, and softball teams for singles. Or it may offer stress-management workshops and seminars on training for a marathon. Many clubs offer a whole array of spa services. You can treat yourself to a massage, facial, mud wrap, salt scrub, aromatherapy bath, or power shower (a super-strong shower that we personally find a little scary). Prices for these services vary greatly, as does the quality of the services. *Remember:* Make sure that your massage therapist is properly licensed. (See Chapter 25 for more tips about massage.)

A number of clubs have gone way beyond day care, building full-fledged kid gyms with tyke-sized weight machines and cardiovascular equipment. The machines are obviously smaller and shorter with a host of safety devices to prevent kids from hurting themselves. This is great. It's never too early to get kids into the habit of exercising (see Chapter 22), as long as you don't force your 5-year-old into an Olympic training regimen. Some clubs offer exercise classes that the whole family can do together, as well as programs such as teen-only exercise classes.

Another popular service is nutritional counseling, including weight-loss support groups, computerized diet analysis, and heart-disease prevention seminars. Prices vary widely, from $250 to over $1,000 for a package of three to ten sessions. Just beware: As with trainers, anyone can call himself a nutritionist, so make sure that you're dealing with a registered dietitian (someone with an R.D. after his name). Most personal trainers don't have an R.D., even though they may consider themselves nutritional specialists. We don't think anyone but a registered dietitian should dispense dietary advice, and that includes chiropractors — giving this kind of advice may even be against the law in your state. Don't let your "nutritionist" hard-sell you any products — including expensive supplements or prepackaged wonder foods that have been designed "especially for your body chemistry."

At many clubs you can also find medical and rehabilitation services, including sports-medicine doctors, chiropractors, physical therapists, and sports psychologists. Be aware that many of these health professionals may not actually be affiliated with the club; they may simply rent office space on the premises. This arrangement helps the health professionals attract more business, and it gives the club added cachet. However, you need to check out the credentials and reputations of the doctors and therapists as thoroughly as you would any others. Don't assume that the club has chosen the most-qualified health professionals; it may simply have picked those who will pay the highest rent.

Braving the Gym Alone

Going to the gym for the first time can be stressful, especially if you're new to working out. But at some point, you have to take a deep breath and dive in. Here are strategies for feeling at ease in your gym:

- **Take a friend.** Going to the gym with a buddy can make you feel more comfortable and less self-conscious. You two can pretend to discuss the stock market while you figure out how to start up the elliptical trainer.

- **Go at off-peak hours.** This way, no one will be breathing down your neck to use a machine, and you'll have more attention from the staff if you need some reminders. Gyms usually are busiest from 7 to 9 a.m., noon to 2 p.m., and 5 to 7 p.m. If you can't go during off-peak hours, choose the morning because most gyms aren't as packed as they are in the evening, and the morning crowds tend to be fairly regular. You'll get to know other faces, and they'll get to know yours.

Monday is always the busiest day in any gym — everyone's trying to atone for sins they committed over the weekend, like eating too many Ding Dongs. Things trail off by Thursday or Friday (but don't wait until then to work out).

✔ **Don't feel embarrassed if you can't lift much weight.** Hey, you're a beginner. Besides, using only one plate on a weight machine doesn't mean you're lifting nothing. Plates weigh anywhere from 5 to 20 pounds.

✔ **Don't overdo it.** If you push too hard, you may feel so sore that you won't want to come back. The morning after your first few workouts, you should wake up feeling a little achy and tender — but not so sore that you can't stand upright. The discomfort usually is at its worst about 48 hours after your workout — a phenomenon known as Delayed Onset Muscle Soreness. Don't be alarmed: Most people are sore after their first workouts, even if they're careful. This is because your muscles aren't used to the extra work.

Delayed Onset Muscle Soreness is caused by microscopic tears in the muscles that you exercise. These tears fill up with fluids and waste products, and until the muscles recover, you're going to be in a little pain. The good news is that, after the muscles repair themselves, they're stronger and harder to tear. So after a few weeks of working out, you won't get really sore except after especially tough workouts.

✔ **Don't expect to master the equipment right away.** You can't learn Italian in a week, right? It takes a while to become proficient with the vocabulary, customs, and nuances of exercise as well. Even if you've spent several sessions with a trainer, you're not likely to remember how to use each and every machine. Refer to your notes, ask a member of the gym staff for help.

✔ **Make friends.** Knowing other members can give you more encouragement. One good way to meet someone is to ask for a spot — in other words, ask somebody to assist you while you do a weight-lifting exercise. Smile and look approachable. Someone may ask you to spot him. For instructions on how to spot and be spotted, see Chapter 13.

In general, when you talk to people at the gym, stick to topics related to working out. Ask if they're done using a particular machine or bench. Ask how to do a certain exercise. The worst approach is to go up to people in the locker room when they're naked, stick your hand out, and introduce yourself.

✔ **Don't worry about people staring at you.** Most people are far too absorbed in their own workout to pay attention to anyone else. But if you really want to block out your fellow gym members, wear headphones; you don't even need to turn them on. Just make sure your headphone wires don't get caught in any weight machines.

✔ **Wear comfortable clothes.** Go for maximum comfort and minimum embarrassment, but don't wear anything so baggy that it impedes your movement or can possibly get caught in some moving part. Don't wear something that exposes you to the world when you climb on some strange contraption. You may end up spreading your legs in front of 30 strangers, none of whom are your gynecologist or proctologist.

✔ **Ask for help if you need it.** Liz knew a guy who was pretty proud of himself for finally making it to the gym. He got through his first workout only to slice his Achilles tendon on the shower door. He lay there in agony for quite a while before calling for help because he was so embarrassed, not to mention naked. The injury required six stitches, and the guy hobbled around on crutches for six weeks. It took several weeks after that for the staff to coax him back to the gym. He finally returned, although he now takes his showers at home.

Health-Club Etiquette: The Unwritten Rules

Every type of club has its own customs, like the secret handshake you and your buddies used back in fourth grade. Or the secret code word that Howard Cunningham used to get into the Leopard Lodge on *Happy Days*. Health clubs don't have secret code words, of course, but you may feel more at home if you know a few of the unwritten rules. Here are some tips on how to act in certain situations:

✔ **If someone's using the weight machine that you want,** ask whether you can *work in*. That's a term for alternating sets with another person. Asking to work in is perfectly legitimate; no one has the right to camp out at one weight machine for a half-hour.

Working in with someone is convenient if all you have to do is switch the pin in the weight stack. But it's awkward if you have to readjust the seat or add or subtract weight plates. In those cases, waiting until the person is done is a better choice.

✔ **If someone is standing over your shoulder waiting to use the machine that you're on,** kindly ask that person to work in with you. Or tell the person how much longer you plan to use the machine. Say something like, "This is my last set. Then it's all yours."

✔ **If you need help adjusting a machine or you forget how to use it,** turn to a staffer or a gym member with a kind face and say, "I'm new here. Can you help me?"

✔ **If someone's doing an exercise that you want to learn,** find an appropriate break in that person's workout and ask him to show you the exercise. Most people are happy to help — in fact, they'll probably be flattered that you asked.

✔ **If you aren't 100 percent sure that you can safely complete your repetitions,** ask someone to spot you.

If you're embarrassed to ask for a spot, think about a guy named Anthony Clark, whose photo hangs on the wall at Dave's Power Palace, a gym in Carson City, Nevada. Clark lost control while doing a squat (an exercise we explain in Chapter 14). He dumped his barbell forward, and the barbell landed on the weight rack — with Clark's neck sandwiched in between. Fortunately, Clark's two spotters came to the rescue, and he managed to survive unscathed. Chances are, this isn't going to happen to you; after all, the guy was squatting 992 pounds. But the point is, be careful out there.

✔ **If someone's hitting on you and the feeling isn't mutual,** heck, we don't know. You're on your own here.

Major no-nos

Most of the following rules are common sense, but they're violated so frequently that we feel compelled to mention them.

✔ **Don't forget your towel.** No one likes to sit down in a pool of sweat. Always wipe off your equipment after you finish.

✔ **Don't fill up your entire water bottle when someone else is waiting for the drinking fountain.** Let the other guy get his drink and then resume filling up your bottle.

✔ **Don't grunt.** You may as well announce over the loudspeaker, "Hey, everyone, look over here! I'm lifting more weight than I can handle!"

✔ **Don't leave your dumbbells on the floor.** Always put weights back on the rack and in the right order. Don't stick the 15-pound dumbbells where the 10-pounders are supposed to go.

✔ **Don't leave barbells or machines loaded up with weight plates.** You can't assume the next person can or wants to lift the exact same weight you just lifted. Some men leave the bench press loaded up with a 45-pound plate on each side of the 45-pound bar — as if the minimum any human being would bench-press would be 135 pounds. If you see someone do this, you have every right to ask him to remove the weights. You don't have to be all that polite about it, either.

✔ **Don't sit on a machine or bench that you're not actually using.** Between sets, allow others to work in. And don't block the aisles between machines, either.

✔ **Don't drop your weights from 3 feet in the air.** Always place them gently on the ground so as not to simulate an earthquake or crush toes. Now and again, Liz sees a guy who performs a bizarre lift: He sets a very heavy dumbbell on the floor, bends over with locked knees, and snatches the barbell into the air while screaming at the top of his lungs. When the dumbbell is above his head, he lets go of the weight. Needless to say, this is very dangerous and distracting behavior.

✔ **Don't interrupt a staff member who is obviously helping or spotting someone else.** You'd want the trainer's full attention if you were the one being helped.

✔ **Don't spit or deposit gum in the water fountain.** Many people don't quite grasp this concept.

✔ **Don't violate anyone else's personal space.** If someone seems to be jamming through a workout, that's not the time to tap him on the shoulder and ask his opinion on school prayer. This rule applies to the locker room, too.

✔ **Don't carry around your gym bag.** That's what lockers are for! Although most gyms post signs prohibiting gym bags on the weight-room floor, many people ignore this rule.

✔ **Don't "borrow" a gym's equipment for use at home.** Nothing is more aggravating to gym members than looking for a jump rope or weight collar that has mysteriously disappeared.

✔ **Don't hog the cardio machines if you've exceeded the posted time limit.** We've seen people surreptitiously cover the console with a towel while they reprogram the machine, hoping that other people won't notice their time is up. That's what we consider the definition of rude.

Locker-room rules

The stories we could tell about bathroom misbehavior could fill an entire book. We've seen a guy get naked and blow-dry his private parts. We've seen people cut themselves shaving and leave a pool of blood for the next person who comes to the sink. We've seen people mistake the shower for a restroom. Remember that you're sharing this space with a lot of other people, so have some consideration! Here are a few rules that should be obvious but, based on our experience, seem to bear mentioning anyway:

✔ Don't take a marathon shower if people are waiting.

✔ Don't leave hair clogging the drain, and don't leave empty shampoo bottles in the stall.

✔ Don't use more than one locker.

✔ Don't hog the mirror or the blow-dryer.

✔ Don't shake baby powder all over the floor.

✔ Close your locker door so the gym doesn't look as though it's been burglarized.

✔ Throw your garbage in those cylindrical and rectangular objects known as trash cans. Would you really just toss your empty pantyhose package on the floor if you were at home? Okay, even so — don't do it at the gym.

✔ Limit the number of towels you use, especially during busy hours, when the club is likely to run out.

TIP

Packing the perfect gym bag

You'll feel a lot more comfortable at the gym if you come prepared. Using 17 paper towels to dry yourself off after a shower is no fun, although Suzanne has found herself in this situation repeatedly. Some gyms provide towels, cosmetics, even workout clothes. Check with your gym so you don't overpack.

Here's a list of gym-bag essentials. A bag with lots of zipper pockets helps.

✔ Membership card

✔ Water bottle

✔ Small towel to wipe sweat off the machines

✔ Large towel for the shower

✔ Padlock for locker

✔ Gym clothes (shoes, socks, shorts, tights, sweats, t-shirt, sports bra or jock)

✔ Plastic bag for wet, dirty clothes

✔ Toiletries (soap, shampoo, deodorant, and foot deodorant for sneakers)

✔ Sweat band, ponytail holder, or whatever you need to keep sweat from dripping into your eyes

✔ Shower sandals

✔ Post-workout snack, especially if you have a long drive home

✔ Basic first-aid kit, including bandages and antibacterial ointment

These items aren't vital, but we highly recommend them:

✔ Weight-lifting gloves (see Chapter 26 for details)

✔ Personal stereo, headphones, and extra batteries

✔ Reading material for the cardio machines

✔ Heart-rate monitor (see Chapter 6 for details)

A Classroom Code of Conduct

An exercise class is a great opportunity to make friends, so don't blow your chances by annoying the people around you, like the guy who sits in front of you and talks during a movie. Here's how to keep everybody sweating in harmony:

- ✔ **If the class requires a sign-up, honor it.** In a group cycling class that Liz taught, a woman signed up, went to the ladies' room, and then returned to find that her spot had been taken by someone else who had arrived late. The latecomer refused to give the first woman back her bike, and Liz had to use Jimmy Carter–like skills to negotiate a peace agreement between the two women.

- ✔ **Don't walk into a class 15 minutes late and make a big fuss setting yourself up — dragging your step, jump rope, and dumbbells across the room in multiple trips as if you're unloading a U-Haul.**

- ✔ **Follow what the instructor says instead of improvising your own routine.** If you can't perform the arm movements in a step-aerobics class, that's fine — just use your legs; but don't distract the rest of the class by belly dancing or practicing the latest salsa step.

- ✔ **Don't talk so loudly that no one can hear the instructor.**

- ✔ **Wear shoes and proper attire.** This is for your safety as well as sanitary reasons, and most gyms have strict rules about what's acceptable and unacceptable. A weight could drop on your foot, or someone could step on your toes. If you wear street shoes, you can damage the floors by digging holes or leaving indelible black marks.

- ✔ **Avoid walking in front of the instructor when entering late or leaving early.** If you do have to leave early, signal the instructor that you're okay so that she doesn't worry that you're going to the restroom to lie down because you're feeling ill.

Chapter 19

Choosing an Exercise Class or DVD

*E*xercise classes have made an evolutionary leap since the early '80s, when legwarmer-clad instructors patterned their routines after the dance sequences in the movie *Flashdance*. Over the last five years or so, there has been a creative explosion in group exercise. In addition to traditional classes like low-impact aerobics and step (which, due to their simplicity, are getting harder and harder to find), you can now try strip aerobics, aeroboxing, and power yoga. Even small aerobics studios offer classes such as firefighter boot camp and Pilates. Some classes also have become more equipment-oriented, using dumbbells, tubes, balls, steps, jump ropes — even treadmills, stair-climbers, and rowing machines.

All this variety has attracted exercisers who have traditionally stayed away from classes. Liz recently peeked into a group cycling class and noticed that every bike in the house was occupied by a man. A decade ago, most men avoided the aerobics studio like it was a pedicure salon.

Exercise classes have matured in other ways as well. For one thing, they're safer. During the aerobics-crazy '80s, exercise classes meant two hours of sadistic military drills — and a steady stream of injuries from the ultra-deep knee bends, jerky moves, and high kicks considered criminal today. Classes are better now because most health clubs and aerobics studios require the instructors to have experience and certification. Many clubs audition teachers, do regular evaluations, and pay attention to participant feedback.

This chapter covers the classes you're most likely to find at clubs and studios. The two exceptions are yoga and Pilates, which have become so popular that we devote an entire chapter to each (Chapters 16 and 17, respectively). For each class described in this chapter, we tell you how much you'll sweat, what you'll gain, and how you'll fare if you're a klutz. Plus, you'll discover how to get the most out of a class while suffering the least amount of embarrassment.

Why Take a Class?

Classes are suited to a certain kind of personality. You'll love 'em if you feed off group energy or if you enjoy following someone else's lead. But if you treat exercise as downtime, you may prefer to exercise on your own.

Beginners will find classes especially valuable. With luck, you'll get an instructor who can teach you a few things about exercise, like how to take your pulse properly and how to use good form when you lift a dumbbell. You'll also develop a certain body awareness that you may not get from walking on the treadmill or pumping weights. You'll probably make friends, too.

Classes are also a great way to learn a new skill. If you want to buy a step for your home, you can get the moves down in a class. Let the teacher correct you so that you know what to watch for when you do the workout alone in your living room. You can supplement this learning process with exercise DVDs.

Getting through when you haven't a clue

Make life easier for yourself: Choose classes with the words *beginner, introductory,* or *basic* in the title. You'll get a much different impression of step aerobics from a slower, simplified beginner class than if you accidentally wander into an advanced class and hear, "Okay, we're going to U-turn right, U-turn left, electric slide four times, then step, hop, turn, and repeat. Got it? Let's go!"

Before the class starts, tell the teacher you're a novice. A good instructor will keep an eye on you and correct your mistakes without making you feel like an idiot. If you don't mind the spotlight, stand in the front — the instructor will be more likely to notice and correct you. If you're shy and prefer to make your mistakes more privately, stand in the back or get lost in the middle. Throughout the class, keep your eye on the teacher rather than a fellow student. And don't compete with anyone. This isn't the time to give your ego a workout.

If you get tired, just march in place. Don't stop cold and walk out in the middle of a class — you risk nausea or even fainting. But don't be afraid to bail if the instructor is a lemon.

Always bring a water bottle to class — you'll drink more often, and you'll avoid the long lines at the drinking fountain. Finally, come back for more, even if the class leaves you feeling like a clod. Skills and fitness take time to develop. You'll feel pretty darn good when you master a class that used to wipe you out.

What to expect from your instructor

Try to watch a class before you take one. A good instructor has the class moving in unison and right on cue, even if the steps are complicated. Terry Walsh, the owner of New York City's Revolution studio, recently taught a promotional low-impact aerobics class in Central Park to more than 200 people. Terry is such a good teacher that she had the entire class moving in unison, as if they were a highly experienced, professional dance troop. On the other hand, if everyone's bumping into each other or several people have stopped completely and are staring off into space, look for another class. No matter what type of class you're taking, your teacher should:

✔ **Ask questions at the beginning of the class.** Some examples include, "Any newcomers?", "Anyone with an injury I need to know about?", or "Is there anyone here who's never tried step before?"

✔ **Include a warm-up and a cooldown period.** The cooldown should be followed by stretching exercises.

✔ **Give clear instructions so you always know where you are and what's coming next.** Your instructor may say, "Two steps right," and then point right with two fingers. She should let you know what moves are coming up next instead of springing a traveling grapevine on you at the last minute. She should also rehearse new or challenging moves before the class.

✔ **Give you plenty of information on technique — but not so much that you feel overwhelmed.**

✔ **Speak in plain language.** The really obnoxious instructors say things like "plantar flex at your ankle joint" — rather than "point your foot." However, a good teacher should educate you. It's perfectly okay for an instructor to say, "Feel this move in your quadriceps."

✔ **Watch the class rather than gaze at himself in the mirror.** He should face the students at least some of the time and occasionally walk around adjusting everyone's form. Liz once bailed on a step class because the instructor did little other than look in the mirror and watch her muscles glisten in the fluorescent light. She never once turned around to acknowledge the existence of the class members, let alone check their form.

✔ **Do a pulse or intensity check during the toughest part of the workout.** This goes for toning and strength classes, too, even if the check is as minimal as asking, "How's everyone doing?"

✔ **Make the class fun.** You don't want your instructor to take your classes so seriously that they become a chore.

✔ **Have an education.** It's a definite plus if your instructor is certified by one of the major national fitness organizations: the Aerobics and Fitness Association of America (AFAA), the Aerobics Instructor from the American Council on Exercise (ACE), the Exercise Leader from the American College of Sports Medicine (ACSM), and Group Exercise Specialist from the National Academy of Sports Medicine (NASM)/Reebok. See Chapter 4 for more information.

The certifications for aerobics instructors usually require less knowledge of muscle mechanics than personal training certifications, but they're more geared toward the skills you need to lead a group, such as motivating students and modifying exercises for different levels. Some specialty fields, such as boxing and Ta'i Chi, are certificates that certified instructors can earn; other specialties aren't. However, some teachers have aerobics-instructor certifications to supplement their specialty.

A word about cost

Class fees vary widely. Some health-club memberships include unlimited classes, while others charge up the wazoo for specialty classes that require the instructor to hold a certificate. Aerobics studios charge $5 to $25 per class, sometimes more for certain specialty classes. At many clubs and studios, you can buy a package of classes — say, ten at once — but be sure to find out if you must use up the package by a certain date. Another option is to buy a month's worth of unlimited class memberships. Some clubs will let you try out a class for free.

Popular classes

Two classes that have the same name may be completely different. One body-sculpting class may use dumbbells; another may use rubber exercise tubes. And, of course, no two teachers have the exact same style. Still, every body-sculpting class has a number of common characteristics. The same goes for other types of classes. Here's a rundown of the most common classes around, roughly in order of their popularity.

A recent trend is the invention of quick fitness classes — intense, 30-minute classes that help people sneak in a workout in the busiest of days.

Step aerobics and BOSU

What it is: A choreographed routine of stepping up and down on a rectangular, square, or circular platform (or, in the case of BOSU, a domed, flexible apparatus). Many classes combine step aerobics with body sculpting, jumping rope, sliding, or funk aerobics.

What it does for you: Gets your heart and lungs in shape and tones your tush. Step aerobics is a terrific cross-training activity for runners, cyclists, and walkers. BOSU is also exceptional at developing balance and flexibility.

The exhaustion factor: Depends on the choreography, the pace, and the height of your step. In general, the more complex the choreography and the higher your step, the tougher the workout. Never use a platform so high that your knee is higher than your hip when you step up. In some classes, you hold weights while you step.

The coordination factor: High. Even basic classes can confound the choreographically challenged. Higher-impact step and BOSU require major amounts of coordination — some instructors make everything so dancy that you feel like you're auditioning for a Broadway musical. Clubs are trying to attract the non-aerobics crowd with classes like Stepping for Athletes. (Translation: This is a class for people, like the authors of this book, who are in decent shape but have two left feet.)

Who digs it: Most everyone. Step classes and BOSU draw a lot more men than do regular aerobic classes. And women like step because it's such a great butt toner. However, if you have back, knee, or ankle problems, you may be better off with another type of class — or at least, keep the platform very low.

What to wear: Some shoe manufacturers (Reebok, Nike, and Ryka, for example) make shoes specifically for stepping. These shoes have sturdy ankle support, are a bit stiff along the sides, and have plenty of flexibility at the ball and cushioning at the heel of the foot. However, a good pair of aerobics shoes with similar features will suffice. Just don't wear running shoes. You may stumble if the waffle pattern on the bottom of the shoe catches on the top of the platform.

Signs of a sharp instructor: Good instructors ask whether anyone is new to step or has any back, knee, or ankle problems. They accommodate newcomers by going over the basics, such as how to place your foot on the platform. Instructors also alert you before every *transition* — step jargon for any type of change in the routine (such as changing directions). In addition, good instructors make sure that you don't lead with the same foot for more than a minute or two. The music shouldn't be so fast that you have to rush your movements to keep up. Instructors should include calf stretches at the end of the class.

Tips for first-timers: No matter how fit you are, always start with the lowest step — don't put any risers underneath. Don't feel intimidated if the guy next to you looks like he's standing on a coffee table. Also, if you find yourself getting confused or behind, forget about the arm movements and concentrate on the footwork for a little while. When step workouts start to feel easy, consider adding a riser.

Body sculpting and core conditioning

What it is: A non-aerobic, muscle-toning class, usually focused on core strength. Most sculpting classes use weight bars, exercise bands, or dumbbells, or a combination of these gadgets. You perform traditional weight-training moves in a class setting.

What it does for you: Gives you strength and muscle tone and lowers your risk of bone loss, but only if you lift heavy enough weights.

The exhaustion factor: Depends on the instructor, the level of class you're taking, and how much experience you have with strength training. Prepare to be sore if you're a novice or if you usually do different exercises.

The coordination factor: Low. Anyone can do this, although it may take a few sessions to learn proper form.

Who digs it: Anyone who wants to firm up. Body sculpting and core strengthening are great if you want to learn the fundamentals before you venture into the gym on your own. We also recommend these classes for people who won't lift weights unless they're in a class.

Signs of a sharp instructor: Instructors should tell you to use moderately heavy weights so that you don't do more than 15 reps per set. (We define reps and sets in Chapter 14.) Watch out for instructors who do dozens of repetitions with light weights: You're not going to build much strength or tone that way. (Some clubs still offer a class called Body Pump, which involves up to 100 repetitions for some exercises. Stay away from these classes.) The instructor should correct your form and remind you where you should feel the exercise. Watch for a warm-up and cooldown, too. Some instructors skimp on these essential workout components.

Tips for first-timers: Prepare yourself for muscle soreness the day or two after your workout. If you want to focus on a particular part of your body, look for a specialty class like Express Abs or Lower-Body Sculpting. Just know that you'll be strengthening (toning) these body parts, not melting fat off them.

Circuit training

What it is: A fast-paced class in which you do one exercise for 30 seconds to 5 minutes and then move on to another exercise. It's like a game of musical chairs: Everyone begins at a *station* (that is, a place where an exercise is done), and when the instructor yells "Time!" everyone moves to the next free station. Some classes alternate an aerobic activity (like stepping or stationary cycling) with a muscle-strengthening activity (like using weight machines). Others focus exclusively on muscle toning or aerobic exercise.

What it does for you: Increases your strength and aerobic fitness and burns lots of calories. However, you don't get the same level of conditioning as you would from doing your aerobics and strength training separately. If you take circuit classes, aim to get in an additional 20 minutes of straight aerobic exercise at least three days a week.

The exhaustion factor: Moderate. Circuit training tends to be intense, but it's completely adaptable to the individual. Beginners use less weight and perform simpler moves than more-experienced exercisers, but everyone gets a good workout.

The coordination factor: Low. Nothing to worry about.

Who digs it: Anyone looking for a good sweat to shake out of a training plateau. Circuit classes also are popular among busy people who want to combine a strength and aerobic routine in one workout. Anyone who wants a really fun and fast-paced workout will like circuit classes.

Signs of a sharp instructor: Good instructors are aware of each class member's level and modify the moves accordingly. Even though you're moving quickly from station to station, the instructor still needs to focus on proper technique. Look for no more than a one-minute rest between stations. Expect a heart-rate check 12 to 20 minutes into the main workout. (Checking your heart rate, or pulse, lets you know if you're pushing yourself too hard or if you're slacking off. Chapter 6 explains how to check your heart rate.)

Tips for first-timers: Pay attention to how you feel. Many people are surprised by how challenging circuit work can be.

Boot camp

These classes are sort of like army training: You commit to eight weeks (one to three days a week), and the instructor works your butt off. We've seen all types of boot-camp classes. Some are patterned after the activities firefighters use to stay in shape (called firefighter boot camp), such as pretending to duck through a window or chop through a door with a heavy stick meant to represent an axe. Others are Marine-style, featuring endless push-up and coordination drills. Some clubs even offer Ballet Boot Camp, combining ballet moves with traditional aerobics-class movements such as kicks, stepping, and abdominal crunches.

If you're already in shape, you'll get even more fit in a boot-camp class. In most of them, you can burn a ton of calories quickly and tone virtually every muscle group in your body. You may also bond with other class members who show up week after week as you do. However, beginning exercisers need not apply.

Choose your boot-camp classes carefully. Some are taught by instructors who have more ideas than credentials. Liz hurt her back in a firefighter's class when she had to drag a 60-pound bag of sand back and forth across the studio a dozen times. The instructor, an actual firefighter, never corrected any of the students' techniques.

Kickboxing (also called aeroboxing)

What it is: A class that takes the moves of a kickboxer's training and choreographs them to music. You'll do some or all of the following: jump rope, shadow-box, forward kicks, punches, and the fancy footwork you see boxers do in the ring when they're trying to avoid taking one on the chin.

What it does for you: Develops anaerobic and aerobic fitness — in other words, power and staying power. (For definitions of aerobic and anaerobic, see Chapter 6.) Kickboxing also improves your coordination, agility, and balance. Most classes build muscle strength, too.

The exhaustion factor: Very high. Kickboxers are reputed to be among the best conditioned athletes. After one of these classes, you'll know why. Most classes are geared toward advanced exercisers, although some clubs offer beginner and multilevel classes, too.

The coordination factor: High. The drills require some fancy footwork and arm work.

Who digs it: Anyone looking for a killer workout with plenty of variety, or anyone who hates his boss.

What to wear: The usual aerobic clothing will do, although some funk-aerobics clothing crosses over into the boxing classes. High-top aerobics shoes are better than running and walking shoes. Cross-trainers are fine. Most gyms supply boxing gloves if they're used in the class.

Signs of a sharp instructor: We recommend classes taught by someone with good kickboxing skills, rather than, say, a step-aerobics instructor who is just futzing around with a few punches and kicks. Some independent kickboxing organizations certify instructors, but most teachers don't have these certifications. They should, however, have at least one of the usual aerobics-instructor certifications described earlier in this chapter, and they should have attended a few kickboxing seminars.

Tips for first-timers: Pay attention to how you feel. If a lot of the moves are bone crunching or the exact opposite of what other instructors have told you to do, skip the moves or modify them. Don't give up. Kickboxing will get easier.

Funk, hip-hop, jazz, ballet, and other dance workouts

What it is: An aerobic routine with choreography borrowed from dance moves. Classes range from simple moves with a little attitude thrown in, to what seems like a tryout for an MTV funk-a-thon or the New York City Ballet. At many urban clubs, you'll find funk aerobics, hip-hop step, and even salsa hip-hop, a funky class spiced up with salsa dance moves.

What it does for you: Develops heart and lung power and really improves your coordination and agility. You teach your body to move in complex ways and use muscles you didn't know you had.

The exhaustion factor: Depends on the difficulty level of the class. Some hip-hop classes are geared toward beginners. Others expect you to be in awesome shape.

The coordination factor: High. If you're a complete rhythm dysfunctional, you'll have a tough time keeping up. Aerobically, you may not be all that challenged, but you'll spend a good deal of the class untangling your feet.

Who digs it: Anyone with a dance background or anyone who likes dance music. If you're a Fleetwood Mac fan, you may want to pass.

What to wear: You can wear your typical sweats and t-shirt, but don't be surprised if you're the only one. Funk classes tend to have their own style of dressing: high-top sneakers, off-the-shoulder tops, baggy shorts, sexy bras, oversized socks.

Signs of a sharp instructor: Good instructors break down complicated moves into a series of smaller ones before putting them all together. They also show you a variety of interpretations to each move and do the moves more slowly and with less attitude when the class is first learning.

Tips for first-timers: If your parents didn't give you the funk gene, definitely take a beginner class and scope out the class first. More than in any other class, novices tend to get left in the dust. But a really good instructor will give enough instruction so everyone can stay together.

High/low-impact aerobics and stripper aerobics

What it is: A traditional dance-inspired routine. With low-impact, you always have one foot on the floor — you don't do any jumping or hopping. High-impact moves at a slower pace, but you jump around a lot. High/low combines the two types of routines. Cardio-striptease is a low-impact workout that combines aerobics with strip-club moves — you've gotta see it to believe it.

What it does for you: Gets you aerobically fit.

The exhaustion factor: Depends on the class. Classes are too varied to make generalizations.

The coordination factor: Moderate to high, especially if you're a new exerciser or if your parents didn't spring for eight years of tap, ballet, and jazz.

Who digs it: Anyone who wants to work out in a group without using any equipment.

Signs of a sharp instructor: Instructors should spell out the terminology, rather than just say, "grapevine left, grapevine right."

Tips for first-timers: Shop around for a teacher you like who plays music you can tolerate. Music can be a great motivator or a major turn-off.

Studio cycling and Spinning

What it is: Group classes taught on stationary bicycles. The most popular studio cycling class is called Spinning, a program invented by ultra-distance cyclist Johnny G. and licensed by Schwinn, which manufacturers the bikes used in these classes. Other studio cycling classes go by the name of Power Pacing and Reebok Studio Cycling. Regardless of their names, group cycling classes follow the same basic pattern: You pedal a stationary bike while the instructor talks you through a visualization of an outdoor workout. ("You're going up a long hill now — you can't see the top yet . . ."). During the class you vary your pace and intensity, sometimes pedaling as fast as you can, other times cranking up the tension and pedaling slowly from a standing position.

What it does for you: Burns lots of calories and strengthens your thigh and calf muscles.

The exhaustion factor: High. Most studio cycling classes last 40 to 50 minutes and are geared toward advanced exercisers. Suzanne's sister Jennifer was so overwhelmed by her first Spinning class that she left after a half-hour. "All I did the whole time was fantasize about getting off the bike, so I finally just did," Jennifer recalls. You always have the option of lightening the tension on the bike so that the pedals are easier to push, and you can stay seated while the rest of the class stands. But you may want to hold off on Spinning until you build more stamina on your own. Or take a beginning Spinning class if your studio or club offers one, as most clubs now do.

The coordination factor: Low. The most complex thing you'll do is stand up on your pedals.

Who digs it: Studio cycling is popular among people who want to be pushed very hard, especially those who thrive on group energy but hate choreography. Cyclists who are cooped up indoors during the winter also gravitate toward these classes.

What to wear: Because most studio-cycling bikes have the same hard, narrow seats as outdoor racing bikes, a pair of padded bike shorts will help keep your fanny happy. Most bikes have water-bottle cages so you can stash your water within easy reach. Wear stiff-soled shoes; walking and running shoes are too soft, so your feet may get numb by the end of the class from being jammed into the toe clips. Some bikes have "clipless" pedals so that you can wear outdoor cycling shoes with cleats that click into the pedals.

Signs of a sharp instructor: Good studio-cycling instructors don't spend the whole class on the bike. They hop off and walk around, correcting form and offering encouragement.

Tips for first-timers: Ask your instructor to help you adjust the height of the handlebars, the height of the seat, and the distance of the seat from the handlebars. Setting up your bike correctly is important for avoiding injury and staying comfortable.

Water aerobics/ballet/yoga and hydro-Spinning

What it is: Water aerobics classes do traditional workouts in waist- to neck-high water. (Some of the more cutting-edge classes use equipment such as webbed gloves to make the workouts tougher.) The resistance of the water makes the workout feel far more intense, while the water cushions you from the impact.

What it does for you: Water workouts gives you moderate fitness. Because water is 12 to 14 times thicker than air and offers resistance in every direction, these classes can give you great muscle tone.

The exhaustion factor: Low. Most people won't find water aerobics as hard as land-based aerobics. Although water is thicker and therefore harder to pull through than air, water really is a gentler medium. Still, we recommend an occasional water workout to get you off your feet and to give your muscles a balanced workout.

The coordination factor: Low. You're forced to move so slowly that you have time to think about each move.

Who digs it: Anyone who likes the water, has injuries, or is in physical rehab. Water workouts are a terrific cross-training activity for runners, cyclists, and maniac aerobicizers. Water workouts are also great for pregnant women, older people, and people with multiple sclerosis, osteoporosis, or other degenerative diseases because moving through the water is much easier on your body.

What to wear: A swimsuit that doesn't creep up your rear end. Wear a pair of old sneakers or special aqua-exercise shoes so you don't scrape your feet on the bottom. Shoes will add more resistance to your workout.

Signs of a sharp instructor: Certification is a definite plus, but water-certification programs are few and far between. A good certification program is offered by the United States Water Fitness Association and by the Aqua Fitness organization.

Safety should be the first priority in any class. A good instructor will identify nonswimmers and insist that they wear life vests at all times during water aerobics. In water running, all class members — even experienced swimmers — wear flotation vests.

Tips for first-timers: Choosing the right class is essential. You don't want to dive in with a group of 90-year-olds with limited mobility unless, of course, you are one. If you're trying to come back from an injury, look for classes with names like Rehab for Runners. Check with the doctor treating your injury to make sure you have the okay to take a class. Also, realize that your target zone is about ten beats lower in the water than on land. (We define target zone in Chapter 8.)

Choosing from Among All the Exercise DVDs

If you think that exercise DVDs are for wimps and disco groupies, you may be surprised to discover just how tough a workout you can get from popping a disc into a DVD player. (Well, not from the actual insertion of the disc, of course; you do have to follow it.) Yet for some reason, exercise DVDs still carry a stigma.

Like health-club classes, fitness DVDs have become safer, more creative, and more specialized. You can buy DVDs for muscle toning, step aerobics, yoga, kickboxing, pregnancy, post-pregnancy, belly dancing, Ta'i Chi — the list goes on and on. Not only are there more high-quality tapes on the market, but because of the Internet, you can now read thousands of reviews, order DVDs more cheaply, and gain inspiration and helpful tips from Internet forums. This section tells you how to choose the winners and avoid the duds. We offer our best-instructor picks, shopping advice, and important tips for using exercise DVDs safely.

Advantages of exercise DVDs

Sure, exercise DVDs don't suit everyone — you may feel silly prancing around your living room alone, mimicking an instructor who says, "You're doing great!" even though he can't see you. But if you're short on time, self-conscious about your body, or taking care of kids at home, DVDs may suit you well. You won't feel pressure to keep up with anyone else, and you can build a pretty extensive DVD library for less than the cost of a yearly gym membership. Plus, you get a lot more instruction from a tape than you can get from a book or magazine. You may even get more creative routines than many health-club instructors can drum up.

How to choose a DVD

Choosing the wrong DVD is hardly the most tragic mistake you can make in life. However, getting stuck with some out-of-focus program taught by an instructor who grates on your nerves isn't any fun. The following tips can help you weed out tapes that aren't right for you and DVDs that are just plain awful.

Read reviews

Amazon.com, the popular Internet bookseller, also sells DVDs and posts reader reviews. An even more informative source is Video Fitness (www.video fitness.com). This Web site is loaded with helpful information — probably because its mission is to inform and inspire you, not to sell products. (The site was recently purchased by FitnessOnline.com, which does sell magazines, books, and equipment, but the Video Fitness portion remains autonomous.) Hundred and hundreds of videos and DVDs are reviewed here — some by more than a dozen different exercisers. In addition to reviews of specific videos and DVDs, you can read general critiques of several instructors.

Scroll all the way through the reviews for each video or DVD, because opinions differ wildly. One reviewer says Denise Austin's voice "has the same effect on me as fingernails on a chalkboard, made even worse by her patronizing tone; she makes me feel like a toddler she's trying to potty-train." Another reviewer adores Denise: "I appreciate her positive attitude. She makes you feel like you are right in the studio, or she is in your house with you."

If you have no idea where to begin, try the Video Fitness "Personal Video Selector," which guides you through the overwhelming choices by asking you a variety of questions and then recommending several videos and DVDs that appear to match your criteria. Also check out the 100 Club, a gallery of "VFers," as Video Fitness enthusiasts call themselves, who own more than 100 videos or DVDs and list their favorites.

Call a consultant

You've heard of jury consultants, management consultants, and wardrobe consultants — well, there are also folks trained to help you sort through the bewildering slew of exercise DVDs on the market. These consultants are the staffers at Collage Exercise Video Specialists (www.collagevideo.com). It's the country's only catalog devoted to exercise tapes — and the only company staffed with operators who have actually sweated their way through many of the DVDs out there. The consultants have watched hundreds of DVDs, and they have TVs and DVD players at their desks so they can review the latest tapes between phone orders. On the Collage staff is a trainer certified by the American Council on Exercise.

In general, you tend to get a more thorough and honest appraisal from the consultants than from the catalog's blurbs. The company rejects tapes that the staff considers unsafe or useless, but among those available for sale, you won't find any bad reviews. After all, they're in the business of selling DVDs. (The blurbs tend to use terms like "bubbly" and "enthusiastic" for instructors that we personally find shrill and annoying.) The consultants are trained to help you find DVDs that will suit your fitness level and personality, but if you prod them for their personal opinions, they'll probably oblige. When we asked one of the consultants about a particular instructor, she said, "She seems so fake. I want to put plugs in my ears and go running the other way."

Rent before you buy

Large movie-rental stores like Blockbuster have a terrific, up-to-date selection of exercise DVDs (although they don't carry many excellent-but-lesser-known instructors). Try out a bunch of instructors. Many have an entire line of DVDs, so if you find a teacher you like, chances are you'll be happy with the whole lot. In the "Our favorite instructors" section later in this chapter, we list some of our preferred instructors.

Inspect the cover

Before you even rent a DVD — and definitely before you buy — take a good look at the front and back of the jacket. You can't always judge a DVD by its cover, but you can find plenty of clues. Pay attention to:

- ✔ **The type of workout:** Make sure that the workout is what you want, whether that's abdominal toning, funk aerobics, or a stepping/body-sculpting combination. Look for a description of the actual moves — don't go by the title or the hype. "Burns Fat," "Pulsating Excitement!" and "A New Attitude" don't tell you anything.

- ✔ **The fitness level required:** Look for a box that says "great for beginners." Don't start with a tape called "For Animals Only." Some tapes offer modifications for all levels.

- ✔ **The equipment required:** Do you need a step? A tube? A weight bench? Three sets of dumbbells? Make sure that you either have what's needed or are willing to buy it.

- ✔ **The length of the whole DVD and the length of each segment:** A 60-minute step aerobics tape may have only 30 minutes of aerobics. The rest may be a warm-up, stretching session, and cooldown.

- ✔ **Instructor credentials:** If the teacher is certified by one of the legitimate professional organizations, you can bet that the cover will say so. Be wary if all you can find is "Internationally Recognized Fitness Expert." See Chapter 4 for details about certification.

- ✔ **The date of the copyright:** Some tapes are timeless classics, but chances are, a DVD produced in the last couple of years will be more in tune with the latest training techniques. Also, choreography is a lot more creative than it used to be, and safety and instruction are given more consideration these days. Even some of the older workouts led by our favorite instructors contain moves considered unsafe by today's standards.

Get a sneak preview

Before you try a DVD workout, sit down on your couch and watch it all the way through. Imagine yourself doing this tape week after week, and consider the following:

- ✔ **Safety:** Use your common sense. Is the instructor doing anything outrageous, like arching her back so much that you can hear her vertebrae screaming for help?

- ✔ **The instructor's style and personality:** Is the instructor upbeat and professional, or is she hyperventilating with excitement? Is she kind and encouraging, or does she refer to "the huge butt you may have?" Does she have a clear, resonant voice, or does she sound like she sucked helium? Some instructors sound like the cheerleader from hell, some do the sex-kitten thing, and others bark orders like a drill sergeant. One well-known instructor blurts out non sequiturs like "Lose those jigglies!"

- ✔ **Instruction:** Does the instructor use good form and give adequate directions? Some instructors look great doing the workout but never explain proper technique or alert you about what to do next. Others go on and on about good form but don't practice what they preach. In one workout, an instructor cautions against jumping around on hard surfaces while she leads an outdoor class on cement! Some instructors are so winded that they can't even get the words out.

  Don't give up on a tape just because the routine seems too complicated: The first time is bound to be confusing. But go with your instinct: Do you think you'll ever get it, or is the instruction just plain lousy?

- ✔ **Production quality:** Does the sound warble? Is the DVD shot in focus? The tape doesn't need to look like an Academy Award–winning feature, but neither should it appear to have been filmed with a camcorder in someone's garage. At the same time, don't confuse slick production with quality instruction.

- ✔ **The music:** Much of the music you hear on exercise DVDs is bland, synthesized garbage. In fact, the music reminds us of a '70s porn soundtrack. (Of course, we don't watch porn, but if we did, we imagine that's what a '70s porn soundtrack would sound like.) Make sure you enjoy the music, or you may frequently opt out of your workout.

- ✔ **The hype:** Everyone progresses at a different pace. To motivate you, instructors can and should say things like, "Most people will feel stronger and look better in about six weeks if they do this workout regularly." They should not say, "You'll lose 30 pounds in 6 weeks if you follow my routine and send away for my world-famous protein powder."

Where to buy DVDs

At supermarkets or megachains like Wal-Mart, you can often pick up tapes for a fraction of the cost that you may pay in a retail store. (Videos and DVDs cost about $9.95 to $29.95.) But these stores don't always have the best selection. They tend to stick to name-brand instructors and celebrity DVDs, ignoring many first-rate but lesser-known teachers. And beware of return policies: You usually can't get your money back unless the product is defective. You can't just say, "I tried this tape, and it stinks."

Fortunately, with the growth of the Internet, you have a lot more shopping options. Here are some of the best places to buy (or barter for) DVDs:

- ✔ **Collage Video** (www.collagevideo.com; 800-433-6769): This catalog carries more than 700 videos and DVDs, probably the widest selection anywhere, including the latest offerings from top instructors who don't have the clout to interest Blockbuster. Each blurb tells you how tough the workout is, how long each segment lasts, what type of music it's set to, how major fitness magazines rate the tape, and what equipment you need.

  Although the prices aren't always the lowest, the service is excellent, and the warehouse is well-stocked. The catalog's official policy is to accept only defective returns; in reality, it'll take back a tape that you simply don't like — as long as you don't abuse this policy.

- ✔ **Amazon.com** (www.amazon.com): The mega-giant online bookseller sells exercise DVDs as well as books (and just about everything else under the sun). Prices are low, service is good, and shipping is free if you order $25 or more. Plus, you can read reviews of each DVD before you buy.

- ✔ **Fitness Wholesale** (www.fwonline.com; 888-FW-ORDER or 330-929-7227): This Internet retailer offers volume discounts and even allows you to "rent" some DVDs; you pay full-price and get a new DVD, but it'll refund part of the purchase price if you return the DVD within three weeks. (The amount of the refund is specified with each DVD.) The selection is relatively small, and you can only read descriptions of the DVDs, not reviews.

> ✔ **Video Fitness** (www.videofitness.com): This Web site doesn't sell DVDs or videos, but you can trade with other videophiles through the site's Video Exchange. You post your DVD "wish list" and a list of your own tapes that you don't like or have outgrown and then negotiate trades with other VFers. No money changes hands.

Your DVD options

Whatever you want to improve, tighten, tone, build, or reduce, there's an exercise DVD out there for you. Chances are, you'll find dozens. Exercise DVDs usually fall into one of the following categories.

Aerobic

This category includes high- and low-impact aerobics, step aerobics, strip aerobics, Spinning, funk, jump rope, and kickboxing tapes. The aim is to keep your heart rate elevated and your calorie burn high. Look for tips on proper form, how to use the equipment, and how to check your intensity level. These tapes should include an easy warm-up to get your blood flowing. The aerobic workout generally lasts 10 to 45 minutes. The cooldown should last at least three minutes and should be followed by a stretching session.

Strength training

Strength-training (also known as muscle toning or sculpting) DVDs use a variety of equipment, including dumbbells, bars, tubes, and bands. Some tapes focus on a particular body area, such as abdominals, thighs, or arms; others tone your whole body. You generally find two types of toning DVDs: gym-style and choreographed. Gym-style workouts typically work one muscle group at a time, doing 10 to 15 repetitions, and you usually need a weight bench.

Choreographed toning routines may work several muscle groups at once or rotate. These routines aren't dancy, but some of them do require coordination. They tend to give you more aerobic conditioning than gym-style workouts, but they won't build as much strength.

Watch these choreographed routines carefully: The instructor shouldn't have you doing a massive number of repetitions. You shouldn't do more than 15 reps per set — perhaps 30 for abdominals.

Toning tapes should explain how to choose the proper weight for each exercise. The warm-up should be well-rounded but have a bit more emphasis on the body parts you use in the main workout. The instructor should provide tips on proper form, how to make the exercise harder or easier, and how to modify a move if, say, you have a back or elbow injury. The cooldown and stretch segments should be similar to those in aerobic tapes.

Combination DVDs

These circuit-training or boot-camp DVDs combine an aerobic workout with a full-fledged muscle-toning routine. The rules for both apply here, so review the two preceding sections.

Stretch, yoga, and Pilates

The introduction should cover how to stretch, how to breathe, and what stretching, yoga, and/or Pilates can do for you. You typically start with simple exercises that prepare your muscles for more-challenging moves later in the workout. The main workout may not be much different from the warm-up, except that the moves are more advanced. Also, you may hold the positions longer. The instructor should tell where you should feel the stretch and offer constant technique reminders. Expect suggestions for people with back, knee, shoulder, and ankle injuries and for those who are less flexible. The cooldown may include meditation or relaxation exercises.

Specialty DVDs

Specialty DVDs include ballet, country line dancing, pregnancy workouts, chair dancing, workouts for those with osteoporosis and arthritis, and routines for those starting out after breast surgery. Some of these tapes are designed to teach you a new skill rather than take you through an actual workout. Use your judgment: If the workout doesn't feel right, return the DVD to the rental store.

Our favorite instructors

These aren't the only good DVD instructors around, but they're among the instructors who we think produce high-quality tapes on a consistent basis. Many of them have their own Web sites. Among our favorite sites are Cory Everson's (www.coryeverson.com) and Cathe Friedrich's (www.cathe.com).

Beginning

Check out these instructors' tapes if you're a beginner:

- Gilad Janklowicz
- Cynthia Kereluk
- Leslie Sansone
- Richard Simmons

Beginning/intermediate

Try a beginning/intermediate-level workout tape from one of these instructors:

- ✔ Kari Anderson
- ✔ Jennifer Kries (The Method)
- ✔ Gin Miller
- ✔ Donna Richardson
- ✔ Kathy Smith

Intermediate/advanced

If you're looking for an intermediate or more advanced program, work out with one of these instructors:

- ✔ Candice Copeland
- ✔ Cathe Friedrich
- ✔ Gay Gasper
- ✔ Lisa Gaylord
- ✔ Kathy Kaehler
- ✔ Karen Voight

Important safety tips

Safety is an important consideration, especially when you don't have much exercise experience and you're working out in an unsupervised setting. Follow these safety tips:

- ✔ **Make sure that you clear adequate space in front of the TV so you don't bang your shins on the coffee table or knock over any lamps.**

- ✔ **For aerobics and strength-training tapes, wear proper aerobics shoes rather than bare feet or socks.** You also may want to buy a board made of springy wood similar to what you find in good aerobics studios. These boards help absorb impact. Gerstung makes a 30-x-60-inch board for about $160 and a 30-x-30-inch board for about $80. In any case, don't jump around on concrete floors.

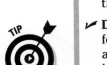

✔ **Even if the instructor doesn't do it on the DVD, gauge your intensity by checking your heart rate or taking the talk test during or immediately following an intense portion of the workout.** We explain these methods in Chapter 6. All our favorite instructors do intensity checks in their workouts.

✔ **Don't try to keep up with the instructors.** They practiced the routine for weeks before it was filmed. Look for someone in the DVD who goes at your pace. Good tapes have demonstrators who exercise at different levels. At the start of the workout, the lead instructor should say something like, "If you're a beginner, keep your eye on Valerie." If you get winded, keep moving by marching in place or walking in a circle.

✔ **If you're just starting out, consider buying a DVD that includes three short workouts rather than one long one.** The shorter workouts last 15 to 25 minutes as opposed to 30 to 90 minutes.

✔ **Remember that your DVD player has a pause button.** Use it if you need to get water.

Chapter 20

Designing a Home Gym

The home-exercise industry is booming. Americans spend more than $4 billion on equipment every year, and it's easy to understand why. You can't beat the commute to your living room, and you can work out at 3 a.m. on Sunday if you really want to. You don't have to pay membership fees, wait in line for the shower, or deal with any unidentified biological matter that doesn't contain your own DNA.

Yet, despite all the convenience, home exercisers have a high dropout rate. The novelty wears off, the bike breaks down, or the 5-pound dumbbell gets used as a doorstop. You can avoid this scenario and the accompanying guilt by designing your home gym carefully. This chapter shows you how.

Planning Your Exercise Space

The inspiration to exercise may have come to you suddenly, but don't make any rash decisions when you buy equipment. You can save yourself time, aggravation, and money by putting some thought into your purchases. Before you even set foot in a fitness store, size up your goals, your budget, and your available space. Here are some specifics to consider before you go shopping.

Looking at the big picture

If you want to get fit at home, be sure to cover all the bases: aerobic fitness, strength, and flexibility. But your home doesn't have to be a palace with high ceilings, racks of shiny weights, and space-age machinery. A complete home gym can consist of a rubber tube, a step, and a handful of videos — equipment that a student on a budget could fit into a studio apartment.

Before you go shopping, think about your goals and consider what type of equipment you're going to need to succeed in all three areas of fitness. Don't just say, "I'll start with an elliptical trainer, and maybe eventually I'll buy some weights." If you plan to get your aerobic exercise outdoors — walking, jogging, or skating, for example — then, sure, spend all of your home-gym budget on weight equipment. Just make sure you have an aerobic exercise plan for the winter. Buying flexibility gadgets needn't be a priority, although in the "Considering Flexibility Gadgets" section later in this chapter, we do recommend buying a cushy mat.

Choosing an inviting spot for your equipment

Where you park your exercise bike can make all the difference between using it to get fit and simply using it as an extra chair for your Academy Awards parties. Put your equipment near entertaining distractions such as the TV or stereo (or away from them, if you want to be away from other family members). And make sure that the spot has adequate ventilation, space, lighting, and climate control; there's a reason that only spiders hang out in cold, damp basement corners.

If you're lucky enough to have a spare room, consider reserving it exclusively for your gym. If you don't have an extra room, at least try to keep all your gadgets near one another. Don't store your dumbbells in the bedroom, your treadmill in the basement, and your stretching mat in the coat closet. Also, plan to keep your equipment within reach. You don't want to hunt through ten drawers to find your favorite exercise DVD. And chances are, anything you store under your bed will stay there — permanently.

We also recommend installing a mirror, preferably in the area where you plan to lift weights. A mirror gives your home gym that health-club feel and enables you to keep an eye on your form. Plus, you can flex your muscles, and no one will think you're a jerk. Over time, you can watch your body slim down and firm up.

Taking careful measurements

Before you buy a major piece of equipment, including a mirror, carefully measure the length, width, and height of your available space. You don't want your dumbbells smashing that new mirror when you raise your arms out to the side. You don't want to bump your head against the ceiling when you press the incline button on your new treadmill. Keep in mind that many equipment stores have high ceilings to accommodate tall equipment.

Measure your door to make sure that you can get your new machinery into the house. Liz ruined a brand-new stationary bicycle when she pounded on the handles with a rubber mallet in an attempt to squeeze the bike through a doorway that was too narrow. One of the handles broke off, which served her right.

Thinking about flooring

If you use exercise DVDs, place your DVD player in a room with a rug rather than a tile or cement floor. The extra padding provided by carpeting helps protect your joints. Plus, there's less danger of slipping.

Don't pump iron on a tile floor, either. If you drop a weight, you'll crack the tile. Carpeting is okay. If you have the luxury of an extra room just for your home gym (and lots of money to spare), consider a rubberized floor. They can run as high as $3,000. Whatever type of floor you have, we recommend putting rubberized mats ($50 to $100) underneath your cardiovascular equipment. This reduces vibration and keeps your floor from getting stained by the globs of oil and other junk that inevitably drip from the underside of a treadmill or other equipment.

Equipment Shopping Tips

After you measure your space, you're ready to hit the stores. The following tips apply to home equipment in general. Check out the "Investing in Cardio Equipment" and "Buying Strength Equipment" sections for suggestions that are specific to aerobic equipment and strength machines.

Shopping around

Prices vary widely, so by all means, bargain-hunt. But remember: A machine isn't a bargain if it collapses with you on it or gives you a hernia. For fancy equipment with lots of moving parts — treadmills, elliptical trainers, stair-climbers, rowers, weight machines, and the like — stick with stores that specialize in fitness equipment. They tend to sell sturdier, more-reliable, and better-designed machines. For simpler equipment like dumbbells, ankle weights, steps, and jump ropes, department stores and sporting goods stores are fine.

If you know the exact make and model you want, you may save money by calling the manufacturer directly. Some manufacturers let you buy direct; others may refer you to a local dealer. But do your homework: Sometimes you can get a better deal from the manufacturer. Other times, going through the dealer is cheaper. You can often save a couple hundred bucks by making a few phone calls.

Buying used equipment is okay, but keep it simple. Stick to gadgets with no motors or complicated designs. The only exception is buying used equipment through an authorized dealer that gives you a warranty. No matter what type of used equipment you buy, ask for a trial period and get all the instruction manuals.

A knowledgeable trainer can save you a lot of research time and may be able to help you purchase equipment. Trainers often get discounts from equipment dealers because they recommend and buy equipment on a regular basis. But ask your trainer if he receives a commission from the dealer or if he'll be charging you a commission; this may eat away at any potential savings. In other cases, a dealer may give you a discount on top of the trainer's commission.

As we explain in the "The Ten Commandments of buying TV fitness gadgets" sidebar, we generally don't recommend buying exercise equipment off TV or the Internet. The picture and real-time video may look fabulous, but when the gizmo arrives at your doorstep, it may be a useless plastic piece of junk. Or it may not even arrive at all, as a friend of Liz's discovered when she ordered a sports watch that never showed up. When the woman tried to check out the Web site again, the URL no longer worked — a tactic that some companies use to evade government regulators.

Buy from the Internet only after you research the product, know exactly which make and model you want, and know that the online dealer is reputable. Liz buys all her athletic shoes on the Internet from a well-known mail-order catalog and saves over 40 percent. Occasionally, she also buys a small piece of exercise equipment over the Internet. For example, she recently found a brand-name heart-rate monitor online for $20 less than the list price.

Taking a test drive

You wouldn't buy a car without taking it for a spin. The same rule applies to exercise machines. Be sure to test every feature. Pull every handle and push every bar. Make sure that a stationary bike pedals smoothly at several tension levels. Try a treadmill on the flat setting and on the incline setting. If the salesperson won't let you give the machine a whirl, say adios.

Looking for safety features

Consider buying equipment with safety features, especially if you have children. For example, to start some treadmills you must punch in a code or wear a special magnet on a string that you wrap around your waist. If you happen to fall, the magnet breaks the connection with the treadmill, and the machine automatically shuts off.

Asking for a discount

High-tech cardio machines and strength machines tend to be marked up about 40 percent above wholesale, so your salesperson probably has some leeway. Asking for a 10 percent discount is perfectly appropriate. You may not get it, but it never hurts to ask. Also, if you're buying several items, ask the salesperson to throw in a complimentary accessory, such as a rubber floor mat to place underneath your equipment. Depending on the square footage, a mat can cost $50 to $200. Some stores will cut your mat to size.

Checking out warranty and service plans

If you're choosing between two similar machines, take the one with the better warranty, even if it costs a bit more. Both aerobic and weight machines should have at least a minimum one-year warranty on all parts.

Find out who's responsible for repairs and maintenance: A good warranty is worthless if no one within 3,000 miles can fix the darn thing. If you buy a machine from an equipment specialty store, chances are someone from the store will come to your house and fix it. Some equipment manufacturers have repairmen on call throughout the country. If you buy from a discount sporting goods store or a TV offer, you may be out of luck.

Investing in Cardio Equipment

Home cardiovascular machines have gotten pretty fancy, and the array of choices can be mind-blowing. Should you go with the elliptical trainer? The rower? The elliptical-rower? The elliptical-rower-stair-climber-treadmill–automatic slicer–microwave oven?

Actually, although the choices are many, we're pleased to report that your chances of buying a high-quality machine are better than ever. Since the first edition of this book was published, the frenzy to market gimmicky cardio machines — riders, gliders, and such — has come to a near halt. (Infomercial producers seem to have switched from hawking schlocky cardio contraptions to hawking bogus weight-loss supplements, which we describe in Chapter 26.)

Which type of home cardio machine is the best? Our answer hasn't changed from the first two editions: The best machine is the one you'll use. That's why testing several machines before you bring one home is so important. You don't want to end up with a space-eating, dust-collecting monster that you can't wait to unload in your next garage sale. This chapter helps you sort through the different options. After you buy your equipment, read Chapter 9, which describes how to use good form on each type of cardio machine.

Treadmills

Treadmill prices have dropped considerably in the past few years, while the quality of some lower-priced models has improved. You can now buy a decent treadmill for under $1,000.

We think self-powered treadmills, the ones without motors, are a waste of money. You typically can't get the walking belt moving unless you incline the machine, but that makes the exercise too challenging for many beginners. Running on these treadmills is impossible — you need an even steeper incline, and the belt tends to stick.

Nor are we fond of treadmills with arm attachments — ski-pole-type mechanisms that you push and pull as you walk or run on the treadmill. Most treadmills with arms are lousy; the rowing motion doesn't match your natural arm swing, so your whole stride is thrown off. (On the other hand, many of the bikes, ladder climbers, and elliptical trainers with arm handles work well.) The big selling point with these double-duty treadmills is the extra calorie burn, but you're not going to burn more calories if the machine slows you down, feels awkward, or exhausts you so quickly that you head for the couch after ten minutes. And if you swing your arms the way you naturally would when walking or running, you're getting that extra calorie benefit, anyway.

Important treadmill features

Treadmills used to be large, noisy, cumbersome contraptions. Now most of them are smooth, streamlined, and quiet. Still, you need to thoroughly inspect any treadmill before you buy it. Here's what to look for:

✔ **A motor to move the walking belt:** Make sure that the belt moves fluidly.

✔ **Safety features:** Don't look twice at any model that doesn't have an emergency stop button and an automatic slow-start speed. A front hand rail is helpful for maintaining balance and is probably safer than side rails, which may actually disrupt your balance if they impede your arm swing. Consider a machine that requires a security code or special magnet to make it go, especially if you have young children. We like the magnet feature for adults, too: If you lose your balance, a magnet that's connected to the treadmill's console pulls off the display panel, causing the machine to automatically shut off.

✔ **Feedback:** Your machine should display the time, distance, speed, and calories burned. Many treadmills also come with a set of preprogrammed workouts and a heart-monitor hookup. (If the heart-rate monitor isn't built into the handrails, you can wear a chest monitor, and your heart rate will appear on the display screen.) Treadmill displays have drastically improved in recent years; you may be able to find one that displays motivating graphics of people exercising at your same pace.

BOSU balance trainers

BOSU balance trainers are a hot new way to get a cardio workout while also improving your flexibility. These fun products are shaped like a dome (see the following figure) that works like a step, but because the trainers are an unstable surface, you challenge your core muscles in addition to getting a great cardio workout. A BOSU will set you back about only $100; $150 with videos and shipping included (see www.bosu.com), and they don't take up much space in your home gym.

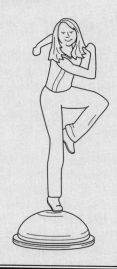

✔ **An incline capability:** Walking uphill adds intensity and variety to your workouts. With most machines, you either turn a crank or press a button to simulate hills. Beware of treadmills that create an incline with hydraulic pistons. These models, often found in department stores, are not likely to support your weight through continued use and tend to break easily and often. If you look at the front of the treadmill on either side and see a metal bar that resembles a bicycle pump (that's the hydraulic piston you're looking at), pass on the machine.

✔ **Programs:** Automatic programs cost an additional $200 to $2,000, but if this feature motivates you, it's probably worth the money. Still, you can create your own varied workouts using the training techniques we describe in Chapter 8.

Our favorite treadmills

Trotter, Star Trac, BodyGuard, Landice, Precor, and True make solid tread-mills with good warranties and service. Precor sells a treadmill for less than $1,000 in certain price-club stores (locations with a dealer service network). The machine has a one-year warranty with guaranteed service. We were pleasantly surprised by its lower-price model, although we don't recommend it for anyone who runs at high speeds more than an hour a day.

Elliptical trainers

Part stair-climber, part treadmill, part stationary cycle, *elliptical trainers* are the hottest trend in cardio machines. Your legs travel in an elongated circular movement, and, on some models, you pump poles back and forth for an upper-body workout. On the best models, you feel like you're doing a sort of rhythmic glide; on the worst, you feel like you're stumbling downhill on your tiptoes.

Unfortunately, most home elliptical trainers we've tried are like most Elvis impersonators: From afar, they resemble the real thing, but on closer inspection, they're nothing but a cheesy imitation. Most of the home units, especially those under $500, aren't as smooth or as comfortable as the more expensive gym-quality models. The home units tend to have a stride length that's too short, too deep, too choppy, or a combination of all three problems. And most of them are so flimsy that we were able to loosen the bolts from the frame and rock them from side to side while taking a test run. This doesn't bode well for durability. Most home elliptical trainers with arm poles are useless because they offer no resistance at all.

The home models we like fall into the major splurge category. The best is by Precor, the company that launched this category. But this machine will set you back nearly $3,500. The Life Fitness home elliptical trainer, for $3,000, comes in a distant but acceptable second. On the cheaper end, Vision Fitness has a $1,500 model that isn't nearly as sturdy as the one from Precor, but it will withstand limited use. Under $500 is an elliptical trainer from ProForm, and although it won't stand up the way more expensive ones will, more and more reliable models are coming available in this price range.

Stair-climbers

We're talking about two foot plates you pump up and down to mimic the action of climbing stairs. Stair-climbers, also called steppers, usually have front or side rails that you hold onto for balance. Their consoles display time, distance, steps per minute (spm), number of flights climbed, and calories burned.

Most steppers have an *independent action;* that is, the movement of one pedal is not affected by the other. With dependent models, the act of straightening one leg to lower the step causes the other pedal to rise. This isn't just a technical detail: Usually, you like the feel of one and hate the other.

Almost all steppers in the $200 to $1,200 range use hydraulic pistons or air pressure to power the pedals. These cheaper steppers are nowhere near as smooth moving as the stair machines people line up for at the gym. Some people don't mind the way they feel, but do stay away from the $200 models, and look for one that doesn't wobble from side to side as you climb. Precor and Schwinn make decent ones at the low end of the price scale.

If you want a gym-quality climber, go with the industry leader: StairMaster (`www.stairmaster.com`). StairMaster makes independent-action machines that use chains and cables to move the steps — and carry price tags of over $3,000. Tectrix makes a respectable clone for about half that amount. LifeStep manufactures the most popular dependent-action home climber in the same price range.

Stationary bikes

Biking is a no-brainer: Park your butt on the seat, plant your feet on the pedals, and away you go, so to speak. You can spend up to $3,000 on a fully-loaded, high-tech super cycle — or $400 for a sturdy, no-frills workhorse. Just keep in mind that every cool feature you opt for jacks up the price.

Before you buy, test-drive both upright and recumbent bikes. *Recumbent bikes* provide back support so that you pedal straight out in front of you. If you have lower-back discomfort, you may appreciate the back support. Recumbents also target your butt and rear thigh muscles at a different angle than upright bikes (the traditional kind, which resemble regular bicycles).

Whichever style you prefer, don't buy a bike from a department store, because quality isn't normally a big consideration in the designs of these products. Some cheap bike seats have been known to collapse with a rider in mid-workout. You don't want to know where the seat pole winds up. Besides, specialty stores carry plenty of inexpensive models.

Important bike features

Two stationary bikes that look similar may feel very different to your derriere and offer different electronic options. So test-ride every bike and do a thorough check of the features:

- **A comfortable, sturdy seat:** Fancy features don't help if you can't sit on the thing for more than five minutes. Some people like a seat that's hard and narrow; others prefer one that's wider and softer. Don't assume that a wide, cushy seat is going to be more comfortable. Extra padding under your rear end is nice to have when you watch TV, but when you exercise, the extra surface area can cause chafing and discomfort. Whatever seat you prefer, it should lock securely into place.

- **Seat and handlebar adjustments:** Make sure that when you sit on the seat, your leg is almost straight at the bottom of the pedal stroke. The handlebars and width of the pedal straps should be adjustable, too. For more details about stationary-bike adjustments, see Chapter 9.

- **Feedback:** You can pay extra for fun features such as preset workout programs, a heart-rate monitor, and games that let you race against the computer. But at the very least, your bike should have a speedometer that displays revolutions per minute (rpm) and miles per hour (mph), an odometer to measure distance, and a timer to keep track of those minutes as they fly by.

  One exception to this rule: Spinning-type bikes. These bikes, primarily used in group exercise classes, are also available for home purchase. They don't have feedback mechanisms, but they have other advantages worth a look. For example, their seat and handlebar positions make the machines feel more like outdoor bicycles. They're relatively inexpensive compared to most other high-quality stationary bikes, and you can buy workout videos specially designed to be used with these bikes. (See a list of some of our favorite bike brands in the next section.) One common complaint is that the seats are uncomfortable, but that's because they're equipped with racing saddles, which are thin and hard. Wearing padded shorts should solve the problem.

- **A way to vary the difficulty:** Look for a knob or button that indicates resistance levels, such as 1 through 12. This way you can accurately measure every workout and track your progress. If 10 minutes on Level 1 used to wear you out, but now you can breeze through 20 minutes on Level 3, you know you've come a long way.

Our favorite bike brands

Here's a brief list of our favorites, but be sure to test-ride any model you're considering to make sure it's comfortable for you:

- ✔ **Non-computerized uprights ($200–$500):** Monark, Bodyguard, Schwinn, and Tunturi

- ✔ **Spinning-type uprights:** Schwinn ($700–$1,200), Keiser ($500–$900), and Reebok ($600–$1,000)

- ✔ **Computerized uprights ($500–$3,000):** Lifecycle, Tectrix, Precor, Combi, and Cateye

- ✔ **Computerized recumbents ($500–$2,000):** Precor, Life Fitness, Body Guard, and Lifecycle

Rowing machines

Forget the rowers with two arms that you pull toward you as you slide the seat backwards. You can never get the tension in the arms quite even, and the entire rowing movement feels sticky and unnatural. If you already have one of these, we're betting it's the most expensive coat hanger you own.

A newer breed of rowers has a chain or cable that wraps around a flywheel. The chain is attached to a handle you pull in a smooth movement toward your chest as you straighten your legs and slide the seat backward. These new rowers do a much better job of capturing the feel of rowing on the water.

Concept II (www.concept2.com) makes an excellent rower that is available through dealers around the country. This machine is so good that the U.S. Olympic Rowing Team trains on it during the off-season. And under $1,000, it gets a Best Buy rating from us. Water Rower makes a good machine that costs a few hundred dollars more. The flywheel churns through a tub of water and makes a sound that's relaxing.

Two cardiovascular bargains

Yes, you can improve your stamina with equipment that costs less than $100. Here are two dirt-cheap yet very effective aerobic conditioning gadgets.

A step

Though essentially nothing more than a glorified milk crate, a step can whip you into shape. Most steps are rectangular, hard plastic platforms; some are springy wood. Good ones have some sort of rubber covering on the top to prevent your feet from slipping. Look for Lego-type inserts called *risers* that snap on underneath to increase the height of the step. Reebok and The Step Company make sturdy steps. In Chapter 19, we recommend several step video instructors to help you make good use of your purchase.

A jump rope

Jump ropes may remind you of pony-tailed little girls in school yards, but don't be fooled: Skipping rope offers some very real, very adult fitness benefits. It strengthens your cardiovascular system, improves your agility, burns tons of calories, and tones your thighs, calves, abdominals, back, chest, and shoulders. You can take your rope with you anywhere, and to use it, you don't need any more space than a small coffee table takes up.

Jump ropes have been subjected to a bit of technology in the past few years. Forget about the frayed cloth ropes you used as a kid. Even leather is history. Many ropes are now made of tough, molded plastic; metal wire coated in acrylic; or space-age polymers with names we can't pronounce, let alone spell. These materials make for ropes that turn faster and more smoothly. Look for features like soft foam or rubber handles, which prevent callusing, and ball-bearing-like swivel action between the cord and handles.

You can get a perfectly good jump rope at a sporting goods store or department store for as little as $3, although you may want to spend $15 to $30 for the fancy features. To size your rope correctly, stand on the center of the cord and pull the ends straight up along your sides. The handles should just reach your armpits.

Many people avoid jumping rope because they view it as a high-impact activity. But if you do it right, it's more like a medium-impact activity on the order of a brisk walk. The secret is staying low. Your feet should barely clear the floor, and you should bend your knees just slightly.

Use a light rope if your aim is to work on skill and agility and to jump fast. Fat, weighted ropes (¼ to ½ pound) work well for building upper-body muscular endurance, but using them for fancy footwork or special tricks is a bit like asking a Clydesdale to run the Kentucky Derby. Buy one of each, and you can mix up your workouts. With weighted ropes, the weight should be in the cord, not the handles.

When you jump, keep your arms relaxed and slightly bent, and keep your upper-body movements to a minimum. Instead of turning your arms in big circles, simply let your wrists swivel slightly. (This is especially important when using a heavy rope; otherwise, you're in for sore shoulders.) Start with a few short sets — about 30 jumps for a light rope, 5 to 10 turns for a heavy rope. Rest by marching in place between sets. Gradually increase the number of sets and jumps per set while decreasing the time you spend marching. Eventually, you'll be able to jump 10 minutes or more continuously (probably less with a heavy rope). Humming the theme song from *Rocky* helps. Building up to long periods of jumping rope is tough, because it's a very intense activity. Jumping rope is best used as a cross-training workout or between body-part exercises while circuit training (see Chapter 15).

The Ten Commandments of buying TV fitness gadgets

In 1984, when the Federal Trade Commission (FTC) abolished limits on the amount of commercial time a television station could air, the commission unleashed a monster: the infomercial. When it comes to fitness products, there's not a whole lot of info in these half-hour commercials that often masquerade as talk shows. Typically, they're filled with exaggerated claims, shameless testimonials, outlandish stunts, and lots of scientific malarkey — all intended to separate you from your dollar.

Try to avoid buying fitness products from TV or a Web site. You have no way to judge the quality of a machine, pill, or gadget. If you do end up purchasing a product that you believe was falsely advertised, file a complaint with the FTC by contacting the organization's Consumer Response Center (877-FTC-HELP or www.ftc.org).

Here are some tips to keep in mind as you watch or read fitness product advertising:

✔ **Don't be suckered by the infomercial audience or "real people" offering testimonials.** Those wholesome folks who whip themselves into a near-evangelical frenzy at the mere mention of the product at hand are usually paid. Often, they've never even tried the product they're gushing over. One acquaintance of Liz gave an emotional testimonial for an exercise video, even though she had never even watched it. "I just wanted to be on TV," she said.

✔ **Beware of the phrase "guaranteed or your money back."** Read the fine print: The manufacturers may promise that you'll lose 4 inches in one month — if you stick to a low-fat diet and a far more extensive exercise program.

✔ **Don't whip out your credit card just because a product isn't sold in stores.** Truth is, most of these gizmos are sold in stores — or they will be on the shelves in a month or two. Sometimes the product is actually cheaper at the store; plus, you can test the product before you buy.

✔ **Don't be impressed by references to Europe, ancient China, or 3,000-year-old secrets.** Bogus fitness products use European research much the same way that "reality" TV shows use Peruvian religious miracles as examples of amazing phenomena: They're too far away for the average person to check out carefully.

✔ **Beware of phrases like "three easy payments" and watch shipping costs.** One gadget claims to cost "Not $60! Not $50!" but "just two easy payments of $19.95." Add in exorbitant (and nonrefundable) shipping and handling costs, and it costs $66.85.

(continued)

(continued)

✔ **Don't be swayed by scientific terminology.** Product manufacturers love to throw around big words, but some of the most impressive-sounding terms have no accepted meaning in the scientific community. Others are misused to hype bogus products.

✔ **Give no credence to celebrity or "expert" endorsements.** Don't think for a minute that a three-time Mr. Universe built his biceps with some plastic contraption that looks like a model of the Starship Enterprise. Athletes and celebs know that fame can be short-lived, and at some point their name may be their only asset. "There's a lot you can talk yourself into," one athlete told us. "You figure, I've gotta make a living. If the public's dumb enough to buy this stuff, that's their problem." Beware, too, of health and fitness "experts" with fancy titles they may have invented.

✔ **Don't be awed by the fact that a product was "awarded a U.S. patent."** You could patent a nose-hair clipper for mice if you wanted to. To get a patent, you need to have an original idea or process, not necessarily a good one.

✔ **Beware of the term "proven."** Many companies cite scientific research without telling you where the studies were conducted. When we inquired about a certain cardio machine, we learned that the calorie-burning studies — which seemed dubious to us — were carried out by a company that the manufacturer owned. This is like admitting your mother was the judge of a beauty contest you won; maybe you were the best looking, but we need to hear it from an unbiased party.

✔ **Hide your credit card between midnight and 4 a.m.** At that hour, everything kinda looks good. Go to bed. If you're tempted to buy an infomercial product, jot down the number and wait before ordering. You may feel differently about that Ginzu Rider in the light of day.

Buying Strength Equipment

There's no shortage of great gadgets to build your muscles at home. There's also, regrettably, no shortage of junk. This chapter covers all your legitimate strength-training options — from $3 rubber tubes to sophisticated, gym-quality machinery. We introduce you to some innovative new products and help you decide which type of equipment is best for your home and your budget.

If you're going to lift weights at home, read Chapters 11 through 14. In those chapters, we explain how to use all types of strength equipment and how to design a strength-training program that'll get you results.

Exercise bands and tubes

Rubber bands and tubes are the absolute cheapest way to strengthen your muscles — you can buy three or four bands for $15 or $20. They're also extremely versatile and great for traveling. Even if you own weight machines or an extensive set of free weights, we recommend throwing in a few bands for variety. (Just know that bands and tubes have their limitations, which we explain in Chapter 13.)

Bands are flat latex strips about 6 inches wide and about 3 feet long, some with handles attached; you hold onto each end or tie the ends around something sturdy, like the leg of your sofa. Tubes come in a variety of sizes and are shaped like very flexible garden hoses, usually with plastic or rubber handles attached. You'll probably like bands for some exercises and tubes for others; you just have to experiment. Because bands and tubes are so inexpensive, it pays to get a variety.

For a few dollars more, you can buy bands or tubes with plastic or rubber handles — a real plus for getting a firm grip on an exercise. Some bands or tubes have built-in ankle and thigh straps. Theraband and LifeLine make nifty band kits that come with a travel bag and several door and bar attachments, priced from $30 to $60. Spri and DynaBand also make quality bands. Because some bands don't come with instructions, we recommend buying a couple of DVDs with band workouts. The following instructors offer quality band workouts: Lynn Brick, Jodi Cohen, David Essel, Donna Richardson, Keli Roberts, and Tamilee Webb.

You also can buy band loops with little foam circles of padding, but you don't really need them. You can just tie your regular band in a circle, which is even more versatile because you can control the diameter of the circle. The smaller the circle, the tighter the tension. You can use a circle to do a number of leg exercises and a few upper-body exercises, too.

Two cautions regarding the use of bands: Check frequently for holes and tears by holding your bands up to the light. When a band is damaged, replace it immediately. And never try to use regular office rubber bands — even thick ones — for exercising. You're just asking to be snapped in the face.

Ankle weights

Ankle weights are great for making floor exercises (like leg lifts) tougher. You'll probably want ankle weights if you like body-sculpting exercise DVDs because at some point, lifting your own body weight will become too easy. As with dumbbells, you can buy an array of ankle weights, from 2 pounds up to 20 pounds. Or you can buy an adjustable set: You insert small weight bars into pockets along the strap. Adjustable ankle weights are a great way to save money. Just know that the weights tend to rattle around. And, it's easy to get lazy; don't neglect to add or subtract weight when you need to. Use ankle weights sparingly if you have hip, knee, or ankle problems. Or, try a pair of weights that strap around your thighs. You may find them awkward to use at first because, well, they're strapped to your thighs, but you get used to them quickly, and they do a good job of distributing extra weight without overloading your knees.

Free weights

Free weights — dumbbells and barbells — are excellent investments: They're simple, versatile, and relatively inexpensive. They do, however, have the highest accident potential; just ask anyone who has dropped a weight on his foot or gotten pinned under a heavy bar. If you're new to free-weight training, please take a few sessions with a trainer. And never do any heavy lifting when you're alone.

On the upside, you won't compromise safety by buying the cheap weights sold at department and sporting goods stores. Weight is weight. There's not much difference between one brand and another. Like meat, free weights are usually sold by the pound. You can pay up to $2 a pound for shiny chrome dumbbells and bars. Gray or black steel will run you 45¢ to $1.50 per pound.

Dumbbells

For a beginner, *dumbbells* (the short weights that you can lift with one hand) should be a higher priority than *barbells* (the long ones that require both hands). Dumbbells (see Figure 20-1) give you more exercise options, and they force each side of your body to pull its own weight.

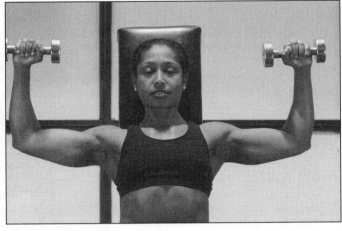

Figure 20-1:
Dumbbells give you a variety of exercise options.

Photograph by Sunstreak Productions, Inc.

When it comes to buying dumbbells, you have two options. The best, most convenient option is to buy several pairs of dumbbells — 5-pound weights, 10-pounders, 12-pounders, 15-pounders, and so on. The cheap choice: Buy an adjustable dumbbell kit. A kit comes with two handles and several weight plates that you clamp onto each end of the handles with a clip or screw-type mechanism called a collar. These kits sell for $30 to $100, depending on the quality and the number of weight plates included.

Owning a whole array of dumbbells saves you lots of time. Let's say that you're alternating shoulder exercises with 5-pound weights and chest exercises with 15-pound weights. All you have to do is put down the 5s and pick up the 15s. With adjustable dumbbells, you constantly have to remove the collar and add or subtract weight plates, which is a huge pain. You may be tempted to use the wrong weight because making the switch is a hassle. Also, locking the weights on securely can be difficult; they can jiggle around or, worse, slide off in the middle of your workout.

A terrific product called PlateMates (www.theplatemate.com) can save you a lot of money on dumbbells. PlateMates are magnets that you stick onto each end of a dumbbell to increase the weight. The magnets come in four weights: ⅝ of a pound, 1¼ pounds, 1⅞ pounds, and 2½ pounds. With PlateMates, you cut down on the number of dumbbells you need to buy. For example, instead of buying a pair of 15-pounders, 20-pounders, and 25-pounders, you can pass on the 20s and create your own 20-pound weights by putting a 2½-pound PlateMate on each end of the 15-pounders. You can stick the PlateMates on the 25-pounders to create 30-pound dumbbells, and so on. PlateMates come in different shapes to accommodate different styles of dumbbells. (However, they won't attach to dumbbells coated in rubber, and the magnets may lose strength over time.) PlateMates cost $19 to $28 per pair. We recommend them in Chapter 25 as one of ten great fitness investments under $100.

If you choose to buy separate dumbbells, realize that you'll need eight or nine different pairs. Although some people use the 10-pound dumbbells for every exercise, this isn't a good idea: A weight that's heavy enough to challenge your back muscles is much too heavy for your arm muscles; a weight that's just right for your shoulders is too light to do your chest any good. If you want to see results, you need to give each muscle the right challenge

For most beginning women, we recommend buying dumbbells weighing 2, 3, 5, 8, 10, 12, 15, and 20 pounds. Even if you can't use the 15s and 20s right away, you'll grow into them pretty fast. The whole set costs between $60 and $150. As for beginning men, start off with 8, 12, 15, 20, 25, 30, 35, 40, 45, and 50 pounds. This set runs $200 to $600.

Shop around and try out different brands of dumbbells. Some have contoured handles that may feel more comfortable than straight ones. Some dumbbells have foam grips; others are coated in rubber. Dumbbells with hexagonal ends are great because they won't roll away. A dumbbell rack is also a good idea. A rack can cost up to $200 but will keep your weights organized and your home gym looking tidy.

If you don't have the space for a whole array of dumbbells but don't want to fiddle with dumbbell kits, either, you have a couple other choices:

✔ **Probell:** Instead of buying six pair of dumbbells, from 5 pounds to 30 in 5-pound increments, you can buy one pair of Probells and get the same versatility. Instead of sliding weight plates on and off, you simply turn a dial to indicate how much weight you want to lift. Through a feat of engineering, the ProBell picks up the requested number of plates.

Just note that ingenuity and space savings come at a price. The steel Probell set costs $199 — about twice the cost of six pairs of no-frills steel dumbbells. But you will save money on the higher end: The $249 chrome Probell costs less than a set of six shiny chrome dumbbells. The Probell stand costs an additional $149. See www.probell.com.

✔ **PowerBlocks:** Each block consists of a series of rectangular, weighted, metal frames, each one nesting inside a slightly larger frame. A series of holes runs along the outside of the frames; you insert a pin inside a hole to select the number of frames you'd like to pick up. You can buy a set of blocks that go from 5 pounds to 90 pounds in 5-pound increments, and you can change the weight instantly. PowerBlocks come with an optional stand and take up about the same amount of room as a telephone table. A 45-pound set sells for about $240; the 85-pound set sells for just under $600. Check out www.powerblock.com.

PowerBlocks rattle around a bit more than ProBells, and their shape is more cumbersome, but PowerBlocks allow you to lift up to 90 pounds with each hand whereas ProBells go only up to 30 pounds.

Barbells

Most people can get along just fine with an array of dumbbells, but you can't beat barbells for power lifts like bench pressing and squatting (see Chapter 14). Plus, barbells add even more variety to your workout. We recommend buying a single bar with a number of weight plates, because buying a whole assortment of bars is expensive. Bars typically run between $25 and $125, depending on the type of steel and where you buy the bar. Bars tend to cost more at specialty shops than at sporting goods stores.

Bars are typically 4 to 7 feet long and come in two sizes: the skinnier *Standard* (about 25 pounds) and the thicker *Olympic* (about 45 pounds). *Plates* (the round weights that you slide onto the bars) and *collars* (the clips that secure the plates) are designed to fit one bar size or the other, so make sure that you buy plates and collars that match your bar. We prefer Olympic bars because they're more comfortable to wrap your hands around — they're also the standard in most gyms.

Purchasing a rack with your barbell is a good idea. Upright racks take up less room than horizontal ones. A one-bar rack can cost as little as $100.

As an alternative to traditional barbells, you can buy a series of lighter bars from 9 pounds to 27 pounds covered with comfortable rubber padding. One popular brand is Body Bar (www.bodybars.com). These bars are good for beginners. They allow you to learn to do barbell exercises without having to use the heavier Standard or Olympic bars. The problem is, you can't clip on weight plates, so you have to buy several bars to accommodate your various muscle groups. They're not cheap either: A 12-pound Body Bar runs about $35. Plus, these bars don't come in heavy enough weights for many intermediate and advanced exercisers.

Weight benches

When you buy dumbbells and/or barbells, buy a bench, too. A bench lets you do many exercises that you couldn't do otherwise. Doing free-weight exercises while lying on your back on the floor is difficult; your elbows may hit the ground before you complete the movement. You also can do several exercises while sitting or kneeling on a bench.

If you're lifting dumbbells lighter than 30 pounds, you probably can get away with a plastic step platform rather than a full-fledged weight bench. With two sets of risers underneath, the platform is high enough and sturdy enough for light dumbbell exercises, but you may want to pad the step with a towel to provide cushioning on your back.

If you're lifting heavier dumbbells or using barbells, buy a real weight bench. A bench is higher off the ground and more stable. We recommend benches that can be easily adjusted to incline or decline so you can challenge your muscles at different angles.

Look for a bench with a thick foam pad covered with Naugahyde or imitation leather. The pad should be sturdily bolted to a steel frame and legs. A bench should be at least a few feet high and shouldn't wobble when you get on and off. A basic flat bench goes for $50 to $300, depending on the quality and thickness of the padding, frame, and legs. We recommend paying a bit more for one that can be set at various inclines because it gives you the ability to vary your exercises. York and Hoist make good ones, but we really love Tuff Stuff benches (from $150 to $450) because they both incline and decline; most benches do one or the other, in which case a bench that inclines is more versatile than one that declines.

Multi-gyms

Multi-gyms are those contraptions that look like a bunch of health-club weight machines welded to each other (see Figure 20-2). Multi-gyms take up a lot of room — usually more than a stereo wall unit — and most require at least 7 feet of vertical clearance space. But many people prefer multi-gyms to free weights or bands because they're so safe and easy to use. Most multi-gyms come with instructions — some even come with videos demonstrating all the different exercises you can do.

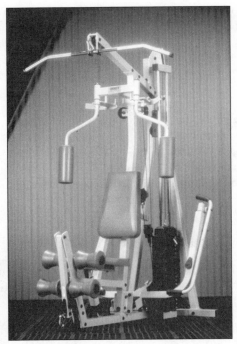

Figure 20-2:
Multi-gyms
are safe and
easy to use.

Photograph by Sunstreak Productions, Inc.

A basic unit has one 200-pound stack of weight plates in 5- to 10-pound increments. This means only one person can use the machine at a time. A basic multi-gym costs $800 to $3,500. If the whole family plans to work out together, you may want a multi-gym with two or three weight stacks, but these can run up to $10,000.

Good high-end brands include Paramount, Pacific, Vectra, and California Gym. For reliable models under $1,000, look at Hoist and Bodyguard.

With the exception of the rather expensive Bowflex systems that many people swear by, we haven't yet found a multi-gym sold on TV or in a department store or discount warehouse that isn't cheaply made. They wobble, they're poorly designed, and the resistance never moves as smoothly as a weight stack. Even some of the TV demonstrators can't help arching their backs on some of the moves. And, sure, you may be able to do 52 exercises with one of these contraptions, but it'll take you about 3 hours just to make the adjustments, which will give you one more reason to blow off your workout.

Take your time shopping for a multi-gym. Try out a whole bunch of different machines, and pay attention to which exercises feel most comfortable. Multi-gyms that look the same sitting on the showroom floor may actually have important differences that you won't notice until you use them. For example, some multi-gyms come with a horizontal chest press; others come with a vertical chest press. You have to decide whether you prefer to lie on your back and press upward, or sit up straight and press forward. Ask the equipment dealer to compare the different ways each multi-gym works each muscle group.

Here's a checklist to consult before you go shopping for a multi-gym. Inspect each machine carefully, and look for the following features:

- **At least the chest/shoulder press, high pulley, low pulley, leg extension, and leg curl exercise stations:** Depending on the brand and model, you may also get chest butterfly, chin/dip, leg press, and abdominal board attachments. If these attachments aren't included with the basic unit, they're usually available as extra-cost options. Keep in mind that most multi-gyms require you to unsnap and rehook cables or arm positions to switch between exercises; making all those adjustments can add extra minutes to your workout and interrupt the flow of your routine.

- **Free assembly:** Pass on any machine that the dealer doesn't put together for you, especially if it comes with an "easy-to-follow" video on how to build it yourself.

- **Weight stacks that move up and down smoothly:** Test several exercises in the store to check for sticking points and levers that don't allow you to fully straighten your arms and legs.

- **A frame made of thick tubular or rectangular steel:** The frame shouldn't shake or wobble when you lean against it. Also, the frame should be painted or powder-coated to prevent chipping and rusting.

- **Upholstery that's sewn on securely:** If you see corners that are curled at the edges, the upholstery probably will rip, tear, or unravel. The same goes for the rubberized padding around the foot rollers and other small parts. If it's made from cheap, thin foam, chances are it will look chipped and beat-up after a few uses.

- **Plates and cables made of quality materials:** Avoid materials that look like they'll snap, fray, or crack.

- **Adjustable seats and arms:** If you can adjust the machine, the whole family can work out comfortably.

- **A good warranty:** The warranty should cover 10 years for the frame, 1 year for moving parts, and 90 days for upholstery. If you ask before you buy the machine, some dealers will give you an extended warranty at no cost. Don't *buy* an extended warranty, however. They tend to be expensive and not worth the money.

Considering Flexibility Gadgets

Most people get by just fine with fundamental stretching exercises that don't use anything but body positioning and gravity. Still, there are some useful tools to help you work on your flexibility. If some of these gadgets get you to stretch when you otherwise wouldn't, they're worth the money. Here's a look at some worthwhile investments:

- ✔ **A stretching mat:** You can use a thick towel or blanket to pad a hard floor, but a mat is a more formal reminder to do your stretches, and you can use it for abdominal exercises and floor exercises, too. Some stretching mats sell for more than $100, but we have no idea why. Just about any mat you come across will suffice. A top-of-the-line mat — one that's cushiony and long enough so that your head isn't hitting your wood floor — shouldn't cost more than $60. Some can be folded in half for storage; others roll up.

- ✔ **An oversized plastic ball:** This is a safe way to improve the flexibility of your lower back. You can drape your body over it forward, backward, or sideways (see Figure 20-3). An oversized ball is also useful for abdominal and leg strengthening exercises. Expect to pay about $30.

The right fit is important. When you sit on the ball, your thighs should be roughly parallel to the floor. However, if you're somewhat inflexible, get a slightly bigger ball. You won't have to bend as far. Also, for stretching, don't inflate the ball all the way; it'll be softer, easier to mold your body to, and less likely to roll away.

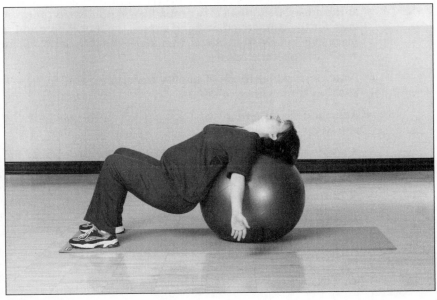

Figure 20-3:
An oversized plastic ball is a nifty flexibility gadget, perfect for exercising during pregnancy.

Photograph by John Urban

✔ **Stretching strap or rope:** Use these nylon bands (Dynamic Stretching Strap or Stretch-Out Strap) when using the Active Isolated method of stretching (see Chapter 6). For $15 to $30 (including a video), you may want to own one, especially if you're too stiff to get into certain stretching poses. For example, if you're sitting on the floor with one leg out and you can't reach your toes, you wrap the strap around your instep and hold a loop in each hand. After holding that position for a while, if you can stretch a little farther, you can let your hands creep up to the loop that's slightly closer to your toes. You can also buy a length of yachting rope at your local hardware store. Just buy a length twice your height.

✔ **The Prostretch:** This gadget is for stretching your calf and shin muscles and the sides of your ankles. The Prostretch is a shoe imprint cast in hard plastic and mounted on one or two curved rockers (wider versions of the rockers you find on rocking chairs). You place your foot on the imprint and drop your heel back toward the floor. Your toes point upward, giving you a terrific calf stretch. If you're not very flexible, you can do this stretch while sitting down. Because the Prostretch supports your entire foot, you get a better calf stretch than if you just hang your feet off the curb, although most curbs won't run you $25.

✔ **Precor Stretch Trainer:** This gizmo is a seat with handlebars and tilting capabilities so that you can lean backward and forward into a stretch. A combination of your body weight and gravity helps control the intensity of the stretch. By switching arm and leg positions, you can stretch nearly every muscle in your body without getting out of the seat. For example, to stretch your hamstrings, you place your leg up on the front of the seat and then lean back. (This mimics the stretch you do on the floor when you place one leg out in front of you then reach for your toe.) The handlebars have wrist straps so that you don't go flying backward if you lose your balance. The gadget also has an adjustable safety pin to prevent less-than-graceful mounts.

At $700, the Stretch Trainer isn't cheap, but it's helpful for people who have trouble getting on and off the floor gracefully. It lets you stretch effectively without having to ask three close friends to help you stand up when you're done stretching. Visit the manufacturer's site at www.precor.com.

Part VII
Exercising for All Ages and Stages

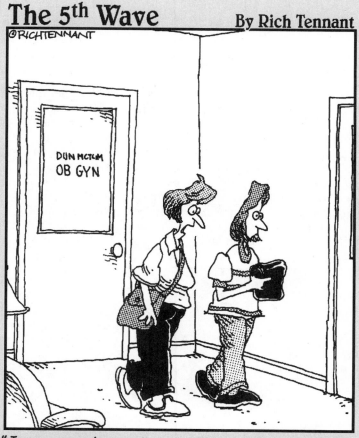

The 5th Wave   By Rich Tennant

DUN MCTUM
OB GYN

"I can exercise as long as I avoid becoming light headed, flush, or short of breath. Of course, if I could have avoided those symptoms a few months ago I wouldn't be pregnant in the first place."

In this part . . .

You discover that exercise isn't only for 20-something singles. Not by a long shot. In Chapter 21, you get a basic primer on exercising while pregnant, a growing (no pun intended) phenomenon that leads to healthier moms, easier deliveries, and healthy babies. In Chapter 22, you find out how to make exercise fun and exciting for your entire family, from toddlers to tweens to, yes, even teenagers. And we're not just talking about healthy thumbs from playing video games. Chapter 23 helps you get and stay fit in your senior years, so that you can live out your retirement with health and vigor.

Chapter 21

Fit Pregnancy: Exercising for Two

. . . .

In This Chapter

▶ Understanding why prenatal exercise is so good for you and your baby

▶ Getting the blessing of your healthcare provider

▶ Knowing how hard you can push yourself

▶ Taking important safety precautions

▶ Choosing the best activity for you

▶ Finding the best types of exercise for pregnancy

. . . .

A generation ago, the last place you'd find a pregnant woman was a health club or a running track. In those days, pregnancy was considered almost an illness — a time to rest in bed, not strengthen your hamstrings. Doctors were afraid that exercise would cause birth defects and increase the rate of miscarriage, but they were just guessing. Now that scientists have actually researched these issues, they know it's perfectly safe for most expectant moms to work out — as long as they exercise common sense and don't try to set a world record in the high hurdles.

Not only is moderate exercise safe for the baby, it has also been shown to have tremendous benefits for mom. Compared to unfit pregnant women, regular exercisers tend to have fewer aches and pains, more self-esteem, and more energy and stamina, especially in the third trimester.

Regular exercisers also have more confidence — and perhaps strength — during labor, and they seem to tolerate the pain better. One obstetrician we interviewed says his inactive patients tend to come to the hospital petrified, but his fit patients are fired up and ready for action. "For them, it's like the Super Bowl," the doctor says. "They say, 'Stand back, let me go. I'm going to push this sucker out!'"

Some research also suggests that fit women have shorter labors than unfit women and that they have a lower rate of C-section. But exercise doesn't guarantee you a free ride in the delivery room. Even if you swim or walk until the day you give birth, you still may have the labor from hell. Some women are simply fated to a prolonged, agonizing labor, while others usher their little ones into the world relatively quickly. However, regardless of the labor experience, fit women do seem to bounce back from pregnancy a lot faster than their inactive counterparts.

Is it safe to exercise during pregnancy if you're not already in good shape? Yes, as long as you work out moderately and have your doctor's okay. In fact, some doctors believe pregnancy is a terrific time to start working out. Entering labor in poor physical condition, they say, is like running the Boston Marathon without any training. It only makes sense to prepare your body for the mega-workout to come.

In this chapter, we offer a brief overview of a fit pregnancy, along with several safety precautions. For an in-depth look at the research supporting prenatal exercise, we recommend *Fit Pregnancy For Dummies,* by Catherine Cram and Tere Stouffer Drenth (published by Wiley), along with *Exercising Through Your Pregnancy,* by James Clapp III, M.D., a top prenatal exercise researcher and strong advocate of prenatal workouts.

Be sure to get your doctor's permission before embarking on a prenatal exercise program. Some high-risk conditions do rule out exercise during pregnancy.

Understanding the Benefits of a Fit Pregnancy

In this short section, we fill you in on how staying fit during your pregnancy makes the entire 40 weeks easier to manage, brings you and your baby tremendous benefits, makes labor and delivery easier than for non-exercisers, and helps you go back to your pre-pregnancy weight and size after your baby is born.

Read *Fit Pregnancy* magazine

If you expect to stay fit when you're expecting, you can find no better source of information than *Fit Pregnancy,* the only magazine devoted to the concerns of pregnant women (and new moms) who exercise. A quarterly created by the editors of *Shape, Fit Pregnancy* (also at www.fitpregnancy.com) is full of great exercise ideas.

The magazine also provides the latest news on the research front. In addition, diet and nutrition are regular topics in *Fit Pregnancy,* as are sex and health issues such as genetic testing and infant vaccinations. *Fit Pregnancy* also rates exercise books and videos, maternity workout clothes, and running strollers.

Here's just some of what you'll be doing if you stay fit during your pregnancy:

- ✔ **Reducing back pain and soreness:** As you likely already know, your baby's growing size puts pressure on your hips, butt, and back, which can lead to stiffness and soreness. When you exercise during pregnancy, you improve your posture and get your back, hip, and butt muscles in shape, thus reducing back pain and soreness.

- ✔ **Gaining enough but not too much weight:** We can't stress enough that you absolutely need to gain weight during your pregnancy, because of the extra fat stores, body fluids, and blood your baby needs to grow properly — not to mention the weight of the child! But many women gain too much, and take years to lose that weight (or never do). Recent studies show that women who regularly exercise right up to the end of their pregnancies gain nearly 8 pounds less than non-exercising pregnant women, but were still well within the normal weight-gain limits for a healthy pregnancy.

- ✔ **Getting good sleep:** If you're having trouble sleeping during your pregnancy — as many women do — exercise can help you sleep more soundly at night and feel more awake during the day.

- ✔ **Reducing delivery complications:** Several studies show that women who exercise have fewer complications during delivery and generally need fewer drugs for pain relief.

- ✔ **Reducing time spent in labor:** One of the most stunning benefits of getting and staying fit during pregnancy is that labor is significantly shorter (by about one-third). Also, women who exercise tend to go into labor about five days earlier than women who don't exercise, making pregnancy that much shorter.

- ✔ **Having a leaner child:** Studies show that women who exercise regularly during pregnancy have leaner (not low-birth-weight) babies, and this leanness continues by age 5. This starts your baby off on the right fitness foot from Day 1. See Chapter 22 for additional tips on helping kids get and stay fit.

- ✔ **Quickly returning to your normal weight:** Women who exercise during pregnancy have less weight to lose after they deliver and find that the weight comes off more easily than for women who don't exercise.

Working with Your Healthcare Provider

If you're pregnant, consult with your healthcare provider before starting an exercise program. Discuss your goals and the type of activity you plan to do, and get an okay from your physician or certified nurse-midwife before you to get started. The health of your child is more important right now than your fitness goals, so if your healthcare provider tells you not to work out, heed his warnings.

That said, some healthcare providers are still living with generations-old ideas about exercising during pregnancy. If you've educated yourself on the topic and feel as though your pregnancy would not be comprised by working out, give a copy of *Fit Pregnancy For Dummies* to your physician, and then meet with her to discuss the possibility. Reassure your physician that you're willing to heed any and all warning symptoms, but if the pregnancy is otherwise proceeding well, you'd like a chance to try to exercise during your pregnancy.

Great Activities to Consider During Pregnancy

Many of the activities listed throughout this book are safe to do during your pregnancy, including those in the following sections.

Walk this way

Some women walk for exercise until the day of delivery. Runners may want to switch to a walk-run program or an all-walk routine if they find that running is just too hard on their lower back and knees. As your pregnancy progresses, avoid steep hills, which make your heart rate soar and may put more pressure on your lower back.

Pay special attention to your walking posture. Stand tall, with a natural S-curve to your back, and your shoulders back and down, not hunched. Lead with your chest. Keep your arms relaxed, and move them forward and back instead of swinging them across your body. Don't walk in very hot or humid weather, because your heart rate elevates more rapidly and your body overheats more quickly. And don't walk when the ground is icy, because your sense of balance is not what it used to be. If the weather sends you indoors and onto a treadmill, hold on to the rails (but not with a death-grip). Treadmills require more balance than walking on the ground.

 Make sure that you wear supportive walking shoes. Because you weigh more than usual, your joints are under extra stress, and they need all the shock absorption they can get. Your feet may swell to the point where you need shoes a half-size bigger than usual.

Getting into the swim of things

Some pregnant women find walking uncomfortable, particularly in the third trimester, so they switch to lower-impact activities such as swimming. In fact, some pregnant women say that the only time they feel really comfortable is in the water.

Water workouts are great because you don't have to worry about your balance. The water supports your weight and the weight of your baby, too, taking the stress off your lower back. Water also reduces the effect of gravity, lessening pressure on your joints. And nothing is more calming and soothing than gliding through the water; swimming can even help reduce pregnancy-related swelling. Plus, you can't possibly fall while you're in the water.

Meanwhile, you can still get a great workout. You can run in the pool, swim laps, and tone your muscles with special equipment like webbed gloves and foam dumbbells. As your pregnancy progresses, you may need to modify your water workouts. Using a kickboard may become uncomfortable because it forces you to arch your back, which can trigger back pain. The frog kick (used in the breaststroke) may also cause discomfort. Don't forget to drink water — you can get dehydrated even in the pool.

Prenatal low-impact aerobics or yoga class

Many health clubs and hospitals offer exercise classes specially designed for pregnant women and brand-new moms. Some classes stick to aerobic workouts; others include strength training, even yoga. Naturally, the exercises are adapted to the limitations of a pregnant body — including the loss of balance, shifting center of gravity, increased joint laxity (looseness), and reduced stamina.

Guzzle water and don't overheat

Pregnant or not, don't exercise without a water bottle close at hand. When you're responsible for someone else's life, too, it's especially important to stay healthfully hydrated. Dehydration is the number-one cause of cramps, particularly in your legs, and it can increase your blood pressure and heart rate, among other things. Always drink before you get thirsty — by the time your body demands, "Water, now!" you're already at a fluid deficit.

Exercise in a well-ventilated area and make sure you wear clothes that breathe. Your baby's temperature depends entirely on your ability to cool your body. Extra-high body temperature irritates the fetus and can lead to premature labor. And keep drinking that water, which cools your body internally.

As a pregnant woman, you do have a built-in mechanism that allows you to reduce exercise-related heat stress. In fact, fit women tend to begin sweating at a lower temperature than inactive women. Still, this adaptation only works to a point, so use common sense.

Participants love these classes because the atmosphere is so much more supportive than it tends to be in regular classes. You don't find a maniacal drill-sergeant instructor yelling, "Okay, today's leg-lift-'til-you-drop day." And you don't find class members in two-piece leotards showing off their sculpted abs.

"It was so great to be working out with other women who were as big as a house!" says our friend Dana, who switched from regular step aerobics to a prenatal aerobics class in her third trimester. "Before, I was always the one who had to stop early because I was too winded or my back hurt." Prenatal exercise classes offer camaraderie and a chance to swap war stories about hemorrhoids, swollen ankles, and husbands who — try as they might — just don't get it.

Continue lifting weights

If you've never lifted weights before, pregnancy isn't the time to start an unsupervised strength program. But if you know what you're doing in the weight room or you're experienced using dumbbells at home, you have no reason to quit your routine. And as long as you make the appropriate modifications, there are plenty of great reasons to stick with it. (We don't want to discourage novices from strength training during pregnancy, but you need to work with a trainer who's very experienced with pregnant women or join a supervised, prenatal weight-training class at a health club.)

Activities to avoid

Certain activities just don't mix with pregnancy, and that list usually includes the following:

✔ Scuba diving, due to the intense underwater pressure, which is harmful to your baby.

✔ Water-skiing, during which you may fall. In addition, if less-than-clean lake or ocean water enters your vagina, you risk getting an infection.

✔ Contact sports, like soccer, volleyball, basketball, and hockey introduce a major risk of falls and contact injuries.

✔ Downhill skiing, figure skating, horseback riding, and mountain biking, all because of the risk of falling.

✔ Cross-country skiing, rowing, and (sometimes) running, because these can be very difficult activities that can overtax your body.

Remember: Check with your healthcare provider for the final word.

Liz's friend Holly lifted weights through both of her pregnancies. Although she had to adapt her routine to avoid machines that she had trouble getting in and out of, she maintained her strength throughout the nine months. The combination of her buff arms and big belly was an inspiration to other pregnant women.

Lifting weights during pregnancy not only keeps you looking terrific but helps cut down on general aches and pains and may even counteract some of the shoulder and back pain that can be caused by enlarged breasts and a growing uterus. Everyday activities won't take as great a toll, and when the big day comes, you'll have more strength to pick up your new bundle of joy (not to mention the diaper bag, stroller, car seat, bottles, and toys that you'll be lugging around).

You do need to adapt your weight-training program to your ever-changing body. You may prefer machines to free weights, because they offer more support and require less balance. Of course, some machines won't fit you anymore. When you're seven months pregnant, you can't exactly lie on your stomach and do hamstring curls. A couple of equipment manufacturers have taken care of this problem by designing a hamstring-curl machine that you use on your side. But most gyms don't have special pregnancy equipment, so ask a trainer to show you more-practical alternatives to your regular routine. Many gyms have standing or seated hamstring machines.

Give special attention to the muscles that are bearing the brunt of your temporary burden, such as those in your knees, ankles, and lower back. But if any exercise starts to feel uncomfortable, stop doing it. Any time that you feel dizziness, nausea, or a pulling in your abdomen, hips, pelvis, or elsewhere, choose a different exercise.

When you're pregnant, your goals in the weight room should change. Don't focus on sculpting your muscles or setting a personal best in the bench press. Instead, aim to maintain your strength and enjoy the movement. Your last few repetitions of each set should be somewhat challenging, but they shouldn't require all-out oomph. Expect to reduce the amount of weight you lift toward the end of your pregnancy, when you may have less energy. Breathe steadily and pay close attention to your form. Don't grip the handles too hard — gripping too hard raises your blood pressure, which shoots up anyway when you exercise.

Monitoring Your Prenatal Workout Routine

Until 1994, the American College of Obstetricians and Gynecologists (ACOG) insisted that a pregnant woman should not let her heart rate exceed 140 beats per minute. Many fit women found this guideline too restrictive; well-trained athletes have exercised during pregnancy with heart rates as high as 190, and without complications. However, most physicians, fearing malpractice suits, were reluctant to approve more-demanding exercise programs. In 1994, the ACOG released new guidelines, eliminating the heart-rate limitation and making many pregnant jocks happy.

However, for a fitness novice, the 140 heart-rate guideline is a good one. (See Chapter 6 for details about monitoring your heart rate.) Pregnancy is not the time to figure out how fast you can run on the treadmill. If you don't want to be bothered with heart-rate calculations, simply use the talk test: Don't exercise so hard that you can't hold up your end of a conversation. Ask your doctor for guidelines tailored to your fitness level. In general, let your body dictate how hard you push yourself, and cut yourself some slack. "I used to get down on myself because I couldn't exercise at the same intensity when I was pregnant," says our friend Elise. "I'd have to stop and rest all the time in my aerobics class. But finally I realized that going hard wasn't the point. I said, 'Hey, at least I'm here!'"

Throughout any prenatal workout, look for the following signs of overtraining and report them as soon as possible to your healthcare provider:

- ✔ **Pain:** Anytime you begin an exercise program, you experience some soreness. However, if exercise hurts in any way, stop exercising and call your healthcare provider.

- ✔ **Fatigue:** If you find yourself feeling overly fatigued throughout the day — and not just when you're exercising — take a day off and relay this information to your healthcare provider at your next appointment.

- ✔ **Overheating:** If you find yourself sweating a great deal, getting excessively hot, feeling faint, getting nauseated while working out, and/or becoming lightheaded, stop exercising, drink plenty of fluids, rest, and call your healthcare provider.

    Never work out during the hottest times of the day and avoid indoor exercise in an area that isn't well ventilated.

- ✔ **Dehydration:** Getting dehydrated is bad for you — and your baby. Keep a water bottle with you throughout much of the day, and check the color of your urine — the lighter and clearer the better — each time you go to the bathroom. (Keep in mind, however, that early-morning urine tends to be dark or orange even if you are hydrating enough, so don't use early-morning urine as a guide.) If your urine looks gold-colored or orangey, you need to drink more fluids. If adding more water to your daily routine doesn't help, ask your healthcare provider for advice at your next appointment.

The key to exercising during pregnancy is modifying your workout routine whenever anything doesn't feel quite right. In addition to the general signs of overtraining just listed, also look for the following warning signs. If you experience any of these, call your healthcare provider immediately.

- **Contractions:** Contractions are a positive sign only if you're within a week or two of your due date. Otherwise, contractions may indicate premature labor.

- **Dizziness:** This could be a sign of *anemia* (low red-blood-cell count that results in weakness and fatigue) or other conditions.

- **Dyspnea:** If you're experiencing *dyspnea*, you may have shortness of breath or rapid and shallow breathing.

- **Headache:** Although many pregnant women report an increase in headaches during their pregnancies (often brought on by fatigue and stress), if you experience a severe headache or a less severe one that doesn't seem to go away, contact your healthcare provider. Headaches can be an early sign of *preeclampsia* (pregnancy-induced high blood pressure).

- **Increased swelling in your legs:** This could be a sign of preeclampsia, which is characterized by high blood pressure and fluid retention and can be quite serious. It could also indicate *deep-vein thrombosis*, a blood clot that develops in a vein.

Don't lie on your back after the first trimester

Starting around the fourth month, you may feel dizzy when you lie on your back. This means that your little one is pressing on your *inferior vena cava,* a major vein that carries blood to your heart. You can modify exercises in a number of ways to avoid this dizziness. For example, if you want to do abdominal exercises on your back, place a folded towel or small blanket underneath one hip. This shifts your body slightly, rolling the baby off the vein. Also, you can do several pregnancy exercises with your back against the wall or while standing or sitting in a chair. In addition, you can do gentle

exercises with a *physioball* — a large, inflated ball that looks like a sturdy beach ball.

One friend of ours took a physioball with her into the delivery room. When she went into *back labor* (when the baby presses heavily against your spine, creating agonizing back pain), she placed the ball against the wall and pressed her back against it. By rolling the ball around on the wall and allowing it to massage her back, she was able to work through most of the pain. She did get some funny looks from the nurses, but when they saw it was working, they thought it was a great idea.

✔ **Muscle weakness:** Muscle weakness can take a couple of different forms: total-body weakness (in which you feel weak all over) or specific muscle weakness (such as your right arm or the left side of your body).

✔ **Vaginal bleeding and/or leaking of amniotic fluid:** Leaking blood or other fluids can be the result of several complications, including *placenta previa* (in which the *placenta,* the organ that grows in your uterus to provide nutrients for the fetus and eliminate its waste, blocks all or part of the cervix), *placenta abruption* (separation of the placenta from the uterus before delivering your baby), premature labor, and miscarriage.

✔ **You can't feel your baby moving:** If your baby's normal movements (that you usually begin feeling between the 18th and 22nd weeks) have diminished or stopped, your baby may be experiencing problems. Keep in mind that your baby will probably be calm during exercise, but you should start to feel several movements again within 20 to 30 minutes after you stop.

Keep Exercising after the Baby Arrives

Working out may seem like a pretty tall order when you're getting two hours of sleep a night and your body feels like it's been through the spin cycle. But even short, easy workouts like a ten-minute walk help you sustain energy (at a time when you really need it), and exercise may help you sleep better at night. Exercise also can help you cope with the depression that sometimes results from sleep deprivation.

But don't rush back into exercise. There's no need to force yourself into anything at a time when a walk to the bathroom may seem like an athletic feat worthy of an Olympic medal. As soon as you feel ready (a few days or weeks after delivery and only after checking with your doctor), try to start a simple routine, such as daily walking. Gradually work up to brisk walks with your baby in the stroller. Consider buying a baby jogger or a special cart that will attach to your bicycle so you can safely take your screamer along for the ride.

Six weeks after an uncomplicated birth — or sooner if your doctor okays it — you can begin more vigorous activity, like swimming, running, or lifting weights. Just make sure you start back slowly. Your abdominal muscles have been stretched, which means they aren't supporting your back as much as they were before you got pregnant. Check with your doctor before you begin your routine again.

Postpartum exercise makes you feel better, but don't expect it to speed up the weight-loss process. The research is inconclusive, but it appears that if you eat regularly and exercise after giving birth, you go through the same weight-loss patterns as women who don't exercise. In other words, it still takes about six months to a year to return to your pre-pregnancy weight and body composition. But you can start regaining your aerobic fitness a lot faster.

Chapter 22

Kids, Tweens, and Teens: Fun Activities for the Whole Family

Statistics on childhood obesity are startling: More than one out of every seven kids in the United States is overweight or obese, and that number climbs every year. As a result of too little exercise and too many calories, these kids are also developing serious diseases: high blood pressure, adult-onset diabetes, and arthritis, for example.

The most effective way to combat poor fitness in your kids is to take a dual approach:

✔ **Tap into your child's natural love of activity.** Kids love to play, indoors or out, and all that "playing" is really just exercise. Ultimately, any kind of activity is exercise (running, climbing, playing tag, skipping, dancing, swimming), so getting kids, especially young kids, to be active isn't usually a problem.

If *you* think of exercise as drudgery, however, and if you present exercise to your kids in this light, you'll likely turn off any natural desire they have for a high level of activity. If you regularly play with your kids — from kicking a soccer ball around to jumping rope to hiking — and make it a priority, your kids will be hooked on exercise within just a few weeks.

✔ **Turn your kids on to healthy foods.** When you stock your fridge and cup-boards with the healthiest, freshest, most delicious foods you can afford, your child's acquired taste for fats and sugars will quickly disappear. Many parents believe that if they don't offer their kids all the pizza, cookies, and salty snacks they want, their kids will go hungry. And, sure, if you fill your cupboards with tofu and green tea, you'll likely encounter resistance. But having access to whole fruits, easy-to-grab veggies, fat-free yogurt, low-salt and high-fiber snack foods, and a range of other healthy foods helps "train" your child's appetite in the direction of nutritious foods.

Try to get outside with your kids every day, at least for a few minutes. Sure, driving home after a long day and finding your child waiting to ride bikes or shoot baskets is tough. But spending time exercising with your child is a wonderful way to get to know and connect with your child and, just as importantly, turn your child on to the routine of regular exercise.

Getting Your Toddler Outdoors

Getting your toddler outdoors is like getting a bird to fly — it's just so natural that many kids wouldn't dream of not doing it. Consider, for example, the following outdoor games kids are motivated to play (and notice that they all do qualify as "exercise" because they build stronger, leaner bodies):

- Playing soccer, Wiffle ball, and kickball
- Climbing trees, monkey bars, and jungle gyms
- Jumping rope
- Playing hopscotch
- Riding a tricycle
- Taking adventure walks in the woods (also known as hiking and snowshoeing)

Yet a toddler who is used to spending most of the day watching TV may think the outdoors is a foreign country, where she doesn't dare venture. It's up to you to change that mindset, showing your child how much more fun playing is than watching Nickelodeon.

Taking your kids along on your fitness routine

Working out with a baby is pretty simple: Put your baby in a playpen and start your aerobics DVD, or set her in a baby seat and pedal your bike for an hour. When she weighs just 15 or 20 pounds, sleeps a lot, and is happy just to be in the same room as you, your workout options are fairly broad.

But life can be different with a toddler. Your 2- or 3-year-old feels very grown up, and she wants to come along with you, at her untimed, relatively unmotivated pace. If you bring her along, you may feel as though your workout will suffer, but if you leave her at home, you're missing a tremendous opportunity to get her hooked on lifelong fitness. What's a fit parent to do?

Bring her along. Although you may decide to supplement with an extra workout on your own a few days per week, you can "work out" with your toddler and still stick to your exercise goals. You just have to change your mindset about what defines "exercise." If you're a runner, what about playing 20 minutes of tag, instead, in which you do most of the running around and take long loops around your yard? If you like to walk, what about alternating ten minutes of power walking with your toddler in the running stroller with five minutes of strolling hand-in-hand with your child, and repeating this three or four times? If you normally do aerobics, what about putting on some danceable music and cutting a rug with your child?

Focusing on fun

Your mission, should you choose to accept it, is to help your child decide how she defines "fun," and proceed accordingly. Don't get too tied up in exercise as you may define it — no toddler ever needs to work out on an elliptical trainer or treadmill. But skipping, hiking, dancing, playing pool games, practicing gymnastics, playing soccer, and doing a host of other activities keep kids moving.

Avoiding fast food

Recent studies at Children's Hospital in Boston found that children consumed enough extra calories (calories above what they need for normal growth) during fast-food meals to add six *extra* pounds per year. In ten years, that makes your child 60 pounds overweight! This study of over 6,000 children also found that kids who eat fast food also tend to eat more fats and sugars and fewer fruits and vegetables, than kids who don't eat fast food.

Avoid making fast food a family "treat" — you can do better making healthy choices at a sit-down restaurant or cooking meals at home. In fact, toddlers love to help cook meals with you, and with just a little training from you on kitchen safety, they can handle a variety of easy food-preparation chores.

When you have to eat fast food, choose grilled chicken sandwiches, turkey subs with whole-wheat bread, baked potatoes (with low-fat sour cream and crunchy veggie toppings), and salads (minus the cheese).

When it looks like exercise, smells like exercise, and tastes like exercise, it's probably exercise. You won't fool your child by taking an inherently boring activity — say, running on a treadmill or swimming laps — and repackaging it by calling it a game. The point is to actually play a game (soccer, say, or sharks-and-minnows) with your child and dispense with adult ideas about exercise. You may enjoy power walking, but your child probably won't; instead, you can both build strength and become more energized by playing a game of duck, duck, goose with you and the neighborhood kids.

Focus on fun, and you and your child will both get a great workout in the process. Don't worry about technique or pace; instead, just keep moving and having fun. If your child tires after 10 or 15 minutes, that's okay; you and your child may be able to get in three 15-minute, no-pressure game-playing sessions every day, and when totaled, that's an impressive amount of exercise for both of you.

Although you can certainly suggest games and activities, let your toddler have the final word on which activity you choose. You may end up playing hopscotch every day for a month, but if you force your desires and expectations on your child, you risk suffocating her natural love of activity. Let her call the shots, and you can just go along for the ride.

Finding Time with Your Preteen

As your child grows, playing becomes less "cool." In elementary school, many kids take three recess breaks; by middle school, this drops to one or even zero. Hanging out at the mall with friends, not jumping rope on the playground, is the order of the day. So, how do you get your tween to exercise?

The answer lies in how you present exercise to your child. If you say, "Come on, sweetie, let's go run for 40 minutes in 30-degree weather," your kid is likely to run to the house of a friend whose parents stock entire boxes of Hostess Ding-Dongs. The trick with tweens is the following:

 ✔ **Make it fun, not drudgery.** Let your child choose the activity you'll do together and just go along for the ride. Have some suggestions in mind, however, so that you don't spend half an hour trying to decide how to spend your half-hour exercise session together.

 ✔ **Make it cool.** The definition of *cool* depends on your child, so ask. You may even want to seek your child's advice on how to dress for your workouts, just so you don't mortify him if his friends see you together.

Making good school lunch choices

Keep this rule in mind: You can *always* prepare a more nutritious sack lunch for your child than she can get at school. The "hot" in "hot lunch" is not synonymous with "healthy." It's just hot. And kids can make their own lunches, too, starting at around second grade. Make them together for a while, and then let her take over for herself.

Even when your child takes her own lunch, though, she still may be beckoned by incredibly unhealthy choices in her school's vending machines. If this is the case at your child's school, get involved and lobby your school district to offer only healthy foods to children. Meet with the principal or superintendent, attend school-board meetings, start a petition — do what you have to in order to give your child healthy food options throughout the day. If the Los Angeles and New York City public schools can cut unhealthy foods out of their vending machines, so can your school.

✔ **Involve as many of your tween's friends as possible (as long as you've followed the preceding rule about making it cool).**

✔ **Encourage participation in school, church, and community sports teams.** Chances are, you can find a team that's playing soccer, basketball, t-ball, football, hockey, and any number of other sports in your area. Tweens usually have a lot of fun in organized sports, meeting other kids their age, developing athletic skills, and discovering the ins and outs of working as a team.

Leaving the car behind

If you have a tween, chances are, you spend a lot of time playing chauffeur to your child and her friends. An exceptional way to help your child become healthier is to substitute walking or bike riding for many of these car-intensive errands. Going to dance lessons? Hop on your bikes and ride the 2 miles to the studio. Heading to the bookstore or library? Stroll there and back. If you live too far to comfortably walk or ride, consider packing your bikes into your car, parking a mile or two away, and pedaling around while you do errands together.

Whether you're heading to school, the park, or a friend's house, use the car as your last option. When you do drive, park as far away from the building as possible to give you and your tween a chance to stretch your legs a bit. Be sure she understands that you're not just being the least cool parent in the world by parking way off in one corner, but that exercise is important to you, and you want to use your legs to get you around whenever possible.

Cutting back on TV and video games

After a hard day at work, you just want to sink into the recliner, grab the remote, and veg out, right? Well, maybe. Taking time to relax each day is, of course, absolutely necessary in life. But spending hours in front of the TV is often more a matter of habit than necessity, and your kids will follow your lead. Watching TV and playing video games is fun — no doubt about it — but so is playing a game of pick-up basketball, taking a walk through town, playing touch football, riding bikes, and climbing trees. If you can limit the amount of time you spend in front of the TV — and we're talking about really limiting it, say, to a half-hour per day — you can open up precious hours to play, talk as a family, finish homework, read quietly, and so on.

It's no great irony that, as TV viewing increases, so do obesity levels.

Connecting with Your Teenager

By their teenage years, your kids have settled into a routine — often one of two routines: as active teenagers who participate in several school sports or as fairly inactive teens. If your teen is of the inactive variety, or is active for one or two school sports seasons but not year-round, you can help your child become more active by taking a few simple steps, discussed in the following sections.

Planning new traditions

Does your family's routine center around food and comfort, or are you an active family that heads out the door whenever possible? Whatever your current routine, talk to your teen about some new traditions you can put into place.

- ✔ Is Saturday morning a time for sausage and pancakes? What about replacing that with a brisk walk to the local coffee shop or a bike ride around the city?

- ✔ Are birthdays usually celebrated with a heavy meal and rich birthday cake? What about taking your teen out of school at lunchtime on his birthday and heading to the nearest city or state park for an afternoon hike, complete with a picnic lunch?

✔ When you go to the mall, do you and your kids spend more time in the food court than you do strolling around? If so, consider eating before heading out the door and/or walking two laps around the entire mall before heading into any stores. Or reward yourselves for getting through your holiday shopping by stopping at the Y for a swim or a game of pick-up basketball.

✔ Is the time between Thanksgiving and New Year's Day a routine of too many cookies and candies, rich holiday meals, and inactivity? What happens if you just don't buy or make any holiday treats, focusing instead on stocking up on holiday fruits, such as sweet, delicious Clementine tangerines or Pink Lady apples? And how about if you spend holiday mornings taking a brisk walk (with snowshoes, in certain climates) or going sledding? Can you invite your teen's friends over for a basketball or Ping-Pong tournament on Thanksgiving afternoon?

"Tradition" doesn't have to be synonymous with "unhealthy habits." Instead, talk to your teen about how, together, you can change your routine in fun, creative ways. Although you may not be able to pull your family away from the traditional Thanksgiving football game, you may be able to get your kids to toss a football around with you during halftime.

Letting your teen find his groove

If your teen is active in school sports, you're facing one of parenting's toughest tests. You have to fully support your child by purchasing equipment and paying for camps and other sports fees, attending as many events as possible, giving rides to and from practices, and so on. But after that, you have to back off. No matter how badly you want your child to be the next city swim champ or earn a sports scholarship to college, no amount of cajoling, pressuring, or forcing your teen through extra workouts will make that happen.

Few kids will grow up to be the next Mia Hamm or Tiger Woods. If your teen wants to devote herself to one sport and pursue it passionately, support that without reservation — you'll spend countless dollars and hours supporting your child in that endeavor. But if she loses interest or decides to try a variety of sports, allow her to enjoy that process, because along the way, she'll develop lifelong friendships and internalize valuable lessons about teamwork and etiquette. Very few kids who are forced into one particular sport stick with it very long.

If your child opts out of school sports completely, you have a rare opportunity on your hands to work out together, if she agrees. Choose any activity that appeals to both of you (from yoga to in-line skating and everything in between), make sure you both have the best equipment you can afford, and focus on having fun together — not so much on heart rate, workout intensity, and calories burned.

TIP

Healthy eating, teenage-style

To encourage healthy eating among the teenage set, you have to master snacks. The term *snack food* probably conjures images of chips, cookies, and bite-size pizza treats, but a snack is, technically, just something to tide you over between meals. Although no teenager is likely to come home from school and lick his lips at the prospect of a steaming plate of broccoli, you can provide a variety of healthier snacks that your teen will go for. Here are some examples:

- Veggie pizzas made with low-fat cheese

- Soups and chili made with poultry breasts, ground turkey breast, and other low-fat meats

- Fat-free or low-fat ranch dressing with carrot and celery sticks, broccoli crowns, cherry tomatoes, and any other veggies he likes

- Grapes, apple chunks, orange sections, bananas, peaches, pears, plums, and any other fruits that appeal to him

- Dried raisins, dates, prunes, and any other dried fruit without added sugar

- Crackers low in fat and salt and high in fiber, rice or corn cakes, a non-trans-fat popcorn

- 100 percent juice drinks

- Natural peanut butter on whole-wheat crackers, apples, or bananas

- String cheese and whole-grain RyKrisp crackers

- Low-fat or fat-free pudding cup or yogurt

- Trail mix

- Low-fat ice cream sandwiches

- Frozen yogurt

- Low-fat chips and salsa

- Hummus and whole-wheat pita, cut into wedges

- Nuts or sunflower seeds

- Low-fat hot chocolate or latte

Chapter 23

Staying Active as You Age

Your senior years are what you've looked forward to all your life: retirement, relaxation, and all those lovely 10-percent-off discounts! But many seniors suffer through a variety of ailments and health problems, losing vigor and strength too quickly.

The secret to aging slowly and with good health is fitness. By staying active as you age, you reap substantial benefits, from looking and feeling young to staving off life-threatening diseases. In this chapter, you discover those benefits, find out how to get started, and take in a few safety tips.

Keeping Yourself Young with Exercise

If you're among the many seniors who think fitness is only for a younger crowd, think again. The *Journal of Gerontology* recently released a study showing that people over age 60 can train just as hard as younger folks and derive the same benefits from exercise as people far younger.

The benefits of beginning or continuing to exercise in your senior years are phenomenal, not the least of which is making you feel 10 to 25 years younger. Consider the extent to which your life can be enhanced by the combination of cardio workouts (like walking or cycling) and strength training (lifting weights) several days per week:

✔ You have more energy.

✔ You experience less depression and anxiety.

✔ You have an easier time losing weight.

- ✔ You increase bone density, build muscle strength, and slow the muscle deterioration that comes with age.

- ✔ You improve your balance, which may prevent the falls that cause hip fractures.

- ✔ You reduce lower-back pain (this is especially true if you're lifting weights).

- ✔ You boost your immune system.

- ✔ You lower your blood pressure.

- ✔ You substantially cut your risk of heart disease, arthritis, diabetes, colon cancer, and Alzheimer's and dementia.

- ✔ Your mind is more alert.

- ✔ You can be more independent in your daily activities.

If you saw a pharmaceutical advertisement that listed even half of those benefits, you'd be lining up at your doctor's office for a prescription. So here's your exercise Rx: See your doctor for a checkup, and then, no matter what your age or experience with exercise, begin doing small amounts of cardio exercises (see Part III), strength training (see Part IV), or a combination (see Part V), three to five days per week. As your soreness wears off and your fitness improves, lengthen your workout times, improve your pace, and increase the amount of weight you're lifting. And be sure to stretch daily (see Chapter 6).

Knowing Where to Begin

Do you find the idea of exercise daunting and just don't know where to start? You're not alone: 85 percent of all seniors don't exercise regularly. If that sounds like you, you've come to the right place: this book. Just about all the information throughout this book applies to you, and you can visit the chapters that make the most sense to you. So, if you've never worked out before, flip to Chapter 2 for information on assessing your current fitness, and then jump to Chapter 3 for tips on setting workout goals.

One of the major reasons seniors don't stick to a workout program is a lack of immediate results. Don't fall for this trap! Getting fit does take time, but if you're doing a combination of cardio and weight training, you may notice small differences in just a week or two. After a month, your clothes may fit better, and within two or three months, your grandchildren will wonder how you're able to keep up with them. Exercise is its own fountain of youth, and while the magic potion does take a little time to make its way into your system, if you find an exercise you enjoy and stick with it, you'll be whistling a happy tune before you know it.

Cardio workouts for a healthy heart

Because cardio workouts (short for *cardiovascular,* the system that includes your heart and lungs) help lower your heart rate, improve your lung function, and make you feel more energized, be sure to include cardio as a part of your overall workout plan. Chapter 8 explains what is and isn't a cardio exercise, how hard to push yourself when you're exercising, and how many minutes or miles you need to work out to reap the benefits.

If you want the lowdown on cardio machines, like treadmills, elliptical trainers, stair climbers, and indoor bikes, move over to Chapter 9, which outlines those machines in detail. That chapter also helps you combat boredom, giving you tips on how to keep from staring at the same spot on the wall for 20 solid minutes.

If you want to combine a cardio workout with resistance training (see the following section), consider trying circuit training, which we discuss in Chapter 15.

Finding a gym that caters to you

You won't find many seniors-only gyms, but with a little effort, you can likely find a gym that caters to your unique needs. Chapter 18 is all about finding and choosing the right gym, so if you're interested in joining a gym, take a few minutes to peruse that chapter. When visiting local gyms, ask the following questions:

✔ **Does anyone on staff carry any senior-fitness certification or other designation?** Several of the governing bodies that certify personal trainers (see Chapter 4) offer training in senior fitness, and you want to have access to a trainer who has taken advantage of these educational opportunities.

✔ **Do any of your classes specialize in senior fitness?** From water aerobics to Pilates,

yoga to marathon-training groups, some health clubs offer special classes and group activities for seniors. If your local gym doesn't offer senior classes, check with your local YMCA, community health program, running or walking specialty store, and local churches.

✔ **Do you offer senior discounts?** Hey, if you're paying 25 percent less for a movie, you should also get a discount on your gym membership, right? Don't be shy about asking for discounts. They may not be advertised, but if you ask, you may just receive a substantial discount on your membership fee.

Resistance training for strength

If you figure weight lifting is only for young, hot, bodybuilder types, get yourself to Chapter 11, which explains the surprising benefits of resistance training. The bottom line? Adding two or three days of weight training makes you stronger and allows you to eat more calories without gaining weight. And no, for most people, weight training doesn't create bulging biceps and puffed-up pecs. You will tone and sculpt your muscles, however. If you're unsure how to use weight-training equipment, flip to Chapter 13. Chapter 14 helps you design your own strength-training program.

One of the major benefits of resistance training is that you improve your overall strength, which gives you more independence in your life. From carrying in groceries from the car to moving furniture around when it suits you, having greater strength allows you to do more without waiting for your son-in-law to show up.

Pilates for balance

Each year, one in four people over age 65 experiences a serious fall, which can lead to an injury that limits your mobility. Thankfully, beginning and maintaining a fitness routine reduces your chances of falling and makes you more likely to "catch" yourself if you do fall. Both cardio workouts and weight training can improve your balance, but Pilates, the subject of Chapter 17, puts special emphasis on your body's *core* — that is, your abdominal, back, hip, butt, and other nearby muscles — which, when strong, can greatly improve your overall balance.

Consider taking a Pilates class or using a Pilates video one or two days per week. This form of exercise can be challenging to master at first (see Chapter 17 for examples of the exercises), but it builds core strength and improves balance so well that you may wonder how you ever lived without it. Also check out Chapter 19 for information on BOSU, a cardio workout that's well known for developing balance and flexibility.

Stretching and yoga for flexibility

Stretching, whether through the stretches in Chapter 6 or through a yoga routine (see Chapter 16), can prevent your ligaments and muscles from shortening, which is the primary cause of walking like the Hunchback of Notre Dame. We recommend stretching or doing some simple yoga exercises every day, even on the days you don't otherwise exercise. After you get yourself into the routine, you may find that stretching — and the wonderful relaxation you feel as a result — is your favorite part of your day.

Staying Safe

Before beginning an exercise program, make an appointment with your health-care provider, just to cover your bases. As you get yourself into a workout routine, keep the following safety tips in mind:

- ✔ Always warm up and cool down (see Chapter 8); stretch as often as possible (see Chapter 6).

- ✔ Check that you can carry on a conversation while exercising. If speaking is difficult, reduce your intensity or stop exercising.

- ✔ Never hold your breath while exercising, especially while lifting weights.

- ✔ Keep yourself hydrated (see Chapter 7). Remember that by the time you feel thirsty, you've started to become dehydrated.

- ✔ In hot weather, wear high-tech fabrics that let heat escape, and always wear sunscreen and a baseball cap or visor.

- ✔ During winter, layer your clothing so you can remove layers as your body heats up.

- ✔ When you have a cold or — worse yet — the flu, take a few days off of your exercise routine.

- ✔ Stop exercising if you feel any of the following:

    - Nausea, faintness, lightheadedness

    - Racing pulse or any abnormal heart rate

    - Cold sweat

    - Chest or neck pain or tightness

    - Muscular pain

    - Excessive fatigue or weakness

Using exercise as a social event

Exercise is a great way to meet and spend time with people of all ages, especially if you join a gym or a fitness group. If you don't have a gym in your town, check with your local community center to see what classes or workout groups meet in the area — or start your own running or cycling club with friends and family. From meeting new friends at the gym to walking with your grandchildren a few days per week, you can use exercise as an opportunity for social interaction.

Part VIII
The Part of Tens

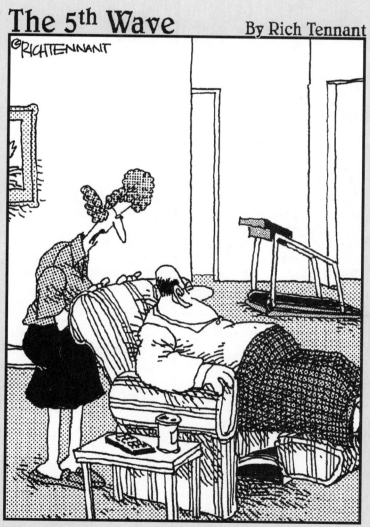

The 5th Wave   By Rich Tennant

@RICHTENNANT

"You know, anyone who wishes he had a remote control for his exercise equipment is missing the idea of exercise equipment."

In this part . . .

We carry on the *For Dummies* tradition of grouping key information in fun, easy-to-skim lists of ten. Just in case you're not sure why exercise is worth your time, Chapter 24 presents ten (well, actually far more than ten) reasons to break a sweat. Chapters 25 and 26 fill you in on the best and worst ways to spend your fitness dollars. Finally, Chapter 27 gives you ten great strategies for staying motivated to work out.

Chapter 24

Ten Great Reasons to Break a Sweat

*Y*ou already know that exercise is important; otherwise, you would have spent your money on Twinkies instead of this book. But when you start a workout program, it's always helpful to remind yourself why — why you're hoisting hunks of steel when you could be lifting beer cans, why you're creating more laundry for yourself by sweating up your gym clothes.

Even if you're already a committed exerciser, you probably have moments when your best intentions are stifled by excuses not to work out. You're too tired or too busy, or the dog ate your dumbbells — we've heard 'em all (and used a few ourselves). Any time you experience one of these moments, flip to this chapter. Better yet, make a copy and tape it to your fridge. One glance at this list, and you'll snap right out of your funk.

Exercise won't prevent ingrown toenails or freeway congestion or the proliferation of bad reality TV shows, but as we explain in this chapter, the simple act of moving your body can work wonders. Here are ten great reasons to work out.

You Reduce Your Risk of Medical Problems

Perhaps the number-one reason for working out is that you'll be healthier. The reasons in the following list alone are enough for you to lace up your shoes and head out the door:

✔ **You're more likely to live a long life.** In an eight-year study of more than 20,000 men, those who were lean but unfit had twice the risk of death as fit, lean men. Even *fat* men who had a history of working out (yes, it's possible — if you eat more calories than you burn off throughout the day, you can still gain weight) had a lower death rate than those who were lean but unfit.

✔ **You have more energy.** People who complain that they don't have enough energy to exercise fail to realize that working out gives you energy. In one study, middle-aged women who lifted weights for a year became 27 percent more active in daily life than before.

✔ **You won't have to count sheep.** After a 12-week aerobic and strength-training regimen, research subjects reported falling asleep faster and sleeping longer than before they'd started exercising, probably because of hormonal changes. Sedentary folks who start exercising regularly boost the amount of time spent in *slow-wave sleep,* the phase of sleep believed to be the most restorative. They also report waking up less often during the night.

✔ **You stay lithe and limber.** As little as five minutes of stretching a day helps keep your muscles mobile and helps you stay agile. Reaching for your purse in the back seat, bending over to pick up a towel off the bathroom floor — being limber is important for countless everyday tasks.

✔ **You improve your balance.** In just three months, 80-year-olds who performed balance exercises — like walking a straight line and standing on one foot — gained the level of body control typical of people three to ten years younger. With improved balance, you have a zippier walking gait as you age, and less shuffling means fewer falls and fractures.

✔ **You're less likely to catch a cold.** Moderate exercise strengthens your immune system. People who walk regularly report cold symptoms on fewer than half the days that couch potatoes report symptoms.

✔ **You can offset the decrease in immune function that weight loss appears to cause.** Research suggests that dieting alone causes a drop in disease-fighting cells but that a program of aerobic exercise and weight training makes up for this loss.

✔ **You're more likely to stop smoking.** People who exercise vigorously while trying to kick the habit are twice as likely to stay away from cigarettes as wannabe ex-smokers who don't work out. And those who exercise as they try to quit smoking gain only about half the weight that non-exercisers do.

✔ **You increase your volume of plasma.** Regular exercise increases the liquid component of your blood, thereby thinning your blood and reducing your risk of developing dangerous clots.

✔ **You lessen the symptoms of PMS.** Exercise may reduce the bloating, lower-back pain, headaches, and anxiety that often accompany premenstrual syndrome. And regular exercisers may be less likely to experience PMS at all.

✔ **You may give birth more quickly.** Research suggests that fit women have labors one-third shorter than women who don't exercise, although the evidence isn't conclusive. Fit women also have a lower risk of premature labor and low-birth-weight babies, and they have less post-partum depression.

✔ **You ease symptoms of menopause.** Highly active menopausal women are significantly less likely to experience hot flashes than their sedentary counterparts. Menopausal exercisers also seem to experience a mood boost after an aerobic workout.

✔ **You strengthen your bones.** Both men and women start losing bone mass between ages 30 and 40. Lifting weights can not only halt the decline but in some cases can reverse it, drastically reducing your risk for osteoporosis. Weight-bearing activities like walking and running also help keep your bones strong.

✔ **You build up bone density for the future.** Young exercisers amass a reserve of bone mineral that may reduce their risk of developing the weak bones that plague their grandparents. A study of elite tennis players found that even after the athletes cut back on their competition, the bone density they had gained earlier remained.

✔ **You're less likely to get a stress fracture.** A study of military recruits found that those with below-average leg strength were five times likelier to develop *stress fractures* (tiny bone fractures) and other overuse injuries during nine weeks of basic training.

✔ **You're less prone to carpal tunnel syndrome.** If you strengthen your wrist and arm muscles, you're less likely to develop this condition, common among people who do repetitive-motion tasks such as typing and scanning items at the grocery checkout stand.

✔ **You can relieve arthritis pain.** Not only can arthritis patients safely participate in exercise programs, but they often are rewarded for their efforts with pain relief and increased mobility.

- **You're less likely to get injured at an impromptu game of touch football or ultimate Frisbee.** By keeping your muscles strong and flexible, you can avoid that nasty hamstring pull or torn rotator cuff that sends you back to the couch with a bag of ice.

- **You're less likely to injure your joints.** When your muscles are strong, they offer more support to your bones and joints. So, you're less likely to twist an ankle stepping off a curb or injure your elbow by carrying a heavy briefcase.

- **You're likely to recover faster from an accident.** If, God forbid, you get into a car wreck or other serious accident, your fitness will serve you well. Frail and weak people have lower survival rates and take longer to recover.

- **You can ease the pain of varicose veins.** The walls of varicose veins have been stretched, allowing blood to pool in the legs. Exercise helps relieve the resulting swelling and aching because the contraction of calf muscles causes blood to shoot upward.

- **You can ease lower-back pain.** Strengthening your abdominal and lower-back muscles can do wonders to ward off lower-back pain and reduce discomfort in people who suffer this pain chronically.

- **You may avoid back surgery.** In one study, most of the back-pain patients who had been recommended for spinal surgery by a physician were able to avoid surgery by following an aggressive strengthening program. Sixteen months after completing the exercise program, only 3 of the 38 patients required surgery.

- **You hold down your blood pressure.** People who exercise regularly have about a 30 percent lower risk of developing heart-threatening hypertension than people who don't work out. Exercise may also help lower blood pressure in people who are already hypertensive.

- **You're less likely to need gallbladder surgery.** Confirming earlier studies on men, new research suggests that women who exercise cut their risk of needing gallbladder surgery by nearly a third. Doctors have known for years that obesity increases the risk of gallstones, but now a sedentary lifestyle appears to be a factor as well.

- **You help keep your prostate healthy.** Three hours of walking per week may reduce the risk of benign prostatic hyperplasia, a condition that leads to prostate enlargement and urinary-tract problems.

- **You're less likely to get diabetes.** Staying fit can drastically reduce your chances of developing non-insulin-dependent diabetes by lowering blood-sugar and blood-fat levels. And if you do have diabetes, exercise — with the permission of a doctor — can help control the symptoms.

- **You're less likely to get colon cancer.** Moderate daily exercise, such as an hour-long walk or a half-hour jog, may reduce your colon cancer risk by as much as 46 percent, perhaps by affecting chemicals inside your intestines.

✔ **You may reduce your risk of breast cancer.** Although the evidence isn't conclusive, research suggests that physically active women are less prone to breast cancer than women who don't work out.

✔ **You lower your risk of coronary heart disease, the number-one killer in America.** People who don't exercise are as likely to develop heart disease as people who smoke. Exercise can also reduce your cholesterol count, particularly your LDL ("bad") cholesterol, although if you're genetically prone to high cholesterol, exercise alone may not keep your count in a healthy range.

✔ **You're less likely to have a stroke.** Burning more than 1,000 calories per week through exercise (say, walking four hours a week) is associated with decreased stroke risk. Burning between 2,000 and 3,000 calories per week may lower your risk even more.

There's a financial benefit to exercise, too. Sure, you have to invest in athletic shoes, a gym membership, and whatever gizmos you need for your favorite activity, but think of all you'll save on doctor's bills and prescription medications by staying healthy. You even save the country money. Perhaps reducing the national debt isn't your major priority in life, but exercising regularly can be a patriotic gesture: Obesity-related diseases cost the nation $100 billion a year.

You Can Control Your Weight

Sure, you can lose weight simply by dieting, but much of that weight will be muscle, not fat. Weight training prevents your muscles from wasting away as you slim down, and aerobic exercise is the most efficient way to burn calories. Check out the other weight-control benefits of exercise:

✔ **You rev up your metabolism.** No pill, powder, or herb can do it, but weight training can. For every pound of muscle you pack on, your body burns an extra 30 to 50 calories per day — not a huge figure, but perhaps enough to help prevent weight gain as you age. Make that 10 pounds of muscle, and you're talking about an extra 300 to 500 calories per day!

✔ **You can eat more without gaining weight.** When you burn an extra 2,000 calories a week on the stair-climber, you can afford to try the fresh peach cobbler or the extra helping of Thanksgiving stuffing.

✔ **You're likely to keep the weight off.** Most people who lose weight gain it back within one to three years, but that's because they don't exercise. Among those who succeed at keeping the pounds off, more than 95 percent work out regularly.

You Improve Your Looks

No amount of exercise can transform Rosie O'Donnell into Cindy Crawford, but with the right workout program, you can shape a rounder derriere, firm up your arms, and tone your legs. And that equals the following benefits:

- ✔ **You can wow 'em at your high school reunion.** Were you the nerd in high school everyone ignored? Were you the captain of the Latin club and second tuba in the marching band? Well, get on a fitness program and *you'll* be the popular one at your next class gathering.

- ✔ **You'll look better in sleeveless shirts.** Heck, with toned arms, you may even land a job on TV or in the movies — á la Jennifer Garner, Sarah Jessica Parker, and Jennifer Aniston.

- ✔ **You're more likely to visit a nude beach.** Okay, maybe not, but research does show that exercisers report having more confidence about their bodies than sedentary people do.

You also look and feel younger. In one study, postmenopausal women who lifted weights twice a week for one year had the strength and bone density levels of women 15 to 20 years younger.

You Gain Psychological Benefits

A truckload of research shows that you have a better sense of well-being, also known as *runner's high,* following a workout. Both aerobic and weight-training sessions seem to offer this boost, as well as a number of other psychological benefits:

- ✔ **You gain confidence that spills over to the rest of your life.** The sense of accomplishment that comes from being able to run 5 miles or do 10 push-ups just may give you the confidence to make that presentation to your most important client or to ask that good-looking bank teller out on a date.

- ✔ **You improve your memory.** In a six-month study of previously sedentary men and women ages 60 to 75, those who walked three times a week scored 25 percent better on memory and judgment tasks, such as recalling schedules and quickly differentiating between vowels and consonants and odd and even numbers.

- ✔ **You experience less stress.** More than 150 studies prove it: Regular exercise makes you less tense and better able to cope with events that might otherwise transform you into Cruella de Vil or Scrooge.

✔ **You can calm your mind and improve your breathing.** Activities such as yoga, Pilates, and stretching provide the perfect antidote to life in the era of cell phones, beepers, faxes, call-waiting, call-forwarding, and conference calls. Learning to breathe deeply can help you control stress and anger.

✔ **You gain perspective.** You notice a lot more about your neighborhood when you walk, jog, or bike down the street than when you whiz by at 30 miles per hour in your car. And although you can get a swell view of New Zealand from behind the window of a bus, the thrill doesn't compare to climbing a glacier or cycling past flocks of sheep.

✔ **You feel happier over the long-term.** Not only does a single workout make you feel better, but regular exercisers enjoy long-lasting psychological benefits.

✔ **You may become less depressed.** Research clearly shows that exercise can help clinically depressed men and women of all ages. A review of 80 studies found that depression appears to diminish after 4 weeks of regular exercise, although the greatest improvements were found after 17 weeks.

✔ **You have a healthy outlet for your anger.** Instead of yelling at your boss, you can get your aggressions out during a kickboxing class — burning calories and improving your health at the same time.

You Enjoy Social Benefits

Going for a walk or a bike ride with a friend or your spouse is a good way to catch up on the latest gossip, weigh in on the day's news, and stay current with each other's families, friends, and pets.

You also boost your chances of finding a mate. Tired of the bar scene or Internet dating services? Join a running club, a kickboxing class, or a soccer team, and you're sure to meet like-minded people. You may even meet your significant other at the gym or through a bike club.

Even if you're not on the hunt for a spouse, getting into a new fitness activity is a great way to widen your social circle. When you hook up with a hiking club or a softball team, you meet interesting people of all ages and from all walks of life whom you may not have had the pleasure of knowing otherwise.

You Improve Your On-the-Job Performance

Whether you're a massage therapist, a trial attorney, a trombone player, or a ball-field groundskeeper, you'll benefit from the increased energy, concentration, and stamina that you get from regular exercise. Here's why:

✔ **You can better cope with shift work.** Working the graveyard shift at 7-Eleven? Swing-shift on patrol? Exercise can help temper the health problems, including sleep disorders, common to people whose work shifts toy with the body's natural rhythms.

✔ **You master the art of teamwork.** When you join a softball team, cycling club, or walking group, you bond with your teammates and find out what it takes to play nicely with others. These skills may come in handy at the next office conference, PTA meeting, or neighborhood-watch meeting.

You also have more job opportunities. You can't be a firefighter, a police officer, or a lifeguard if you flunk the physical. And if you have your sights set on being a bouncer, big, strong muscles are pretty much a prerequisite.

Finally, you save your company money. Employees who take advantage of corporate-wellness programs tend to have fewer doctors' visits and fewer absences from work. Companies have saved millions by giving their employees incentives to exercise.

Your Family Benefits

When you exercise, you have more options for family togetherness. Sure, you can all sit in the living room and watch slides of Aunt Marie's 1974 vacation to Venice, but a fit family can also shoot hoops on the driveway, go hiking in the woods, or play softball. When you and your family exercise, you find all sort of benefits:

✔ **You have more confidence if you're a new father.** In a study of 87 new dads, those who exercised expressed more confidence in their new role than fathers who didn't work out. Although scientific studies haven't yet focused on new mothers, the benefits surely work for mom, too.

✔ **You set a good example for your kids.** Want your kids to grow up healthy and strong? You can be a great role model by exercising regularly. This is especially important in an era in which childhood obesity is at an all-time high.

✔ **Kids are likely to perform better in school.** Compared to sedentary girls, active girls have better grades, a lower drop-out rate, and a greater likelihood of attending college.

✔ **Kids can succeed in science.** Marie Curie may not have run any marathons or spiked any volleyballs, but research shows that high school girls who play sports are more likely to get good grades in science classes than their nonathletic peers.

✔ **Kids discover abilities they never knew you had.** Maybe your child has the tennis talent of the Williams sisters, but it has been hidden all these years. Maybe your child's body is built for power-lifting but she just never realized it. Chances are, your kids have a real knack for some type of athletic endeavor — whether it's running, softball, or aerobic dance — but they won't know until they try.

✔ **Kids can become more resilient during childhood.** Research shows that kids who participate in sports are more likely to bounce back from disappointment and adversity than children who aren't active. Fit kids are also less likely to feel stressed out.

✔ **Kids are less likely to start smoking.** Boys and girls ages 12 to 16 who spend much of their leisure time doing physical activity are significantly less likely to start smoking than low-activity groups.

✔ **Kids are less likely to get pregnant as teenagers.** Teenage female athletes are less likely to get pregnant than girls who don't participate in sports. They're also more likely to have their first sexual experience later in adolescence than nonathletes.

✔ **You can keep up with your grandkids.** Wouldn't it be nice to toss around the pigskin with your granddaughter without your arm getting sore and tired? Regular workouts can give you the strength and stamina to be a worthy opponent for family tennis tournaments and basketball on the driveway.

Your pet can get fit, too. Take your pooch for longer and more frequent walks, and he'll live a longer, healthier life. Plus, dogs thrive on activity. They much prefer to trot around and take in the sights than impersonate a throw rug that happens to be alive.

You Satisfy Your Competitive Urges

Participating in a local 5K road race or vying for a trophy in the company golf championship is a healthy outlet for your competitive spirit. Even racing against the clock can be a satisfying pursuit. Plus, you perform better in all sports. A dead-on jump shot or wicked tennis serve carries you only so far. Regular exercise gives you the stamina and agility to outlast your opponents on the court or on the field.

At the same time, you can help find a cure for leukemia, multiple sclerosis, or breast cancer. Nationwide, hundreds of athletic events raise money for important medical research. You can run, walk, bike, swim, even snowshoe — all in the name of having fun and saving lives.

And don't forget that, when you compete, you get cool stuff. Run a 10K or ride in a bike-a-thon, and you score all sorts of unique t-shirts, caps, water bottles, sweat bands, and socks that you won't find at Gap or Target. These items lend you an air of mystique and athleticism, plus they're pretty useful. Not bad for a $15 or $20 entry fee.

You Have Fun

When you discover an activity you love, whether it's step aerobics or indoor rock-climbing, you stop thinking of exercise as drudgery and look forward to lacing up your athletic shoes. Exercise is like recess was in grade school — a time to stop being serious and just get out there and play.

You also have infinitely more travel options. Instead of taking yet another cruise or bus tour or parking yourself at the craps tables in Vegas, you can bicycle in Vermont, kayak in Alaska, or hike the Grand Canyon. And back on the home front, instead of sequestering yourself indoors for four months this winter and piling on the sweaters to hide extra poundage, you can snowshoe, ski, snowboard, skate — invigorating activities that can prevent winter weight gain and give you an edge for snowball fights with the neighborhood kids.

You Enjoy Life More

Sure, this is kind of a catch-all category, but the bottom line is that life is more fun when you're fit. Check out these additional benefits to working out:

- **You're more creative.** In one study, subjects who did aerobic exercise scored higher on creative thinking tests than did subjects who watched a video. That's not surprising: Many people come up with their best ideas while on the run.

- **You can catch up on your reading.** Does your living room resemble a newspaper recycling facility? Are you burdened with guilt for not even opening the 14 magazines you subscribe to? Kill two birds with one stone by reading on the stationary bike or the stair-climber.

✔ **You sharpen your math skills.** When you load weight plates onto a bar-bell, you have to do some fast calculations. (Quick: How much weight is a 45-pound bar plus two 10-pound plates and two 5-pound plates?) The math gets even more challenging when you convert miles per hour on the treadmill to how many minutes per mile you're running.

✔ **You're more useful around the house.** You don't need help unscrewing that stubborn jar of pickles, hoisting that 10-gallon jug of water, or pulling apart the sofa bed for your houseguests.

✔ **You're more productive.** Can't garden for more than 20 minutes without stopping to rest your achy knees? Can't get all your errands done in one shot because you need to take a break? Do you avoid visiting your friend who lives in that fourth-floor walk-up? When you're fit, none of this is a worry.

✔ **You're likely to watch less junk TV.** When exercise is part of your life, you don't have time to sit around with the remote, bouncing around from *Survivor* to *CSI* to *Desperate Housewives*.

✔ **You have an excuse to go shopping.** You can buy an endless number of nifty gadgets without feeling guilty, such as a heart-rate monitor, a set of dumbbells, a titanium bike seat, or a windproof ski vest.

✔ **You enjoy retirement more.** Not that we don't love Scrabble and gin rummy, but fit seniors have more activity choices, from golf to gardening to world travel.

✔ **You discover a lot about your body.** When you lift weights, you become intimately acquainted with your muscles and their individual job descriptions. You notice that your back muscles are called for duty when you pull a bar toward you, and you realize that your chest muscles kick in when you push a bar away from you.

✔ **You get to learn a whole new language.** Reps, sets, pecs, lats, target zone — when you hang out at health clubs or build a library of exercise videos, you quickly become fluent in the language of exercise. Your friends will be impressed!

✔ **You develop a greater appreciation for the athletes you watch on TV or cheer for at sporting events.** You don't understand just how tough it is to hit a 90-mph fastball, duck a lightning-fast left hook, or cycle 100 miles uphill until you try these sports yourself. After you start working out, you'll watch events like the Tour de France and the New York City marathon with a whole new outlook.

Chapter 25

Ten Great Fitness Investments under $100

*Y*ou can spend thousands of dollars on high-tech exercise machinery, but some of the most valuable fitness products around cost less than $100.

In this chapter, we recommend simple products and services that can turn pain into pleasure and drudgery into fun. These ten cheap fitness investments are sure to pay you back many times over. We list them roughly in order from cheapest to most expensive.

A Water Bottle

You're a heckuva lot more likely to down your eight to ten glasses a day if you carry around a water bottle — at the gym, at the office, or in front of the TV. If you have to hop off the treadmill and traipse halfway across the room to the water fountain, you won't. Honestly, you have no excuse not to own a water bottle. They're often offered as freebies when you join a gym or buy a bike, and even if you have to break down and pay for one, you're still only out $5.

Although water bottles are the ultimate indoor exercise accessory, there's an even better product for outdoor workouts: a hydration pack. It's an insulated pouch that you wear like a lightweight backpack when you're cycling, walking, hiking, skiing, or snowshoeing. You fill the pouch with water; to drink, you bite down on the end of a flexible tube that hangs over your shoulder. Camelbak, the inventor of the hydration pack, even makes a nifty winter version that has an insulated tube that won't freeze. Research suggests that hydration-pack users drink more fluids — and drink more frequently — than water-bottle users. This makes sense because biting down on a tube is much more convenient than reaching down to grab your water bottle. Hydration packs cost $40 to $100. Many come with extra zipper pockets to store food, money, extra bike tubes, and so on.

A Good Pair of Socks

You probably put quite a bit of thought into purchasing your athletic shoes, shorts, jackets, skates, skis, and helmets. But socks? Nah. Chances are, you grabbed a six-pack at the discount store without considering anything but the price.

It may seem ridiculous, but there are socks designed for almost every sport, and usually they're worth the extra money. Socks act as a buffer between your foot and your shoe, so they help prevent blisters, calluses, and other shoe-friction problems. For each sport, you use your feet differently and wear different shoes, so it only makes sense to wear different socks. There's even a difference between running socks (extra padding across the toes and bridge of the foot) and walking socks (more padding in the heel).

Suzanne used to cycle in the same cotton socks she'd wear to the movies. It wasn't until she scored a pair of freebie biking socks at a fundraiser that she realized the difference: Socks designed for cycling wick away sweat and let her feet breathe. And when it rains, her feet don't freeze. She now gladly pays $7 for Air-eators, her favorite brand.

Experiment with different types of socks, and before you invest in a whole new wardrobe of socks, buy a single pair to test. In general, we prefer light-weight synthetic sock materials such as CoolMax because they breathe better and dry faster than cotton or wool socks. We also like SmartWool socks ($7–$15), which are made from high-quality wool and specially treated so they dry quickly and hold their shape well. Two other sports sock brands that we like are Wigwam and Thorlo.

Stretching Mat

Sure, you could stretch on a rolled-up towel or plush carpet, but how often do you actually do it? A mat not only makes stretching more comfortable but also reminds you to do your flexibility exercises. For about $7, you can get a perfectly functional stretching mat made of flexible plastic. (The $7 ones are too stiff to roll up, but they fit pretty neatly in a closet or under a bed.) If you're willing to pay $30 or more, you can get a mat that folds up and has a cloth covering.

If you do a lot of yoga (see Chapter 16) or meditation, try a "sticky" mat, which costs from $15 to $40. These mats are made of soft, thin plastic coated with a sticky film that helps keep you steady during moves that require balance. Brands we like include Frelonic and Airex.

Weightlifting Gloves

Lifting weights (see Chapter 11) does countless good things to your body — shaping your muscles, boosting your strength, and thickening your bones, to name a few — but pumping iron isn't kind to one particular area: your palms. After a few months of gripping dumbbells and weight machines, the skin on your hands starts to feel like sandpaper. You can prevent major callus buildup by wearing weightlifting gloves, sold at most sporting goods stores for $15 to $20.

Gloves not only protect your palms but also give you a better grip on the weights. Suzanne is convinced that she can do more pull-ups while wearing weightlifting gloves than while gripping a slippery bar with naked hands. She's so enamored of her gloves that she keeps them in her backpack when she travels so that she's all set to work out if she unexpectedly walks past a gym. Suzanne likes gloves with Velcro wrist adjustments so that she can tighten and loosen the gloves as needed.

A Workout Log

You may think tracking your workouts in an exercise diary is obsessive; who needs extra paperwork? But a workout log offers proof of your commitment to exercise. Nothing is more motivating than seeing your accomplishments on paper.

Jot down as many details as you can think of without making yourself feel like a court reporter at a deposition. (Chapter 3 lists the particulars worth noting.) A workout diary need not be a fancy affair — a notebook from the drugstore will suffice. Personally, we're partial to store-bought logs designed especially for the purpose of tracking daily workouts. They lend a sense of importance to what you're doing, and many are filled with good training tips and inspirational quotes.

You can purchase workout diaries for less than $20 at bookstores, sporting goods stores, and the Internet. Some logs are designed for specific activities — like walking, cycling, and weight lifting. You also can buy all-purpose logs that provide space to track weight-training exercises, cardiovascular workouts, stretching, and nutrition notes.

PlateMates

When you start a weight-training program, increasing your weights by the smallest increment possible is important. PlateMates, shown in Figure 25-1, can help fill in the gaps. These ingenious weight magnets adhere to each end of a dumbbell and save you the cost of buying extra weights. They come in four weights: ⅜ pound, 1¼ pound, 1⅞ pound, and 2½ pounds. Prices range from about $19 to $28 per pair. Stick a pair of 1¼-pound PlateMates on the end of your 5-pound dumbbells and voila — you have 7½-pounders. Now stick 'em to your 10-pounders, and you have 12½-pounders. You can buy a handy carrying case for the weights (about $9) so that you can take them to your health club as well.

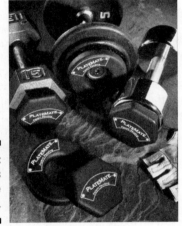

Figure 25-1:
PlateMates
can save
you big.

Photograph by Sunstreak Productions, Inc

A Gym Bag

You'd never consider boarding an airplane carrying your shirts, pants, shoes, toothpaste, hairbrush, and shampoo all in your hands. Yet many people arrive at the gym juggling all sorts of paraphernalia, including car keys, membership card, tape player, towel, water bottle, and magazines. Perhaps this is because they don't realize how sophisticated gym bags have become. The best ones have pockets for everything — small compartments for a wallet or membership card, medium-sized zipper sections ideal for a radio/CD player or workout gloves, and mesh pouches for your stinky clothes so that mold doesn't start to grow. Many bags have special features for different sports. In-line skating bags have special pockets to hold your skates. Soccer bags have compartments to separate your muddy, grassy cleats from the rest of your items. Swimming bags are designed to accommodate your fins, paddles, and goggles; good ones have a waterproof compartment to throw your suit in when it's wet.

You can get a good bag for less than $50. Look for sturdy, easy-to-wash fabrics such as thick nylon. Canvas tends to rip and soil easily. A gym bag should have a rigid bottom so that when you place it on the floor, it stands upright. This helps keep your items in place. We also like bags with both shoulder straps and handles so that you can choose how to carry your bag. If you tend to walk home from the gym at night — or even just from the club to the parking lot — look for a bag with reflective stripes or glow-in-the-dark panels.

A Heart-Rate Monitor

Heart-rate monitors are the training tool of choice for both serious and recreational exercisers. Because your heart rate is directly proportional to how hard you're working, a monitor is a great way to determine your exercise intensity. We especially recommend these gizmos for beginners who are just learning how to push themselves, and for people training for a competition who want to get a sense of what it feels like to work out at near-maximum pace. (See Chapter 8 for details on how to put your monitor to good use.) A monitor is also especially valuable if you're a home exerciser. You don't have the roar of the crowd to keep you going, or the wide assortment of equipment to occupy you; your heart rate gives you something tangible to focus on. Prices range from $59 for a simple model to $400 for one that lets you download information to your computer, create graphs of your training intensities, and cross-reference this information with every variable from the weather to the type of shoes you wear.

A Personal Training Appointment

Hiring a personal trainer sounds like hiring a personal chef — an extravagance that's swell for Oprah but unrealistic for the rest of us. But we're not talking about a lifetime commitment here. You can hire a trainer for a couple of sessions, either at home or at a health club, to get you started on a program tailored to your goals and your fitness level or to update your current routine. Trainers cost between $25 and $100 per session. If you buddy up with a friend or two, your sessions may cost less.

If you plan to be a short-timer, inform your trainer of your intentions so that he can cover more in a shorter period of time. And think specifically about your goals for these few sessions. Do you want to learn a routine you can take on business trips? Do you want training advice for a summer cycling vacation? Do you want a program to help you lose fat? Act like you're taking a crash course in Italian two weeks before you move to Rome: Be prepared to soak up a lot of information. Arm yourself with questions and take notes. By the end of your session(s), make sure you know how to adjust each machine, grip each handle the right way, and perform each exercise using the correct technique. And consider scheduling follow-up sessions once a month or so to check your progress, stay up-to-date, and continue to improve your skills. Also find out whether your trainer is willing to answer quick questions via e-mail as part of the overall cost.

A Massage

Okay, you've been exercising for a solid month. You deserve a reward, and besides, your legs feel a little sore. What better way to treat yourself than with a rubdown?

Massage loosens up kinks in your muscles, relieves stress, and helps you relax. Research suggests it may even speed your body's recovery from a workout or injury by increasing blood flow and, therefore, delivering more oxygen and nutrients to your muscle cells and restoring muscle and joint mobility. Massage may also make you more mentally alert. In one study, subjects who had been massaged were able to do math problems in half the time, and with half as many errors, as subjects who weren't touched.

Although we're not all that motivated to improve our algebra skills, we like massage for a more important reason: It feels *soooo* good. Depending on where you live, an hour-long massage can run you between $35 and $100. Sessions in your home usually cost a little more, to compensate for the driving time and the fact that the therapist has to lug a big, heavy table to your door.

In most states, massage therapists are required to pass a certification exam. Chances are, any therapist who works at a club or spa is fully licensed and certified, but it never hurts to ask. For a home massage, get a recommendation from a doctor, trainer, or friend you trust. You may think "bad massage" is an oxymoron, but you can get rubbed the wrong way. A rock-climber friend of Liz's had his arms massaged by someone who practically mauled him. The guy was so bruised and in pain that he couldn't climb for two weeks.

Chapter 26

Ten Fitness Rip-Offs

*A*t a fitness-equipment trade show not long ago, we mentioned to an infomercial executive that a certain abdominal gadget appeared to be flimsy and useless. "I wouldn't disagree with you," the executive said, smiling. "But we've sold 20,000 units in the first month."

You oughta be insulted. The fitness industry has no shortage of hucksters, and they count on the public's naiveté — and hunger for a quick fix — to keep the money rolling in. They sell exercise gizmos that, off the record, they admit are useless. They use scientific mumbo jumbo to promote products based on nothing more than wishful thinking. They pay celebrities big bucks to go on TV and lie.

The Federal Trade Commission, the government agency that monitors truth in advertising, is aware of these scams and has boosted efforts to nail companies making fraudulent health and fitness claims. However, the advertising police are not unlike big-city cops: They only have the manpower to hunt down the most egregious offenders. And with the rise of the Internet, fitness crooks have proliferated.

All of this means that you need to be a very savvy fitness consumer. In this chapter, we give you the lowdown on ten products that we consider to be a waste of money. We also offer tips on judging other fitness products that you may come across on TV infomercials, on the Internet, in magazine advertisements, and in fitness-equipment and health-food stores. Our advice, in a word: Beware!

Anti-Cellulite Products

The products: Creams and gels intended to eliminate *cellulite,* the puckery fat that forms on the butt, hips, and thighs of most women and some men. What are the magic ingredients? Cellasene pills contain, among other things, gingko biloba, sweet clover, grapeseed bioflavonoids, and dried fucus vesiculosus (a kelp-like seaweed found off the Atlantic coasts of Europe). Lipofactor cream is made of "biotechnologically derived elements a/y." We have absolutely no idea what this means, but this phrase is repeated all over the Internet.

The reality: Talk about scientific mumbo jumbo! No legitimate research exists to show that any pill or cream can reduce cellulite. Physiologically speaking, cellulite doesn't even exist. The term is marketing hype for plain old fat that clumps at various points on your body. The ripple effect is caused by a network of connective tissue fibers that attach muscle to skin and compartmentalize the fat like stitching on a quilt. You reduce cellulite the same way you reduce any fat: through a healthy diet and regular exercise. However, you may never lose the ripples. For some people, they're a genetic fact of life.

Metabolism Boosters

The products: Pills and powders intended to speed up your metabolism so that your body burns more calories during the course of the day without requiring you to increase activity. Several of these supplements — such as Ultra Burn, CitraLean, and Hydroxycut — contain HCA (hydroxycitric acid), a form of citric acid found in fruits. Others contain chromium picolinate, a form of the mineral chromium, or ephedra (also called ma huang), an herbal stimulant. Some combine almost every ingredient known to mankind.

The reality: Solid research shows that chromium picolinate has little nutritional value. Only two legitimate, published studies have even tested HCA in humans, and the results were contradictory. (Animal studies have shown the substance to be toxic, causing rat testicles to atrophy.) As for ephedra, the FDA has fielded more than 800 reports of medical problems from this stimulant, including heart attacks, strokes, seizures, and a nasty side-effect known as death. Ephedrine can be especially lethal for those with high blood pressure. It is banned in California.

Amphetamines and over-the-counter stimulants can indeed rev up your metabolism, but even if you can withstand the side-effects (such as increased blood pressure and heart rate), your body tends to adapt to these substances, so the effect is likely to be short-lived. The only safe and lasting way to boost your metabolic rate is to increase your muscle mass by lifting weights (and even that, as we explain in Chapter 11, isn't going to have a magical effect).

Fat Blockers

The products: Pills intended to prevent your body from absorbing the fat you eat. Chitosan — a substance that forms the hard shells of shellfish and insects — is a popular ingredient. Another is pyruvate, a substance that occurs naturally in the body and is involved in energy production.

The reality: Sure, it would be nice if you could enjoy fried chicken, mounds of mashed potatoes and gravy, butter, rolls, ice cream, and cake — all without gaining weight. But guess what? You can't! We don't know whether pyruvate and chitosan are beneficial for weight loss. We do know that both Fat Trapper and Exercise in a Bottle can run you as much as $300 a month — a whopping $3,600 a year. That's ten times the cost of many gym memberships. If you're serious about dropping body fat, stay away from high-fat foods and get plenty of the type of exercise that doesn't come in a bottle.

Effortless Exercisers

The products: These contraptions are the player pianos of exercise machines. They move whether you're holding on or not. Consider the Stretch-A-Cizer, essentially a chair with a handlebar mounted above the seat back. "All you do is sit on the seat and hold onto the exercise bar while it goes through the motions," explains an Internet ad for this $1,200 electric contraption (freight prepaid!). Also in this category: the Chi Machine Aerobic Exerciser. You lie on your back on the floor, place your ankles on the machine's contoured footrest, flip a switch, and let this $460 gizmo toss you around like a fish out of water. "This is not a 10-kilometer run kind of workout, where one gets all sweaty and exhausted," the Chi Machine Web site reports. "Instead you lie down, relax, [and] have a 'workout.'"

The reality: This is all a bunch of baloney. We don't think we have to tell you why you won't get thin by lying on the floor and having electrical impulses shoot up your spine so you flop around like a fish — even if you do this five times a day for 15 minutes, as the Chi Machine literature recommends.

Electronic Muscle Stimulation Machines

The products: Metal boxes that deliver a low-impulse jolt of electricity to muscles that are covered by electrodes. This jolt is supposed to tone and tighten muscles.

The reality: The only way to strengthen your muscles is to work out. We think the reason electrical stimulation gizmos have such staying power is that electrical stimulus or transcutaneous electrical nerve stimulation (TENS) machines do have legitimate medical uses: They're used by highly trained doctors and physical therapists to manage pain and help rehabilitate certain injuries. But they can cause serious injury from burns and electrical shocks when used by laypeople.

Spot-Reducing Gadgets

The products: Abdominal gizmos, neoprene "waist trimmer" belts, neck toners, "reducing" shorts — there's no shortage of products that profess to melt the fat on a particularly blubbery spot on your body. In response to a crackdown by the Federal Trade Commission, many abdominal-gadget manufacturers have stopped making the direct claim that their products will cause weight loss in the abdominal area. However, they haven't stopped implying that this will happen, firming and flattening abs, melting excess fat, and so on.

The reality: The concept of spot-reducing is bogus; you can't pick and choose where on your body you'll lose fat. Abdominal exercises can only strengthen your abdominals (and many of them don't even do a good job of that). To lose that gut, you have to embark on a sensible eating and exercise program — an approach that will reduce your overall body fat. Some of this body fat is likely to come from your midsection.

Weight-Loss Clothing

The products: Vinyl and synthetic rubber exercise suits that make you sweat like it's August in New Orleans.

The reality: It doesn't matter whose heat you use: Reducing inches by sweating profusely can put you in serious danger. People have died from wearing vinyl and rubber suits after working out in the heat or wearing the clothing over a long period of time. Cause of death: extreme dehydration or a form of blood poisoning brought on when chemicals from the suit escape into the bloodstream. We think suggesting that these suits can be worn for "the most strenuous activities" is particularly appalling. The more strenuous the activity, the more important it is to wear clothing that lets your skin breathe.

Four-Minute Workouts

The product: ROM, a popular infomercial machine that looks like a combination stepper and indoor bicycle. The idea is that the machine offers such a phenomenal cardio and flexibility workout that you can get into the shape of your life in just four minutes per day.

The reality: No four-minute cardiovascular workout will give you significant strength-training or weight-loss benefits. Certainly this contraption is no substitute for ten gym machines. And it doesn't burn nearly three times the calories of a treadmill. (Machines don't burn calories; people do. The number of calories you burn per minute depends on how hard you push. Some machines do allow you to work at a more intense pace than others, but the Romfab claim is totally unfounded.)

Gym Cardio Machine Knockoffs

The products: Cheapo treadmills, stair-climbers, and elliptical trainers that profess to work and feel exactly the same as the cardio equipment found in health clubs. You can find these at sporting-goods stores, online, and in mail-order catalogs.

The reality: You simply can't buy sturdy, high-tech aerobic machinery for the price of dinner at a fancy restaurant. Top-quality machines cost thousands of dollars for a reason: They're based on years of scientific research and the study of body biomechanics. The angle of movement, the placement of the seat, how far your legs can move — all these important features are based on solid engineering. That's usually not the case with cardio knockoffs. After a while, you may find that your back hurts or your knees ache because of poor design.

What's more, these contraptions aren't as sturdy as the gym versions. When you step on the treadmill at the gym, you don't feel the walking belt sink or the handrails wobble. Suzanne almost toppled over while testing one of these at a trade show. And several people have filed lawsuits after allegedly hurting themselves on cheapo machines while trying them out in the store.

One more caveat: Cheap cardio machines usually don't come with good warranties — usually 90 days or less — compared to 1 to 3 years for high-end machines. See Chapter 20 for tips on buying high-quality cardio machines for your home.

Hand Weights

The products: Dumbbells that weigh 1 to 5 pounds and are designed to be held while running, jogging, power walking, and doing step aerobics. Many of these products claim to combine strength training with aerobic conditioning in one workout, while causing you to burn extra calories.

The reality: People who power walk with weights in their hands look quite serious and impressive, but the truth is, these weights aren't doing them any good. Research on walkers shows that carrying hand weights burns only 10 to 15 percent more calories — a mere 20 to 30 calories over the course of an hour, at least half of which come from exaggerating your arm swing, not from the weights. (To put this in perspective: Speeding up from a 3-mph pace to a 4-mph pace burns an extra 54 calories.)

Research on aerobic dancers suggests that you may actually burn fewer calories holding hand weights than holding nothing at all. That's because weight-holding exercisers must keep both arm and leg movements tight and controlled. In other words, you don't move your body as much or as far because if you flail the weights around, you get thrown off balance. As a result, you burn fewer calories.

Also, swinging hand weights vigorously can place undue stress on delicate upper-body joints such as the shoulder, elbow, and wrist. Due to a concept called torque, there are points in your arm swing when a weight exerts up to ten times the usual force on your joints. In other words, a measly 3-pound weight will place up to 30 pounds of force on those delicate joints. Plus, this force is delivered in a jerky manner, which can do a lot of damage.

Finally, realize that you're not going to build strength with these weights. Any dumbbell that's light enough for you to carry around while walking is too light to strengthen your muscles. As we explain in Chapter 13, to build strength you need to lift weights that are heavy enough that you can perform no more than about 15 repetitions of an exercise.

Chapter 27

Ten Ways to Stay Motivated

For some people, the motivation to work out comes naturally. These people have the same passion for exercise that others have for wine tasting or watching NASCAR or following the stock market.

But for most people, the inspiration to work out comes and goes. And the truth is, even the most dedicated fitness buffs go through periods when they just don't feel like lacing up their cross-trainers and heading to the gym.

So what separates those who can pull themselves out of the exercise doldrums from those who succumb to feelings of inertia? There's no single strategy. Instead, successful exercisers tend to rely on a whole repertoire of tactics. Here are ten of the best ways to keep yourself motivated. Try all these strategies. At least one is bound to work for you.

Train for an Event

Suzanne once interviewed an Olympic weightlifter who described himself as a "pretty lazy guy." "If I wasn't training for the Olympics," he said, "I probably wouldn't even work out."

Even if you don't aspire to hoist 424 pounds overhead before thousands of screaming fans, committing to an event can jump-start your workout program. The options are countless — a 5K walk, a 10K run, a mini-triathlon, a 100-mile bike ride. The minute you mail in your entry fee, you have a whole new sense of purpose. And the feeling of accomplishment you get from completing your event is like nothing else.

If you're a novice, an excellent option is to join a training program organized by a charity. You'll have the double motivation of getting in shape and knowing that you're raising money for a good cause. Here are two of the best national programs:

- ✔ **The Leukemia Society's Team in Training** (www.teamintraining.org): This program prepares even complete beginners to run or walk a marathon or bicycle a *century* (100 miles). Each week you and your teammates meet with an experienced coach. You're also paired with a local "Honored Patient" who cheers you on throughout your training. On the day of the event, you wear a special wristband with the patient's name.

- ✔ **AIDS LifeCycle** (www.aidslifecycle.org): You get all the flat-tire seminars, training tips, and camaraderie you need to complete one of nine annual AIDS Rides, three- to seven-day cycling tours that cover 50 to 80 miles per day. Many participants don't even own bikes when they sign up.

  "Every week on the training rides you see people of all different shapes, sizes, and ages training for the same cause," says our friend Tracy, who has completed the San Francisco–to–Los Angeles AIDS Ride four times. "That gives you the psychological momentum to keep going." Finishing the ride along with 2,000 other cyclists in matching shirts is exhilarating, Tracy says. "People are honking their horns and lining the streets for miles with posters, balloons, and banners. You feel like a celebrity."

Keep Your Goals in Plain Sight

The "lazy" Olympic weightlifter mentioned in the preceding section keeps a picture of the Olympic rings next to his bed. Some people tape their goals to the bathroom mirror or refrigerator. Suzanne knows a swimmer who writes his goals on his kickboard. Liz has a client who enters her workout goals into her computer's screen saver so that she sees them scrolling by every time she takes a break from typing.

Whether you write your goals on the side of your shoe or in your training diary, glancing at them on a daily basis helps keep you focused and motivated. What if you don't have specific goals to write down? Turn to Chapter 3 ASAP.

Work Out with a Club or a Team

Back when Suzanne rode her bike alone, she'd roll along at a leisurely pace, get bored after about 20 miles, and head home before she was even tired. Some days she was so uninspired that she'd keep pushing the snooze button on her alarm until it was too late to work out. But these days when the buzzer sounds, she flies out of bed, blends up a fruit smoothie, and heads out for a ride. The difference? She hooked up with an informal group of 15 cyclists who meet on a street corner three days a week in suburban Los Angeles. Now her rides are so much fun that Suzanne doesn't even mind sitting in traffic for 50 minutes to get to the starting point. Plus, by riding with a group of cyclists who are much faster than she is, Suzanne has become a much stronger biker.

Whether you join a bike club, a hiking group, a swim team, or a soccer league, you're sure to gain inspiration from your workout buddies. Don't worry if you're the slowest one in the group; just do as much as you can handle. Eventually, you'll catch up with the rest. Don't sweat it, either, if the group isn't friendly right off the bat. Some groups can be cliquish, and it takes time to break in. If you keep showing up, eventually you'll be one of the gang. If you don't have a group of friends who are interested in working out, check with your local running or cycling store or search the Internet for the name of your town and terms like *workout group*.

Work Out with a Buddy

If you can't find a local club that fits your schedule, set up a workout schedule with a friend. When Liz's friends Patty and Ann trained for a triathlon together, they met at 4 a.m. every morning for a bike ride, followed by weight lifting and yoga. On the weekends they did their runs and swims together. This went on for six months until they completed the event successfully. Both say they couldn't have done it without the other's support and companionship. "The only way I could get my butt out of bed at 4 in the morning was knowing Ann would be there, too," says Patty.

Join an Internet Fitness Community

Not everyone can find workout partners in his neighborhood. But thanks to the Internet, you can gain inspiration from fitness buddies across the country — or even the world. Several fitness Web sites have forums where visitors can chat with like-minded exercisers and develop strong bonds with one another.

Some sites even help you find an e-mail pen pal with similar interests and fitness goals. For instance, at the Fitness Jumpsite (`www.primusweb.com/fitnesspartner`), you can post an ad describing your exercise pursuits and what you're looking for in an e-mail fitness buddy. Postings run the gamut — from a single mom in Australia wanting to lose 50 pounds to a North Carolina college student needing inspiration to lift weights instead of hanging out all night in his dorm downing pizza and beer.

Internet groups are especially helpful for home exercisers. "People who exercise at home don't have the social benefit that you can get at a health club, and in many cases, they don't have any friends or family who exercise," says Wendy Niemi Kremer, founder of Video Fitness (www.videofitness.com), a Web site for exercise video enthusiasts. (See Chapter 19 for more details about the site.) "Video Fitness has become an enormous support group. When any crisis in your life can derail your exercise program, it's nice to have somewhere to go."

Test Your Fitness Regularly

Sure, exercise gives you intangible benefits like more energy and greater self-esteem. But it also helps to translate your progress into raw numbers: how many pounds you can bench-press, how many beats your resting heart rate has dropped, how fast you can run a mile, how much body fat you've lost. (We explain all these tests in Chapter 2.) Track these numbers in a workout log or notebook (see Chapter 3) so that you can keep track of your progress over time.

For your first year that you work out regularly, you may want to get tested every three months. (You make the most noticeable improvements when you first start exercising; then progress becomes less dramatic.) After the first year, we suggest getting tested every six months. If you don't want to spend the time or money on a whole battery of tests, ask a certified trainer to do the part you find most motivating, such as a body-fat test or blood-pressure reading. A heart-rate monitor can be useful for the do-it-yourself tests that we describe in Chapters 2 and 8.

If you're training for a specific event, you may want to do a time trial once a month. For example, if your goal is to walk a mile in a certain amount of time, break out your stopwatch once a month and go all out. If you train properly, each time you test yourself you'll move a bit closer to your goal.

Mix Up Your Workouts

Some people thrive on routine. Suzanne bicycles with a 67-year-old retired racer named Barry who has been riding the exact same route on Saturdays for 41 years. Much to the frustration of his wife, Barry refuses to take non-cycling vacations, because he doesn't want to miss his daily ride.

Most of us, however, need a bit of variety to stay motivated. For this reason, you may want to try *cross-training,* which simply means mixing up your activities. Cross-training means different things to different people. You can vary your sport — running on Mondays, swimming on Tuesdays, hiking on Wednesdays, and so on. Or you can vary your pace and terrain — walking fast and flat one day, slow and hilly the next. Or you can try different equipment — using weight machines one session and free weights the next. If you always use the treadmill, expand your horizons by trying out the elliptical trainer or the rower.

You can also pair activities that focus on different aspects of fitness. For example, do yoga one day to work on your flexibility and engage your mind; the next day run on the treadmill while watching *Law & Order*.

Dress the Part

We're not encouraging you to become a fitness-clothing junkie — or use the lack of a new outfit as an excuse to skip a workout. But buying snazzy new workout shorts or comfy new cross-trainers can really get you fired up to work out. Plus, you feel like a workout pro, and you let your fellow exercisers know you're one of them.

When Liz first started indoor rock climbing, she showed up in running shorts and a t-shirt. She noticed that all the good climbers wore tank tops and long sweat pants cut off at the bottom. Gradually, Liz conformed to the dress code and found out a few things. For one, the "in" crowd was more accepting of her because she looked serious about the sport. But more importantly, Liz realized there's actually a reason rock climbers dress that way: The long sweats protect you from bumps and bruises. Cutting off the elastic at the bottom lets you move your legs and feet more freely. And a sleeveless top makes moving your arms easier.

If you find yourself really digging a certain activity, research the gear and equipment that you see everyone else wearing. A few choice items can put you into the right frame of mind for your workouts.

Keep Yourself Entertained

Combining exercise with life's guilty pleasures can make your workout fly by. Maybe you'll enjoy your treadmill power walk more if you do it while watching reruns of *Sex and the City* or listening to the latest OutKast CD.

These days, you have more opportunities than ever to keep yourself entertained while you work out. Most gyms now have some sort of high-tech entertainment system that gives you access to TV, radio, CDs, and even the Internet. (We describe these systems in Chapter 9.)

If you don't go to a gym, you can carry your own radio or CD player while you exercise, as long as you exercise in a safe environment and remain aware of your surroundings. Portable CD players have improved to the point where they won't skip even if you carry one while running. You can even find underwater tape players for swimming and water aerobics, and some pools pipe in underwater music. For the ultimate lightweight player, though, consider getting an iPod or other MP3 player, which can store hours of music and doesn't require discs.

Read Success Stories

We're not talking about those before-and-after weight-loss ads in which a blubbery guy with a scowl on his face is miraculously transformed — "in just six weeks!" — into a grinning, chiseled hunk of muscle.

No, we're referring to legitimate accounts of fitness success chronicled in magazines and on fitness Web sites. The good ones offer not only inspiration but specific and realistic advice. One woman featured in *Shape* magazine's monthly "Success Stories" column wrote that she had ballooned to 226 pounds at age 23. (Get the magazine at your local newsstand or visit www. shapemag.com.) Fed up, she vowed to her husband that in one year, he wouldn't recognize her. "That's when I got the fire in my belly," she wrote. In addition to cleaning up her diet, she walked a hilly 3-mile route each night after work. "My face was beet red, and I could barely breathe," she recalled. Thirteen months later she had lost 96 pounds. "Best of all, I had gained self-confidence thanks to taking care of myself."

Not all fitness success stories are about weight loss. Some are about overcoming anorexia or starting to exercise for the first time at age 60 after a stroke. You can find success stories in other magazines as well, such as *Fitness, Men's Fitness,* and *Good Housekeeping.*

Appendix

Educating Yourself

• •

*I*t pays to educate yourself, whether you're thinking about buying a stair-climber or you want to exercise with your kids. You'll have more confidence and more fun with your workouts if you read about fitness in magazines or on the Internet, and you can keep abreast of the latest exercise techniques, workout gadgets, and nutrition controversies. And you can get inspirational tips from folks who overcame their inertia. Of course, you also can get completely confused. Use this appendix to educate yourself.

Sifting Through Scientific Research

It seems as though every day in the news you hear about some new study that seems to contradict the one you heard the month before. First, chromium picolinate helps build muscle and burn fat; then, it's a complete waste of money. One day you hear that one set of weight-training exercises builds as much strength as the traditional three; then you hear that three sets are actually better than one. How do you find out the truth?

First, realize that there may not be a truth right now. It often takes decades for the scientific community to reach a consensus. That "startling new report" you hear about on TV may simply be one minuscule piece in a gigantic puzzle — one scientist's best guess. But because of the way news is generated and reported, you may not get the full picture. Scientists sometimes overstate their findings because they want media attention or grant money. In the same way, stories are sometimes inaccurate because an expert passes along erroneous information. When reviewing studies done by scientists, journalists may hype ambiguous results because they need a big story. Or they may get the facts wrong because they had only two hours to decipher a 20-page study full of phrases like "deuterium oxide concentration was measured by using a fixed-filter single-beam infrared spectrophotometer." Finally, when the news media hypes a story as "controversial," the facts get a little lost.

Stuff like this happens all the time. Sometimes readers don't have any way to discern truth from fiction, but you can get a decent handle on the facts by paying attention to the way studies are reported. Consider reading the newsletters and Web sites of the American Council on Exercise (www.acefitness.org) and the Center for Science in the Public Interest (www.cspinet.org), both of which track the way scientific studies are reported — and distorted — in the media. Also check out WebMD (www.webmd.com) and Medline (www.medlineplus.gov). The following tips will also help you sort through the research that you read and hear about.

Look for context

Does the news report mention how the latest research compares to the studies that came before it? The results of a single study may be a complete aberration.

A few years ago, the media jumped on a study suggesting that kids who drank a lot of fruit juice were fatter than children who didn't drink much juice. But the newspapers and TV stations failed to report a key fact: The study hadn't considered the children's exercise or overall eating habits. "Several studies had found before and have found since that you can't blame it on the juice," says registered dietitian Elizabeth Somer, a nutrition book author who frequently appears on *Good Morning America*. "It's lack of exercise and their whole diet pattern that makes kids fat." Somer stood in the studio cringing as the news anchor informed the nation that drinking juice is bad for kids. "They should never have even reported on that study," says Somer, who couldn't contradict the news anchor in her own nutrition segment.

Don't alter your lifestyle on the basis of one study. Many theories are later proven to be wrong. As late as the 1960s, many experts were still telling women that exercise would damage their uteruses.

Consider the source

A health study is more likely to be legit if it comes out of a major university or government agency rather than some mysterious, private institute. Some private companies and foundations do valid research, but many organizations with impressive-sounding names, like Sportlife Exercise Health Sciences Institute, are just facades for companies promoting their products. Look for the term *independent research*. A tobacco study done by RJ Reynolds or a rating of treadmill brands done by a treadmill manufacturer should fall under the category of things that make you go "Hmm."

On the other hand, just because a study was conducted at an elite university doesn't mean it's the gospel. Recently, the National Institutes of Health National Cholesterol Education Program (NCEP) made bold new recommendations for taking cholesterol-lowering statin drugs to reduce the risk of heart disease. Those studies are now under review, however, because, among other reasons, scientists brought to light that eight of the nine members of the panel making the recommendations had undisclosed financial ties to makers of statin drugs.

Don't assume cause and effect

If a study says that eating oat bran is linked to or is associated with low blood-cholesterol levels, this doesn't mean eating oat bran causes low cholesterol levels. Maybe the oat bran eaters are health-conscious and get a lot of exercise. You have to ask, "Was it the oat bran or the exercise?" Also, take any individual study with a grain of salt; when several studies back certain findings, you can be far more sure of their validity.

Look for comparison groups

One magazine article we came across touted the benefits of a powdered food replacement. As evidence, the article cited a study of 28 overweight women who cut their daily calories by taking the powder twice a day instead of food; the subjects also exercised three times a week. After two months, the article stated, "an astounding 100 percent" of the women lost weight and felt better. Astounding? Any overweight person who cuts calories and exercises regularly is going to see results after two months. For the study to have any validity, the researchers should have compared the group taking the powder with a control group of similar subjects who ate the same number of calories and followed the same exercise program but didn't use the product.

Do some math

You often read that a certain habit "doubles" the risk of death or "increases the risk of disease by 50 percent." These figures can be misleading. In a study that followed 115,000 nurses for 16 years, researchers found that gaining 11 to 18 pounds in middle age raised the nurses' heart disease risk by 25 percent. But the number of deaths in the study was so small that a 25 percent increase would mean the difference between 10 deaths in 10,000 people and 12 or 13 deaths in 10,000.

Notice the length of the study

A four-week study doesn't tell you whether a weight-loss pill or exercise regimen is safe or effective. Maybe a pill stops working after two months or a year.

The same goes for exercise programs. Several studies show that one set of weight training exercises builds as much strength as three sets, and these one-set studies have been well-publicized in fitness magazines. But the magazines typically don't mention an important fact: Most of the one-set studies have lasted only three months. Only a handful of studies have tested subjects for a longer period of time, and these have generally shown that after four to six months, people doing one set tend to plateau while those doing three sets tend to continue making strength gains.

Pay attention to the number of subjects

A study performed on a dozen people can't tell you much of anything, but this doesn't stop manufacturers from hyping research conducted with a sample size no larger than your morning workout group. The makers of an anti-cellulite pill, now in litigation, originally launched a massive national campaign to publicize an Italian study purported to show that their pill worked. But the study was conducted on only ten women. (Furthermore, the researchers who took the measurements knew which of the women were using the supplements.)

Don't make too much of animal studies

The way an obese mouse responds to a diet drug may not be the same way you respond. Chromium picolinate, a diet supplement touted on bottles as a "Super Reducer!" received plenty of good press. What you may not have heard is that most of the fat-loss studies have been performed on pigs. Human studies show that the supplement does not help humans lose weight.

Recognize that people lie in surveys

Large studies usually rely on written questionnaires or phone surveys, a method that can lead to very misleading results. Subjects may not remember how many leafy green vegetables they ate last month, or they may exaggerate their exercise habits. According to the *New England Journal of Medicine,* nearly half of all research participants overestimate how much they exercise, and an equal percentage underestimate how much they eat.

Fitness Magazines

Just when the fitness-magazine industry seems to be saturated, along comes yet another magazine devoted to exercise, health, and nutrition. This is good news — we welcome more choices. Even better, fitness magazines are becoming more specialized, so you have an excellent chance of finding a magazine that speaks to you. There's at least one fitness magazine to suit every type of exerciser: pregnant women, African American women, men in their 30s, walkers, swimmers, runners, cyclists, yoga practitioners, and cooking enthusiasts who want to be fit.

But the stiff competition makes some magazines resort to underhanded marketing tactics, including sensational headlines, misleading articles, and uninformed writers. Ask a trainer or fitness-minded friend for magazine recommendations. Also, keep in mind the following tips for judging the fitness information you read in magazines.

Check out specialty magazines

You're more likely to get good fitness information from magazines that specialize in fitness than from general-interest or beauty magazines that mix in an occasional exercise article. This isn't a hard-and-fast rule: Some mainstream magazines run perfectly good fitness stories, and some fitness magazines run perfectly lousy ones. But women's fashion and beauty magazines are notorious for unrealistic promises like "Permanent Weight Loss! A Revolutionary Three-Week Plan."

Be especially wary of magazine pieces that offer fitness advice from celebrities; being a movie star doesn't make you an exercise expert.

Beware of sensational headlines

Stay away from magazines whose cover lines seem way too good to be true, such as "Drop 9 lbs. in 7 Days," which is the fitness equivalent of "Elvis lives." And if the fitness article is next to a story about Burt Reynolds' ghost having a secret rendezvous with a two-headed man, you're probably not getting your information from the right source. Tabloid rags have caught on to the fact that the American public is obsessed with weight loss, so what's one more story about an alien diet or psychics predicting the health regimens that work?

Even reputable fitness magazines run misleading headlines to draw in readers. Suzanne wrote an article for a health magazine debunking the myth that abdominal exercises can give you a flat midsection. But the magazine ran a headline that directly contradicted Suzanne's story: "A Flat Tummy in 5 Minutes a Day."

Know that advertisers influence editorial copy

The editorial and advertising departments of journalistic publications are supposed to be like church and state: completely separate. In reality, health and fitness magazines sometimes abandon objectivity and censor or alter their stories to favor the companies that buy advertisements from them.

Product reviews are a good example. "At one magazine where I worked, we had to sugar-coat our shoe reviews because of advertising pressures," says a writer we know. "With certain shoes, we had to search for aspects that weren't negative and emphasize those. Like if a shoe was incredibly stiff, we'd write some innocuous copy about how the shoe had a good lacing system."

The crumbling bridge between advertising and editorial is perhaps most evident in a growing category of advertising called the *advertorial*. These are paid ads intended to look like regular articles. Typically, the layouts, typeface, and photos are very similar to the magazine's editorial style so readers won't make the distinction. The more manipulative advertorials even have bylines (for example, "By Joe Schmo") so that the ads look like articles that have been written by regular reporters. Most magazines require advertisers to include the word *advertisement* at the top or bottom of the page, but sometimes the type is so small it's easy to miss.

A prominent women's magazine recently ran an advertorial on home exercise equipment. It was designed to look like an editorial product review, complete with a writer's byline and a ratings system. (Surprise — all the products received the largest number of stars possible!) The word *advertisement* was printed in small, light red letters at the top of the first page.

Newspapers

We're glad daily papers have stepped up their fitness coverage, but don't use the dailies as your only source of fitness information. Newspaper reporters tend to be very responsible about attributing information to experts. The problem is, given the reporters' tight deadlines, they often have no choice but to interview the first available expert, who may not necessarily be the best expert (and may not be an expert at all). Magazine writers sometimes run into this problem, too.

Also, newspaper reporters tend to be jack-of-all-trades types who may not have the fitness experience to distinguish a real expert from a charlatan. Only the largest newspapers can afford to have reporters who cover the fitness beat exclusively.

Even though magazine articles are written three to six months before publication, they're often more up-to-date than newspapers. Many newspapers get their exercise ideas from reading fitness magazines. So, if you're looking for articles about fitness trends, training techniques, and exercise equipment, mainstream fitness magazines tend to be better sources than daily papers.

The Internet

Surfing the Internet for fitness information is a bit like entering into automated-phone-system hell: You press one key after another, and pretty soon, you're either totally lost or back where you started. You may have the intention of finding out how to train your abdominals, but with a few unwitting clicks of the mouse, you're downloading porn. Still, if you have the time and patience to look around, you can get some great fitness information online — from descriptions of the major yoga poses to the complete Surgeon General's Report on Physical Activity and Health.

However, you also can get plenty of hogwash. In general, you'll come across more misleading and biased fitness information online than in mainstream fitness publications printed on paper. So perusing health and fitness Web sites with a particularly critical eye is important. Keep in mind that the line between advertising and editorial is particularly blurry on the Internet.

In addition, the "experts" quoted in online fitness articles may not be experts at all. Often, they're people with products to sell. When a mainstream magazine publishes an article on heart-rate monitors, the story typically quotes coaches or university professors. But on one fitness Web site, we found a heart-rate-monitor article that quoted the executive assistant to the president of a heart-rate monitor manufacturer! "Anyone who is concerned about their weight, improved fitness, or athletic competition . . . can benefit from using a heart-rate monitor," said the assistant. We agree, but the information doesn't have a heckuva lot of credibility coming from someone who has a financial stake in the product.

Finally, watch out for outdated information. You may think of the Internet as the most up-to-date of all media, but the Internet often doesn't live up to its potential as the best source for late-breaking information. In an attempt to get Web sites up and running quickly — and to appear loaded with "content" — many sites are cluttered with ancient material.

Use fitness Web sites as a starting point for educating yourself, but remember that the Internet is full of misinformation. Be sure to compare what you read online with what you read in magazines and newspapers.

Index

• *I* •

• *J* •

• *K* •

• *L* •

BUSINESS, CAREERS & PERSONAL FINANCE

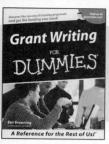

0-7645-5307-0

0-7645-5331-3 *†

Also available:
- Accounting For Dummies †
  0-7645-5314-3
- Business Plans Kit For Dummies †
  0-7645-5365-8
- Cover Letters For Dummies
  0-7645-5224-4
- Frugal Living For Dummies
  0-7645-5403-4
- Leadership For Dummies
  0-7645-5176-0
- Managing For Dummies
  0-7645-1771-6

- Marketing For Dummies
  0-7645-5600-2
- Personal Finance For Dummies *
  0-7645-2590-5
- Project Management For Dummies
  0-7645-5283-X
- Resumes For Dummies †
  0-7645-5471-9
- Selling For Dummies
  0-7645-5363-1
- Small Business Kit For Dummies *†
  0-7645-5093-4

HOME & BUSINESS COMPUTER BASICS

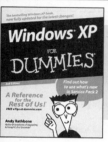

0-7645-4074-2

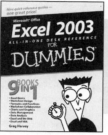

0-7645-3758-X

Also available:
- ACT! 6 For Dummies
  0-7645-2645-6
- iLife '04 All-in-One Desk Reference
  For Dummies
  0-7645-7347-0
- iPAQ For Dummies
  0-7645-6769-1
- Mac OS X Panther Timesaving
  Techniques For Dummies
  0-7645-5812-9
- Macs For Dummies
  0-7645-5656-8

- Microsoft Money 2004 For Dummies
  0-7645-4195-1
- Office 2003 All-in-One Desk Reference
  For Dummies
  0-7645-3883-7
- Outlook 2003 For Dummies
  0-7645-3759-8
- PCs For Dummies
  0-7645-4074-2
- TiVo For Dummies
  0-7645-6923-6
- Upgrading and Fixing PCs For Dummies
  0-7645-1665-5
- Windows XP Timesaving Techniques
  For Dummies
  0-7645-3748-2

FOOD, HOME, GARDEN, HOBBIES, MUSIC & PETS

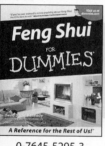

0-7645-5295-3

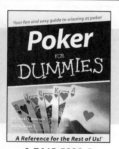

0-7645-5232-5

Also available:
- Bass Guitar For Dummies
  0-7645-2487-9
- Diabetes Cookbook For Dummies
  0-7645-5230-9
- Gardening For Dummies *
  0-7645-5130-2
- Guitar For Dummies
  0-7645-5106-X
- Holiday Decorating For Dummies
  0-7645-2570-0
- Home Improvement All-in-One
  For Dummies
  0-7645-5680-0

- Knitting For Dummies
  0-7645-5395-X
- Piano For Dummies
  0-7645-5105-1
- Puppies For Dummies
  0-7645-5255-4
- Scrapbooking For Dummies
  0-7645-7208-3
- Senior Dogs For Dummies
  0-7645-5818-8
- Singing For Dummies
  0-7645-2475-5
- 30-Minute Meals For Dummies
  0-7645-2589-1

INTERNET & DIGITAL MEDIA

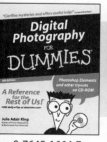

0-7645-1664-7

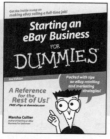

0-7645-6924-4

Also available:
- 2005 Online Shopping Directory
  For Dummies
  0-7645-7495-7
- CD & DVD Recording For Dummies
  0-7645-5956-7
- eBay For Dummies
  0-7645-5654-1
- Fighting Spam For Dummies
  0-7645-5965-6
- Genealogy Online For Dummies
  0-7645-5964-8
- Google For Dummies
  0-7645-4420-9

- Home Recording For Musicians
  For Dummies
  0-7645-1634-5
- The Internet For Dummies
  0-7645-4173-0
- iPod & iTunes For Dummies
  0-7645-7772-7
- Preventing Identity Theft For Dummies
  0-7645-7336-5
- Pro Tools All-in-One Desk Reference
  For Dummies
  0-7645-5714-9
- Roxio Easy Media Creator For Dummies
  0-7645-7131-1

* Separate Canadian edition also available
† Separate U.K. edition also available

Available wherever books are sold. For more information or to order direct: U.S. customers visit www.dummies.com or call 1-877-762-2974.
U.K. customers visit www.wileyeurope.com or call 0800 243407. Canadian customers visit www.wiley.ca or call 1-800-567-4797.

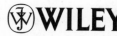

SPORTS, FITNESS, PARENTING, RELIGION & SPIRITUALITY

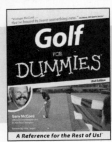

0-7645-5146-9

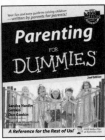

0-7645-5418-2

Also available:
- Adoption For Dummies
  0-7645-5488-3
- Basketball For Dummies
  0-7645-5248-1
- The Bible For Dummies
  0-7645-5296-1
- Buddhism For Dummies
  0-7645-5359-3
- Catholicism For Dummies
  0-7645-5391-7
- Hockey For Dummies
  0-7645-5228-7
- Judaism For Dummies
  0-7645-5299-6
- Martial Arts For Dummies
  0-7645-5358-5
- Pilates For Dummies
  0-7645-5397-6
- Religion For Dummies
  0-7645-5264-3
- Teaching Kids to Read For Dummies
  0-7645-4043-2
- Weight Training For Dummies
  0-7645-5168-X
- Yoga For Dummies
  0-7645-5117-5

TRAVEL

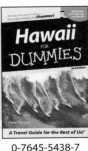

0-7645-5438-7

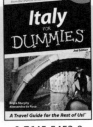

0-7645-5453-0

Also available:
- Alaska For Dummies
  0-7645-1761-9
- Arizona For Dummies
  0-7645-6938-4
- Cancún and the Yucatán For Dummies
  0-7645-2437-2
- Cruise Vacations For Dummies
  0-7645-6941-4
- Europe For Dummies
  0-7645-5456-5
- Ireland For Dummies
  0-7645-5455-7
- Las Vegas For Dummies
  0-7645-5448-4
- London For Dummies
  0-7645-4277-X
- New York City For Dummies
  0-7645-6945-7
- Paris For Dummies
  0-7645-5494-8
- RV Vacations For Dummies
  0-7645-5443-3
- Walt Disney World & Orlando For Dummies
  0-7645-6943-0

GRAPHICS, DESIGN & WEB DEVELOPMENT

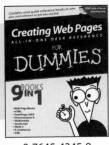

0-7645-4345-8

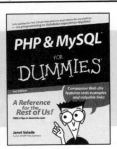

0-7645-5589-8

Also available:
- Adobe Acrobat 6 PDF For Dummies
  0-7645-3760-1
- Building a Web Site For Dummies
  0-7645-7144-3
- Dreamweaver MX 2004 For Dummies
  0-7645-4342-3
- FrontPage 2003 For Dummies
  0-7645-3882-9
- HTML 4 For Dummies
  0-7645-1995-6
- Illustrator CS For Dummies
  0-7645-4084-X
- Macromedia Flash MX 2004 For Dummies
  0-7645-4358-X
- Photoshop 7 All-in-One Desk
  Reference For Dummies
  0-7645-1667-1
- Photoshop CS Timesaving Techniques
  For Dummies
  0-7645-6782-9
- PHP 5 For Dummies
  0-7645-4166-8
- PowerPoint 2003 For Dummies
  0-7645-3908-6
- QuarkXPress 6 For Dummies
  0-7645-2593-X

NETWORKING, SECURITY, PROGRAMMING & DATABASES

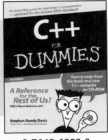

0-7645-6852-3

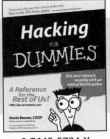

0-7645-5784-X

Also available:
- A+ Certification For Dummies
  0-7645-4187-0
- Access 2003 All-in-One Desk
  Reference For Dummies
  0-7645-3988-4
- Beginning Programming For Dummies
  0-7645-4997-9
- C For Dummies
  0-7645-7068-4
- Firewalls For Dummies
  0-7645-4048-3
- Home Networking For Dummies
  0-7645-42796
- Network Security For Dummies
  0-7645-1679-5
- Networking For Dummies
  0-7645-1677-9
- TCP/IP For Dummies
  0-7645-1760-0
- VBA For Dummies
  0-7645-3989-2
- Wireless All In-One Desk Reference
  For Dummies
  0-7645-7496-5
- Wireless Home Networking For Dummies
  0-7645-3910-8